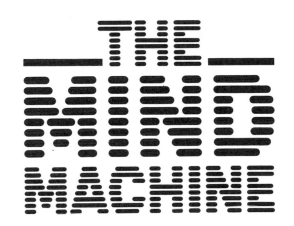

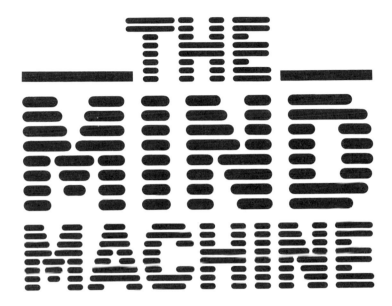

THE MIND MACHINE

COLIN BLAKEMORE

with the help of Richard Hutton,
Martin Freeth and the production
teams of BBC Television and WNET

BBC BOOKS

Published by BBC Books
A division of BBC Enterprises Ltd
Woodlands, 80 Wood Lane
London W12 0TT

First published 1988
© Colin Blakemore 1988

ISBN 0 563 20646 2

Typeset in 10 on 13 point Baskerville and printed and bound
in England by Butler and Tanner Ltd, Frome and London
Colour printed by Technik Ltd, Berkhamsted
Jacket printed by Belmont Press Ltd

Contents

In 1976 I GAVE THE REITH LECTURES ON BBC Radio, on the subject of the brain. It is both sobering and exhilarating to look at the progress that has been made since then – sobering, because it provides ample evidence that any view of science, at any moment in history, is a mere snapshot of a constantly changing scene; exhilarating, because much of the recent research is scientifically and medically important.

When Martin Freeth of BBC Television approached me about the possibility of helping with a co-production with WNET Channel 13 of New York, on brain and mind, it seemed a marvellous opportunity to try to produce at least another snapshot of the excitement and importance of the subject.

This book, based on the BBC series *The Mind Machine*, touches on topics as diverse as addiction, ageing, thought, healing, language and violence. It would have been impossible to write it without a great deal of practical help. First and foremost I thank Victor Balaban, who interrupted his studies at Cornell University and came to Oxford to help with research and unflagging support.

The inspiration for this entire project came from Richard Hutton of WNET, the author and chief producer of the American series *The Brain* and *The Mind*. Serious scientific programmes are rare on American television and they have to be fought for, nurtured and funded against heavy odds. Richard, together with WNET executives George Page and Jack Sameth, did the hard work needed to bring the venture to fruition. Science reporter Bonnie Benjamin's painstaking research over five years laid the foundations for the work of the other producer/directors John Heminway, DeWitt Sage, Vivian Ducat and Peter Bull. I thank them and everyone else at WNET. Richard Hutton, Bonnie Benjamin and Alison Guss helped very directly with five of the chapters.

On the BBC side, Martin Freeth, the series producer, set standards of stamina and dedication that left us all breathless. His vast experience and flair for programme-making underpinned the BBC series. Ian Calvert produced several of the programmes and influenced all of them through his knowledge of science and his concern that the media should do it justice. Martin and Ian helped me enormously with the chapters on addiction and violence. I also thank Jonathan Drori who stepped into a gaping breach at a very late stage and produced two of the films. Behind the scenes, the series was sustained by the hard work and good humour of production assistants Annina Rive and Gay Bain and by the celluloid alchemy of the film editors Keith Raven, Justin Amsden and Chris Bezant. Mick Rhodes, head of BBC's Science and Features Department, gave us crucial help and encouragement when we needed it most.

On a different plane, I am deeply grateful to all the scientists who gave their time and their knowledge to advise and participate in the programmes, and on whose work this book relies so heavily. Any failings in the book, particularly in interpretation, are my responsibility; but any qualities it has are due to the army of brain researchers around the world.

At BBC Books, Susan Kennedy, Kelly Davis, Frances Abraham, Rachel Hardman and Jennie Allen squeezed this book out of me, designed it, researched many of the illustrations and pushed through its publication with a seemingly impossible schedule.

Finally, I must thank my own scientific colleagues in Oxford, my secretaries, Pippa Cann and Sue Saunders, and my long-suffering family, who tolerated, sometimes with amusement, often bemusement, my eccentricity in devoting all my spare time for several months to this project. I think and hope that they respect my conviction that scientists have a responsibility to try to communicate with the public, especially at a time when science in Britain is suffering a crisis of funding and facing a demand from the government to prove its 'relevance'. My main motive for helping with the films and writing this book is to attempt to convey to a broad audience something of the significance of brain research.

The ultimate aim of this branch of science is to understand the human brain – the most complex piece of machinery in the universe. The subject is vast, ranging from the basic physical and biological sciences, now applied to details of how nerve cells work, right through to psychology, anthropology and philosophy. The potential rewards are immense – not only to elucidate, perhaps eliminate, some of the most frightening diseases that affect human beings, but also to understand ourselves, our minds, as products of the stuff inside our heads. The sceptics quote the old adage that if the human brain were simple enough to be understood, we should be so stupid that we couldn't understand it! But I'm an optimist, and I have history on my side in thinking that science can achieve what was thought to be impossible.

In the eighteenth century, the French philosopher and surgeon Julien de LaMettrie was persecuted because of the view expressed in his book *L'homme Machine* that the whole human body is essentially an automaton. Since then, science has inexorably explained the mysteries of bodily function in terms of physics and chemistry. I realise that the mechanistic view of the human mind crystallised in the title of this book will offend some people. But I do not think that such a view reduces human beings to 'mere' machines. It celebrates the richness of the mechanism inside our heads – the machine that makes the mind.

Colin Blakemore *Oxford, September 1988*

BEGINNINGS

Along the northern shore of the Gulf of Corinth, in Greece, the wall of mountains that rises sharply from the ocean is dominated by Mount Parnassos, which Apollo, the god of light, chose as his sanctuary. In the *Hymn to Apollo*, the blind poet Homer tells the story of Apollo's arrival:

> You climbed rapidly, running across the hilltops and you reached the regions of Krissa below Mount Parnassos which is covered with much snow, at the point where it forms a knee to the west and a large rock overhangs the spot, while below a wild valley stretches out; this was the spot where the Lord Phoibos Apollo decided to have a beautiful temple.

This temple, ruined but still beautiful today, lies at the heart of the holiest shrine of the ancient world – Delphi. If you stand in the ruins of Apollo's temple and look up beyond the precipice to the sky above, you can sometimes catch a glimpse of an eagle; a descendant, perhaps, of the pair of eagles that Zeus commanded to fly from the two ends of the Earth until they met, here, at its very centre.

More than 3000 years ago Delphi was already famous throughout the ancient world. It dominated the thoughts of kings and emperors until the end of the fourth century AD when its power was finally lost. But what was the magic of this place? Not its beauty alone, magnificent though it was, but its gift of *prediction*. For this was the home of the most famous and influential oracle of recorded history, the Oracle of Delphi.

By the seventh century BC, the pronouncements of the oracle had become an annual ritual, performed on Apollo's birthday. The Pythia, a peasant woman more than fifty years old, cleansed herself in the Kastalian spring, which still pours from the rocks below the temple, and then, intoxicated by the smoke of burning laurel leaves, she fell into a trance. She answered the questions of the pilgrims in unintelligible tones, which were translated into hexameter verse by the prophets who attended her.

All this myth and mystery seem very remote from the modern world. But we do share something with those pilgrims. They knew about the past and longed to know the future. Like them, we have within our heads the most complex instrument in the universe – the human brain. This fragile lump of jelly is the most valuable thing that anyone will ever possess. It creates its owner's mind: it is the *mind machine*.

• THE SEARCH FOR MIND •

The journey that this book describes takes us inside our own heads, into a world of nerve cells and chemicals on the one hand, and of thoughts and emotions on the other. But the first step is backwards, beyond the birth of Delphi to the conception of humanity. When did people first have minds?

The legends of Homer, passed by word of mouth from one generation to another, are full of fear, hope, jealousy and love. In the *Odyssey* Homer said, 'He saw the cities of many men, and knew their minds.' Two millennia later, we can look at Homer's words and be confident that the Ancient Greeks had minds very much like ours. Further back, in the darkness of prehistory, the signposts become scarcer and harder to read.

Long before Homer's time, people who looked like us had already settled over much of southern Europe. They left no legends, no temples, no written word. But 17 000 years ago, one group left a message, in a limestone bottle; a message painted in earth colours and charcoal on the bright white calcite walls of the caves at Lascaux in south-west France. Those walls are alive with the jumbled images of deer, bison, bulls and horses. The modern visitor stands and stares in reverence – a voyeur peeping through the keyhole of time into the minds of people who lived four hundred generations ago. Don Johanson, American archaeologist and anthropologist, sums up the meaning of this place: 'It's almost as if you're walking into the past and having an opportunity to look at the world of 17 000 years ago through the eyes of the people who actually lived then.'

The Cro-Magnon people of Lascaux were *Homo sapiens*, the same species as you and me – opportunistic people, who had come to terms with the hostile environment at the end of the Ice Age. Like present-day hunter-gatherers, they probably lived in small groups of half a dozen families, pooling their talents and their children as their investment in the future. The seventeenth-century philosopher, Thomas Hobbes, wrote of the lives of such people as 'nasty, brutish, and short', but the magnificence of their art tells us that they already had a sense of beauty and a need to leave their mark on the world. Whatever the practical function of these paintings, the sheer joy in the minds of those ancient artists in creating such magnificent images goes far beyond their pragmatic value.

• THE CRADLE OF THE MIND •

The human beings of Lascaux were descended from stocky, flat-headed people who walked, upright, into Asia and Europe more than a million years ago. Their brains were half the size of ours, but they already knew how to make fire and stone tools, and they must surely have been able to carry food and water. But their most precious possession, the one that gave them an advantage over every other species on this planet, was their ability to communicate inventions and ideas and to conceive of their future.

Almost certainly the true Garden of Eden, the birthplace of mankind, was Africa. We shall never know, of course, why those ancestors of ours, of the species *Homo erectus*, marched out of Africa, across the desert of Sinai. But we do know that their bones and the relics of the things they made are scattered across the whole of the Eurasian landmass, from Heidelberg to Java. A sense of curiosity, a need to know what was over the next hill, must surely have driven them on from generation to generation.

Every species on this earth is a miracle of adaptation, a perfect product of the environment in which it lives. Every species but one, that is. Human beings are the ugly ducklings of evolution. Without their magnificent brains, their gawkish, ill-adapted bodies would have chained them to one narrow niche of existence. The hallmark of humans is their resourcefulness, rather than the perfection of their commitment to any particular place or any specific way of life. We are the great paradox of the living world; we were made by our environment, but our evolution gave us the ability to create our own environment and thus to seize the reins of our own destiny.

The lineage of the human species stretches back 15 million years or more before the march out of Africa, to the time when the tree of evolution branched, separating the lines of humans and apes. This transcendental division may have taken place in the savannah that covers what is now Ethiopia and Kenya. Here, in the East African rift valley, close to the Equator, the upheaval of the earth has thrown up the layers of ash and shale that were trodden by creatures who lived here aeons ago, and yielded the splinters of fossilised bone, worn-down teeth and shattered tools that are our only mementoes of our earliest forefathers.

Richard Leakey, Director of the National Museums of Kenya, turns in his hands a replica of the skull of *Homo habilis*, the predecessor of *Homo erectus*, who lived in this part of Africa between 1 million and 3 million years ago. Its bones have been found on no other continent.

For most of us, who are mere spectators of the science of palaeo-anthropology, the fascination in seeing these fossil skulls is to contemplate the faces that once hung from them, and to wonder how they grimaced or smiled or wept. But Richard Leakey's expert fingers slip *inside* the skull, looking, like the visitors to Lascaux, for messages about the mind written on the walls of the space within. He searches inside the cavity, on the left side of the head:

> In modern humans, that part of our brain that is associated with speech is situated up in the frontal area. It is called Broca's area. If you fill the skull with rubber, you can pull out what we call an endocast form, which gives you the external shape of the brain. If you take an endocast of *this* skull, Broca's area is clearly apparent. Chimpanzees and gorillas don't show Broca's area. This one did. The *potential* for speech was already established.

A perplexing revelation: the brain of this creature, only half the size of ours, apparently had the specialised region that in modern humans controls speech. Yet all the evidence from the fossil record suggests that *Homo habilis* and even *Homo erectus* must have been very slow, limited and clumsy in their vocalisations. If the area of the brain that we use to communicate developed far in advance of the full capacity of speech, did the order and structure that language impose on thought exist long before our ancestors were able to speak to each other? Did *Homo habilis* use this part of his brain to control communication through gestures, as many palaeoanthropologists have suggested? Or did the primitive Broca's area give this creature his ability to manipulate objects, to plan and to construct stone tools? To Richard Leakey, the stone implements that early hominids left behind tell us about their minds:

> Ancestors of ours, living 1.5 to 2 million years ago, were making beauti-fully shaped stone implements. To make a hand axe out of a piece of stone, you have to be able to pick up a stone that contains the hand axe before you make it. You have to see the finished object in the piece of stone. Now, that ability to conceptualise, to abstract, to see something that isn't there, seems to be human.

Although chimpanzees and gorillas have only pint-sized brains, one third the size of ours, they share 99 per cent of their genetic material, the DNA of their chromosomes, with modern humans. That critical 1 per cent has given us our spoken language and in turn our culture, our science and our art. Does this mean, then, that our nearest living relatives in the animal kingdom do not have minds? Could those 1 per cent of human genes be mind-makers?

In 1960, Jane Goodall, a student from Cambridge, was working with Richard Leakey's father, Louis. He suggested to her that the study of chimpanzees in the wild might cast light on the social life and behaviour of our Stone Age ancestors. At that time, little was known of the natural life of apes and the impression gained from observation in laboratories, zoos and circuses was that apes have excellent memories, good vision and remarkable dexterity but that they live shallow, mindless lives.

The work of Jane Goodall in the Gombe Stream reserve in Tanzania has changed all that. She has described the richness of chimpanzee society, the intense bonds that hold family members together, their communication and co-operation. But one discovery above all, made very early in her work, sticks in her memory: in November, 1960, she saw one of the adult males, David Greybeard, 'fishing' for termites by pushing a long grass stem into holes in the red earth mound of a termite nest. This was no chance conjunction of random actions; the chimpanzees would search far from the termite nest for appropriate twigs and stems, cleaning them carefully and putting a stack of spare implements on the ground beside them as they got to work on the termites. Jane Goodall sent a telegram to Louis Leakey, who had defined humans as creatures who made tools to a regular and set pattern. He replied: 'We must either redefine tool, redefine man, or accept chimpanzees as humans'!

Chimpanzees not only share with us intelligent social behaviour but they also have an ugly side to their nature. In 1974, Goodall first saw a band of chimpanzees waging war, attacking and driving out a neighbouring troop. No one who reads Goodall's story can fail to believe that the brain of the chimpanzee can kindle the flickering flame of mind. But chimpanzees did not escape from the forest, did not trek into the hostile unknown of Europe and Asia, did not struggle against the dying Ice Age, built no cathedrals. In Jane Goodall's view, language is the key to the achievements of man:

> Spoken language frees humans from the present. It enables us to make meaningful plans not only for the immediate future, which even a chimp can do, but for next year, or ten years time. It enables us to pass on traditions and cultures to our children.

Chimpanzees cannot speak; that is the one certain fact in the science of communication. But psychologists have now shown that chimpanzees do have the capacity to communicate in symbols, even if they lack the grammatical power of true language. More of that later.

• THE SELECTION OF MIND •

The arrogance of human beings, the deep-rooted belief that people are unique and radically different from the animal world, is easy enough to understand. All species *are* unique; if they were not they would not be independent species. In order to do its biological job of sustaining itself and its genes, any animal must *act* as if the world exists for the benefit of it and its family alone. In people, this fundamental biological imperative of self-preservation has been turned into our anthropocentric view of the universe.

Deep in the network of caves at Lascaux, an artist left the only picture of a human being – a crude stick figure with a bird-like head, toppling under the impact of a charging bison, which is painted with care and accuracy. The person who drew this strange image of abstract man and representational animal surely saw human beings as separate and special. The arrogance of uniqueness was there 17 000 years ago.

The shock that we now face is the notion that even our most treasured possession, our mind, is *not* uniquely human but is merely the highest rung of the ladder of mental function, which stretches down far into the animal world. Evolution, most of the time, moved in imperceptible steps; but every now and then, a tiny structural development produced a qualitative change in function. The wing of a primitive bird was little different in structure (and in the genes that built it) from the limb of its reptilian ancestors. But the bird could do something that the reptile could not have dreamt of; it could fly. Surely the evolution of the human brain, and its product the mind, must have been of this explosive kind. A minor embellishment of structure (that primitive Broca's area, perhaps) pushed the brain off the cliff of evolution and enabled its thoughts to fly.

For Richard Dawkins, Oxford zoologist, evolution is starkly simple: 'The point or the purpose of anything in a living system is to propagate the genes that made it.' Darwin had seen that the pressures of the environment *select* individual animals (or even co-operative groups of animals) on the basis of their *fitness* to deal with those demands. But what *makes* an animal fit, in those terms, is the genes that construct its body. What, then, does a Darwinian reductionist make of the flowering of the human mind? For Dawkins, the mind *is* the actions of the brain, which 'evolved because it made animals more efficient in propagating genes'.

The massive expansion of the brain, and especially the cerebral cortex, that occurred during the evolution of monkeys and apes might have been driven by their tree-dwelling lifestyle. Moving rapidly through a complex world of branches and leaves must have placed enormous demands on the computer inside their head. When early hominids left the forests and ventured out on to the savannah, they carried with them the brains they had inherited from their tree-dwelling ancestors. Like the arm that became a wing, this big brain suddenly revealed that it could do other, wonderful things.

The picture that Dawkins paints seems, at first, chilling. Genes are little more than viruses with which our bodies, their products and servants, have come to terms. They use the bodies that they inhabit merely as vehicles to transport them. And, ultimately, those bodies reproduce the genes that made them. The living animal is a robot and its brain is the computer that controls it.

Let us examine and, I hope, dismiss the fear and outrage that that mechanistic comparison arouses. I know that my heart is merely a lump of contractile proteins with various chemical and electrical properties that make it beat rhythmically. I know that my genes built it and that its actions can be described in simple, physical terms. But that does not make me value it any less. Equally, if the march of brain research helps us to understand our minds as products of our brains, it may eliminate the mystery without destroying the wonder. As Richard Dawkins puts it:

> Humans can fall in love, can have emotions, can enjoy beautiful music, and so on. All those things are fully within the capabilities of the kinds of robots that we are. We are robots in the sense that we are mechanical systems. We are built from the laws of physics.

• AN ATTITUDE OF MIND •

We speak of having a strong mind, of losing it, of making it up. We take the mind for granted, but have only the dimmest notion of what the word means. This book will tell you more *about* the mind, but I cannot promise you complete knowledge or full understanding. I can, though, state a point of view and a principle of belief. I think that all those things that you do when you feel that you are using your mind (perceiving, thinking, feeling, choosing, and so on) are entirely the result of the physical actions of the myriad cells that make up your brain. The brain performs the actions that we explain to ourselves in terms of our minds.

I hope that this materialistic view of the nature of mind will not offend too many readers. In my opinion we are now witnessing a change of public attitude towards the nature of humanity as significant as that which Darwin's theory of evolution brought about. In the last forty years,

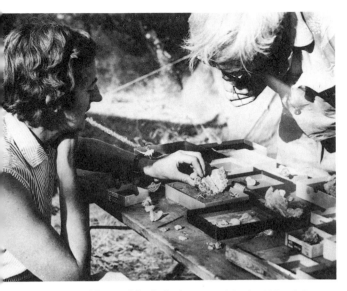

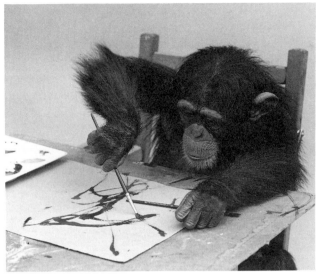

Mary and Louis Leakey at work in the Olduvai Gorge in Tanzania in 1959 (above). They described Homo erectus, *the immediate predecessor of modern man, and the earliest known true hominid,* Homo habilis.

Zoologist Desmond Morris observed the painting of 'Congo', a chimpanzee at London Zoo in the late 1950s (above). The compositions had a simple sense of design, but were never representational.

This scanning electron micrograph (right) shows neurons from the human cerebral cortex. Each has a large cell body (typically 0.01–0.02 mm across), a single fibre or axon, that transmits messages to other nerve cells, and a bush of dendrites – short branches on which the axons of other cells terminate to form synapses. The conventional electron micrograph (below right) shows a very thin, highly magnified section through the cortex of a rat. (The horizontal bar is 0.001 mm long.) The terminal of a nerve fibre (labelled 'I') forms a synapse with a dendrite ('D') of another cell. The terminal is packed with small 'vesicles' containing transmitter substance, which is released to communicate information across the synaptic gap, marked by an arrow. The appearance of this synapse suggests that it is inhibitory; the chemical transmitter would reduce the activity of the next nerve cell. Nearby, another nerve terminal ('E') forms a synapse (probably excitatory) on a 'spine' ('S') – a small knob on a dendrite.

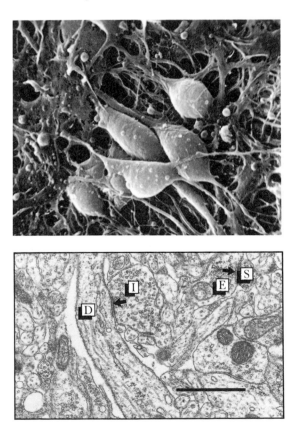

medical science has developed remarkable new treatments for disorders of brain and mind, in the same way that it works its everyday miracles on other organs of the body. Epilepsy is yielding to drugs and tumours to surgery; we are now hearing of the first successes of transplantation of brain tissue in the treatment of Parkinson's disease. 'Mental' illnesses, formerly discussed in hushed tones, as products of the supernatural world or subconscious sexual fantasy, are now accepted by the majority of ordinary people as tragic faults in the chemistry or the structure of the brain.

Take, for instance, Huntington's disease. It starts, often at the prime of life, as an uncontrollable twitch in the face. The jerky convulsions spread, inexorably, to the whole body. Walking, speech and even breathing become difficult or impossible, and most sufferers also undergo a cruel psychological disorder, with failures of memory and judgement, and delusions and emotional outbursts like those of people suffering from schizophrenia. This complex, lethal condition affects one in ten thousand people in the population as a whole. However, it runs in families and in certain isolated communities the incidence is much higher.

Nancy Wexler, American clinical psychologist, has a special interest in this disease: her mother and all of her mother's brothers died from it and there are only two known survivors in her family. She studies an isolated, interbred community around Lake Maracaibo in Venezuela. This single family of over three thousand people nurtures the largest concentration of Huntington's disease in the world. One person out of four dies from it.

The physical ravages wrought by this disease are plain to see in the brain from a dead sufferer. Right in the centre, below the cerebral hemispheres, the fluid-filled ventricles are swollen and the surrounding brain tissue is dead. This region, the basal ganglia, is involved in the control of movement. Scientists such as Wexler now have the techniques to probe below the veneer of the terrible symptoms, beneath the obvious damage in the brain, to the chemical mistake that causes Huntington's disease. Drugs that influence the symptoms, exaggerating them or reducing them, suggest that this illness is due to excessive production or heightened action of dopamine, just one of the multitude of chemical substances that nerve cells use to communicate with each other. There is evidence that schizophrenia too is caused by over-activity of the dopamine system, in other parts of the brain.

Probing further in the network of cause and effect, we see undeniable evidence that a genetic fault underlies the chemical error; each child of a parent with the disease has a 50 per cent chance of inheriting it. Just four years after the start of Nancy Wexler's research in Venezuela, she and her colleagues discovered a marker for the guilty gene, which can be seen under the microscope. This genetic marker allows her to identify the young people who will develop the disease, and to advise them not to have children. This breakthrough was one of the first clear indications of a hereditary factor in a brain disease. Other genetic links are now emerging, for schizophrenia, for depression, for Alzheimer's disease and for many of the rarer neurological disorders.

Genes build nerve cells that communicate in a language of chemicals; the connections of those cells determine our perceptions, our thoughts and our actions; even our emotions and the characteristics that make us individual persons are the products of physical processes in our brains. The mind is what the brain does.

• KNOW THYSELF •

John Searle, a philosopher from the University of California at Berkeley, sums up this changing view of the nature of mind:

> Mind is the name of a process, not a thing. That process is entirely caused by physiological events in the brain. It is not something mysterious that stands outside of the natural world. It's just part of our ordinary biological life.

Recorded philosophy was born in the Ancient Greek colonies of Asia Minor in the sixth century BC, a time when mythological explanations of natural events and of human destinies were widely accepted – when the Oracle of Delphi held supreme authority in the civilised world. The first philosophers made it their profession to question established beliefs; the inconsistencies and physical impossibilities of the events in myths defied any kind of rational account. Yet so much of what happens in the world is clearly a matter of straightforward cause and effect. Order and logic, the philosophers held, should be the basis of explanation.

By 385 BC, when Plato established his Academy in Athens, two diametrically opposed ideas about the human mind were clearly formulated – that it is part of the physical world, and that it is not. Plato himself believed the human soul to be unified and immortal, an indestructible spiritual substance that determines both actions and thoughts, in a separate universe of meaning from the mere body with which it is temporarily married. As the famous motto from Punch has it:

> What is Matter? – Never Mind.
> What is Mind? – No Matter.

Thus the theory of *dualism* was born – a theory that put mind in a separate category from body, not (as modern dualists do) because of frustration at the implausibility of explaining mental processes in terms of the physical actions of the brain, but because of respect for abstract ideas and belief in the unique status of mankind. However, even in Plato's own time, the harsher hypothesis was rearing its head. Democritus argued that *everything* in the universe, even the human mind, is created from the assembly of 'atoms' in the void. The mind, though composed of special atoms, is fundamentally material in its structure.

If the philosophy of mind were a football match, one would have to admit that, in the first half, dualism scored most of the goals. In particular, the 'interactive dualism' of the great seventeenth-century French philosopher, René Descartes, has left its impression to the present day on philosophy and science. He was fascinated with machines; with clocks, with pulleys, and with the automated fountains that were all the rage in the palaces of France at that time. To him, the body, including the nervous system, was nothing more than a machine – detecting events in the outside world through the senses, storing that information, reacting, moving its limbs. All of these things were accomplished solely through the connections of nerves from the sense organs to the brain, their complex organisation within the brain and the flow of fluid out along the nerves to the muscles. Most of the time, the spiritual soul was a silent observer, unseen and unneeded amongst the marvellous tangle of nerves. Only now and then, in situations of moral judgement or deliberate choice, did it somehow interact with the machinery of the brain – a touch on the tiller from the ghost in the machine.

In 1649, Descartes suggested that the mind or soul might exercise its influences through one particular structure in the brain, the enigmatic pineal gland, although he had earlier pointed out that mind and body appear to blend totally with each other. In the *Meditations on First Philosophy* of 1641, Descartes wrote, 'I am not merely lodged with my body, like a sailor in a ship, but am very closely united and as it were intermingled with it.'

Descartes's notion that the complex workings of an animal's brain and even the majority of the actions of the human brain are simply the products of spiritually worthless machinery, freed science from the straitjacket of religious dogma. On the other hand, the notion that all the really *interesting* bits of human mental behaviour (perceiving, thinking, choosing, for instance) are done by a spiritual something that lies outside the methods and laws of science is a form of philosophical surrender. Perhaps there is a force within us, essential to our being, that is beyond the realm of the laws of physics and chemistry. But if that is true it should be accepted only when science has failed to provide alternative, material explanations.

On the lintel of the Temple of Apollo at Delphi was written the motto of the Greek sages, 'Know Thyself'. We feel that consciousness – self-consciousness – gives us that knowledge of ourselves. Descartes reasoned that the *only* thing that he could trust was his own conscious experience. But what do we mean by consciousness, and do we truly know ourselves and our brains through introspection?

• THE LIMITED VISION OF •
THE INNER EYE

Consciousness is a window through which we view the world and ourselves in it. Moreover, it is our most cherished possession. You can buy insurance policies that offer to pay you for the loss of your faculties or your functions; £5000 for one eye or one hand, £10 000 for both. But how could they compensate for the loss of *consciousness*? To be unconscious is not to exist as a person. Yet we know almost nothing of the workings of this searchlight that cuts through the darkness of the human mind.

Many modern-day philosophers, who are inclined temperamentally towards physical explanations of brain and mind, still find themselves in a dilemma when it comes to accounting for the window of consciousness. Some just deny its existence as a *thing* needing explanation; some see it as merely a mistake in our use of language; some say that it belongs to that category of problems (such as the nature of infinity) that simply cannot be comprehended by the human mind. Others again, including John Searle, view consciousness as a *product* of the machinery of the brain, the synthesis of which is possible only because of the very special material from which the brain is made. As Searle puts it:

> The proof of consciousness is the fact that each of us is conscious. If the scientist tells me the table isn't really solid, because it's really composed of a cloud of microparticles; or the scientist tells me the sun *looks* like it sets, but it doesn't really set, it's just an illusion created by the rotation of the earth on its axis; I can accept both of these, because I can see how there's a distinction between appearance and reality. But where the existence of consciousness is concerned, the appearance *is* the reality. If I think I'm conscious, I am conscious.

Computers made by human beings *might*, one day, be made to have conscious experiences, but John Searle contends that they cannot be said to be conscious simply because the programs that they run allow them to imitate, even perfectly, things done by conscious humans. He supports his argument with an allegory: the story of a strange computing machine consisting of a room in which a real, conscious, thinking human being is locked. Through one window are pushed cards with Chinese characters written on them. The person inside has a stack of similar cards with words in English and a huge book of rules, which tells him which English cards to push out through another window in response to the signals in Chinese. He understands neither Chinese nor the function of the rule book. He is simply slavishly carrying out instructions. Moral: the room is a computer, the man its central processor, the rule book a program for the translation of Chinese into English. The 'computer' does its job but is unaware of what it is doing. Thus, Searle concludes, computers cannot be said to be conscious simply by virtue of the similarity of the things that they do to the performance of conscious human beings.

To my mind, this argument contains an essential flaw which is a clue to the real nature and function of consciousness. Searle believes that consciousness has real value and that we manage the important parts of our lives entirely through mental processes. But if consciousness *is* so important, how could any kind of computing machine imitate *completely* the richness of human behaviour unless it too had this essential quality of mental experience?

At the end of his great work, the *Tractatus*, published in 1929, the enigmatic philosopher Ludwig Wittgenstein wrote: 'Whereof we cannot speak, thereof we must be silent.' To a scientist, that seems a very cloistered viewpoint. We have a rich language for the everyday world of the mental, but no precise words to describe the *machinery* of consciousness; surely that does not mean that we commit some kind of philosophical blasphemy to mention the subject in a scientific context. Just as nuclear physicists have had to invent 'hadrons', 'bosons' and so on to give an account of the wonderland of particles inside the atom, so science will have to invent new ways of speaking about the process that we call consciousness in order to describe its mechanism.

But before we understand how it *works*, we can ask what it does. Nicholas Humphrey, zoologist and philosopher, has written that 'Nature has given to human beings the remarkable gift of *self-reflexive* insight'. Well then, if *Nature* made us conscious, the machinery for consciousness must have evolved by natural selection; and in that case, the 'insight into the workings of the brain' that Humphrey believes consciousness gives us must have improved the chances of biological survival for those creatures on which Nature first bestowed this gift.

The clue to the *adaptive* function of consciousness, Humphrey believes, is the complexity of human society. Certainly, the fossil record strongly suggests that the earliest hominids were highly social creatures. The shift from a vegetarian diet to meat-eating put the emphasis on social hunting, with all its demands for planning, co-operation and communication. But another factor may have been much more powerful. Life expectancy was very short, perhaps as low as 20 years on average. But childhood and adolescence were already very long, to allow man's huge brain to grow and mature. The strong likelihood of the death of parents before the maturity of their children would surely have put a premium on the development of cohesive social groups with a commitment to the nurturing of their offspring. Any development of the brain that aided these early people in dealing with the increasingly complex structure of their society would have been beneficial and therefore preserved. Nicholas Humphrey sees this as the clue to consciousness:

> Human beings ... have to have a way of predicting and understanding the *behaviour* of other members of their own species. How do they do that? They do it by employing a mental model, which makes use continually of the kind of information we get when we look with the inner eye of consciousness and see our own minds as being composed of desires, wills, emotions, sensations, and so on. It gives us a conceptual framework for understanding *other* human beings.

This elegant theory prompts two questions. First, why does consciousness use such strange symbolism? For instance, the biological value of finding a partner obviously has to do with the nitty-gritty of procreation. But when you find your perfect mate, you *feel* that you are in *love*, a sensation that tells us nothing directly about the crude necessity of reproduction. Consciousness translates biological necessities into feelings of pain and pleasure, need and emotion.

Second, why does the inner eye see so little? It gives us only a tiny glimpse, and distorted at that, of the world within. Much of what our brains do is entirely hidden from consciousness. When you recognise a friend, you have not the slightest impression that billions of nerve cells have digested the signals from your eyes and distilled them into the wisdom of perception. When you pick up a pen, thousands of calculations set the tone of muscles and adjust the strength of your grip to your knowledge of the weight of a pen and the force of gravity. Most of the actions of the human mind are beyond the gaze of the inner eye of consciousness.

I hesitate to use the word 'subconscious', because the unconscious domain imagined by modern psychology is far from the subconscious world of Sigmund Freud and the theorists of psychoanalysis who followed him. On the shelf of the library in the house in Hampstead to which Freud brought his family in 1938 is the 1875 German edition of the complete works of Charles Darwin. Freud claimed that he was much influenced, like most scientists of his generation, by Darwin's ideas. Yet the curious world of repressed sexuality and black symbolism that Freud thought of as the subconscious mind seems to me to tell us more about the middle-class culture of pre-war Vienna than about the animal origins of mankind. Modern psychology has given us a new concept of the unconscious mind.

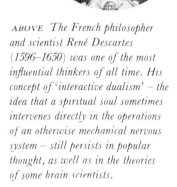

ABOVE *The French philosopher and scientist René Descartes (1596–1650) was one of the most influential thinkers of all time. His concept of 'interactive dualism' – the idea that a spiritual soul sometimes intervenes directly in the operations of an otherwise mechanical nervous system – still persists in popular thought, as well as in the theories of some brain scientists.*

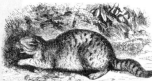

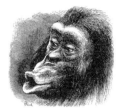

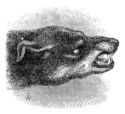

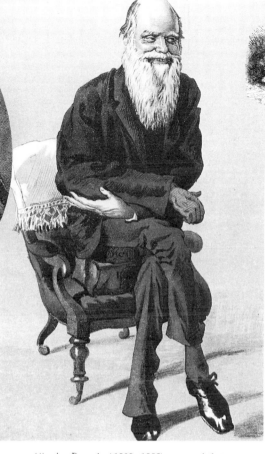

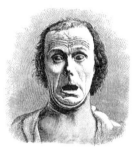

ABOVE *Charles Darwin (1809–1882) proposed that all the components and functions of animals, including the brain and the mind, are the product of natural selection. He was particularly interested in the way in which facial and bodily reactions are used by animals and humans to convey their emotions (right).*

RIGHT *Sigmund Freud (1856–1939) was the father of psychoanalysis and champion of the subconscious mind. Modern cognitive psychology has a different view of subconscious processing and emphasises its role in perception, thought and the control of language and movement.*

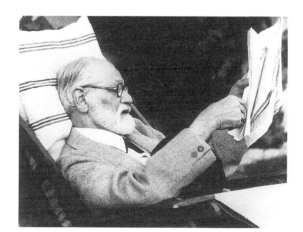

At its heyday, during the Greek wars with Persia, the machinery of prediction that underlay the Oracle of Delphi was enlarged and improved. In a sense, it worked a little like the human mind. The Pythia herself was consciousness in this model of the mind – perceiving, understanding and predicting the future. But behind her was an invisible, subconscious world. A network of spies acted as her eyes and ears. And the prophets who surrounded her secretly weighed the evidence before advising her and translating her incoherent mumblings.

Consciousness explains and predicts, but the view of the world and the future that it gives us depends on mechanisms that are hidden from view. Our perceptions, beliefs, thoughts and memories can be influenced by our states of need or expectation, by our social and political views of the world, or even by the suggestions of a hypnotist.

Brain research and psychology must try to give an account of the mystery of mind in terms of the structure and organisation of the brain. The task is immense but the potential rewards are beyond value. For me, the human brain is the most exciting challenge left for science. To understand the world of physics, from the atoms to the stars, is wonderful. But to understand the organ that allows us to understand would be little short of a miracle. The human brain makes us what we are. It makes the mind, which has driven people to build theatres, temples and palaces, to invent religion, philosophy and science, drama, music and art, to explore the entire planet and even to escape from the environment that created those people.

THE UNFOLDING MIND

ALBERT EINSTEIN was once a single cell. So too was Adolf Hitler. We all start our long journey to mindfulness as that tiniest unit of life – a fertilised egg. At birth, a human being has a brain with more nerve cells than it will ever have again, but the baby has probably not yet had a single conscious experience. In a few years this child, with its brain, will have mastered language, will understand the complex rules of social culture, will be aware of the world, the past, the future and itself.

• THE BEGINNING •

An ovum is fertilised by a sperm. Each is an envelope containing a vital message – a genetic story written in the strange four-lettered language of DNA. To live for ever is the ultimate prize of all the great religions of the world. Yet we are all immortal in the sense that the DNA, which makes us what we are, passes from generation to generation.

For a few hours the fertilised egg appears dormant. Then it divides. Its chromosomes split and replicate themselves to make a full set of forty-six for each of the new cells. The ritual of division repeats itself again and again; eight days after conception the embryo is a mass of several hundred cells. Any one of the central clump of cells, which will form the fetus itself, could be removed and development would continue quite normally. Then, suddenly, the cells of the embryo start to become committed to different paths of development.

About nineteen days after fertilisation comes the first step in the formation of a brain. A patch of cells in the surface of the ball becomes receptive to a chemical signal, produced by the layer below. In the fraternity of cells that form this plate, a gene switches on to synthesise a substance that makes their membranes stick together. Within a few days this neural plate has folded in on itself to form a tube. From this small cylinder will grow the entire brain and the rest of the nervous system. One end of the tube begins to thicken; it will be the brain. The other, thinner end will develop into the spinal cord. The cells of the primitive brain begin to multiply rapidly: some will become neurons, the nerve cells themselves; the others become glial cells, which guide the growing neurons, support them and nourish them.

The pace of cell division becomes frenetic, as if the genes were racing against time to make astronomical numbers of neurons in preparation for birth. Each new wave of nerve cells crawls along a guiding framework of glial cells to reach its destination in the growing brain. Successive generations of cells migrate past the layers of neurons that were born earlier and have already come to rest. It is this curious inside-out pattern of migration that leads to the characteristic layered structure of so many parts of the brain. Once a nerve cell begins its journey, it stops dividing and it resonates in subtle and mysterious ways to the changing pattern of chemical environments through which it moves. The genes of the cell react to these signals by turning on new chemical programmes that drive the cell irreversibly to its particular destiny. Differentiation, the process by which the cells of the body, all containing precisely the same genetic message, become specialised to perform their particular tasks in the body, remains one of the deepest mysteries in biology. It depends on an intimate interplay of genes and environment, responding to each other with perfect timing. Nowhere are the consequences of differentiation so remarkable as in the developing brain.

• A TIME OF DANGER •

By the eighth week after conception, the apparently reckless proliferation of neurons and glial cells has somehow, almost magically, produced a structure with recognisable shape. Here the stem of the brain, there the cerebellum, and on top the cerebral hemispheres, pushing out the growing skull. It is during this period that developing brains are most vulnerable to damage. On 6 August and 2 September 1945, atomic bombs exploded over Hiroshima and Nagasaki. Radioactivity shows no respect for the mere flesh and blood that protect a growing fetus. Among the survivors of the blasts were more than a thousand pregnant women: some of their children, now in their forties, were born with defects of the nervous system and they are still mentally retarded. William Schull and his colleagues at the Radiation and Sex Research Foundation in Hiroshima found that the mothers of all the most severely affected children had been between eight and sixteen weeks pregnant when the bombs exploded. The children of mothers who were more advanced in their pregnancies, or less than two months pregnant, suffered milder forms of retardation or none at all. This identified a period of great vulnerability in the growth of the brain, between eight and sixteen weeks of age, when radiation has a particularly cruel effect on the fetus.

This window of sensitivity coincides with the period of most rapid creation of nerve cells – up to a quarter of a million every minute – and their widespread invasion of the developing cerebral cortex. For the brain to function correctly, neurons must be in the right place to form the right connections and carry out their predestined tasks. Radiation probably affects not only the production of nerve cells but also their crawling journey along the web of glial fibres to their ultimate destinations, forcing them to stop short of their intended targets.

In 1970 Christy Uland, then a resident doctor in the Department of Pediatrics at the Children's Hospital in Seattle, Washington, noticed a curious similarity among some of the infants that she was studying. They were small for their age; they had flattened faces; and they were all mentally retarded. They looked as similar as the members of a single family but they were not related. The only thing that they had in common was alcoholic mothers. Kenneth Jones and David Smith of the Child Development and Mental Retardation Center in Seattle called this complex of symptoms the *Fetal Alcohol Syndrome*. It is now known to be the third most common form of birth abnormality after Down's Syndrome and neural tube defects, such as spina bifida.

Sterling Clarren at the University of Seattle has been studying baby monkeys to try to understand when and how alcohol, which easily crosses the placenta and enters the bloodstream of the fetus, affects the developing brain. Baby monkeys are naturally curious but if their mothers have been given alcohol during pregnancy, the babies are absurdly hyperactive and disturbed in their behaviour, rather like human infants with Fetal Alcohol Syndrome. Clarren discovered that alcohol affects the developing brain throughout gestation but *early* exposure is far more devastating in its results. Once again, the finger of evidence points to that critical early period, when the fetus is about two months old, as the time of greatest vulnerability.

The probable cause of the mental deficiencies became apparent when Sterling Clarren had the opportunity to study the first autopsied case of a baby who had had the disease and died. The brain was very small, but there was more wrong with it than its size alone. In a normal human brain the surface of the cerebral hemispheres is deeply infolded, so as to cram the vast area of the cerebral cortex into the space under the skull.

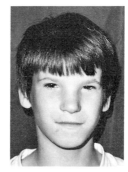
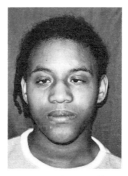

Two young boys, suffering from Fetal Alcohol Syndrome, show the impact of this condition on the appearance of their faces

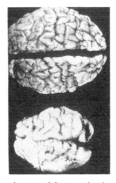

A normal human brain (top) and the damaged brain (bottom) of a child who had suffered from Fetal Alcohol Syndrome.

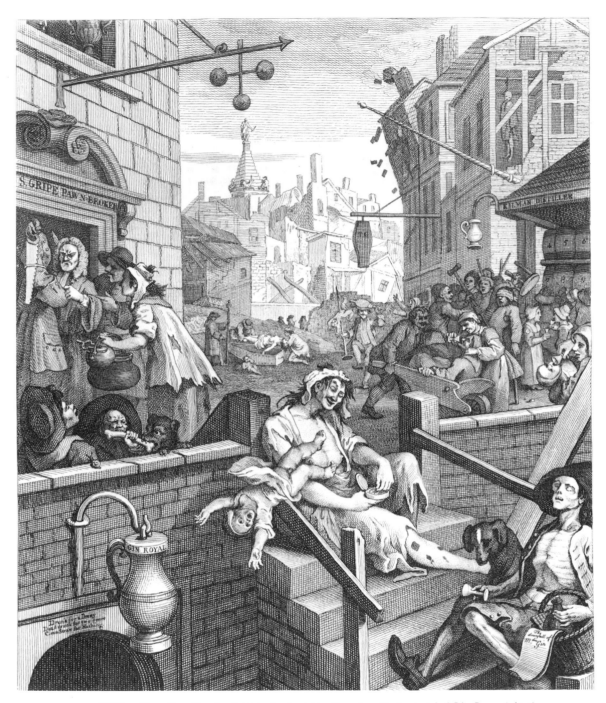

William Hogarth, critic of social injustice in eighteenth-century England, etched Gin Lane *(above), published in 1751. Depicting the evil influence of alcohol, it shows a mother pouring gin into a baby's mouth. In fact, a baby's brain is most sensitive to the effects of alcohol long before birth.*

But in the alcohol-injured brain, the fluid-filled ventricles within the brain are far too large, the layer of nerve fibres (white matter) under the cortex is abnormally thin and the infoldings of the cortex itself are much too shallow. So, both the total area of the cortex and the amount of connection that it receives are reduced.

The microscope reveals further evidence of devastation and disorganisation. The layers of the cortex are deformed and distorted, as if there had been no signal to tell the migrating neurons when to stop. Many of them continued on past their proper destinations until they broke through and erupted on to the surface to become a tangled, scrambled mass.

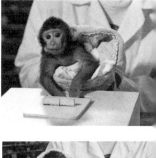

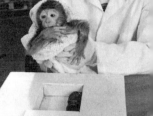

• DEATH AND TRANSFIGURATION •

It is halfway through gestation. In many parts of the brain, the waves of migration have ceased: the brain begins to stabilise itself. The immature, unformed nerve cells have reached their destinations and begun to differentiate. They will vary in size, in shape, in the chemical substances that they produce and use to transmit signals. But most of all, they will differ in their connections with other nerve cells. If any one process is responsible for the genesis of mind, it is the formation of connections in the brain. In the middle months of gestation that process is fast and furious. But the making and breaking of connections continues, not just until birth but into childhood and, in subtle ways, throughout life.

Each differentiating neuron sprouts a thin finger that pushes rapidly into unknown territory, feeling the chemical world around it. This will become the axon or fibre of the nerve cell. At its growing tip, tiny twitching hairs probe the territory ahead, searching for cells with the right tastes on their surfaces, gripping and pulling the growing axon towards its target. The axons of certain cells, the motor neurons in the spinal cord and in the brainstem, force their way out into the body where they seek the muscles that they will ultimately control. When these connections are made and the motor neurons start, spontaneously, to transmit impulses, the fetus begins to twitch, to kick, and eventually to *breathe* – sucking the fluid around it into its lungs, practising for the time, months ahead, when it will take its first gasp of air.

Within the brain itself, neurons connect to neurons, and those to others, and on and on to form networks of breathtaking complexity. The sense organs – the eyes, the ears and the multitude of other receptive cells around the body – send their fibres into the central nervous system. Within the sensory pathways inside the brain, development proceeds in a cascade, from the outside towards the centre. The ingrowing sensory fibres find their central targets, clusters of nerve cells interposed on the way up to

Research at the University of Seattle has defined the sensitive period for the effect of alcohol in monkeys and has shown that their behaviour is affected like that of children with Fetal Alcohol Syndrome. A normal baby monkey (top) is naturally curious and will immediately reach for a toy that has been hidden from view. A monkey whose mother was exposed to alcohol during pregnancy (bottom) is inattentive and uninterested.

the cerebral cortex. At each level the invading axons stimulate a phase of growth and development in the receiving structure. When the fibres in each optic nerve, connecting the eye to the brain, reach their first target, called the lateral geniculate nucleus, it is little more than a homogeneous ball of cells. More than half of the optic nerve fibres cross over to the opposite side of the brain, so each lateral geniculate nucleus receives a mixture of fibres from the two eyes. Their arrival galvanises the unformed mass into a new phase of development; its cells differentiate and redistribute themselves to form layers, each layer receiving fibres from only one of the eyes. This perfectly timed sequence – the arrival of fibres followed by the formation of layers – is no coincidence. The ingrowing axons themselves stimulate the lateral geniculate nucleus to enter this new stage of anatomical development. The brain uses its own activity to help to construct itself.

One of the most surprising of recent discoveries is the fact that death, on a massive scale, plays a crucial part in the development of the brain, long before the child is born. Some weeks *before* birth there are far more cells in the brain than there will be in the newborn child, and their connections are more widespread too. The *death* of nerve cells and the *removal* of connections both play vital parts in the perfection of the brain. The genetic programme that orchestrates the construction of the nervous system seems to play safe by building in extra cell divisions and by encouraging the immature neurons to form exploratory connections to distant parts of the nervous system. Both the unneeded cells and the unwanted connections are eliminated as the brain becomes refined to its ultimate state.

The factors that regulate the death of cells and the rearrangement of connections are numerous. Some of the changes seem to be written in the inbuilt blueprint of the genetic code – a code that can kill as well as create. But others depend on the individual battle fought by each growing fibre for space in the crowded brain. The optic nerve of a monkey, some weeks before birth, contains more than 2 million fibres; twice the number that it will keep as an adult. If one eye is missing at this stage, the remaining eye retains more nerve cells and more optic nerve fibres than usual. Presumably fibres from the two eyes normally fight with each other for space on their target cells in the brain – a deadly game of musical chairs in which the losers die.

The literal death of neurons is not the only mechanism that the developing brain employs to remove unwanted connections. Some cells, especially in the cerebral cortex, send out their fibres to unusual targets but then, at some specific stage in development, withdraw those connections and make new ones instead, without the cells necessarily dying. Giorgio Innocenti at the Institute of Anatomy in Lausanne discovered that this process of switching connections plays a major part in the

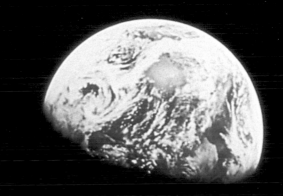

Earth – the world that created the mind machine inside our heads. Every other species on our planet is essentially trapped in one particular style of life, perfectly adapted to one corner of the earth's environment. But human beings, through the power of their brains, have changed their own world, explored every hostile corner of the earth and even escaped from the environment that created them. In 1968, the astronauts on the Apollo 8 spacecraft saw this view of their own planet rising above the horizon of the moon.

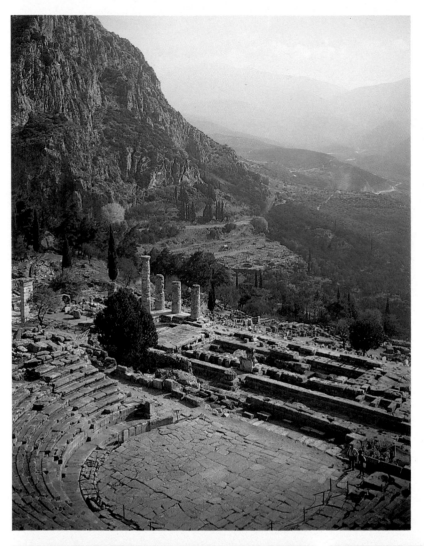

LEFT *Delphi was the holiest spot in ancient Greece – centre of the world, home of Apollo, symbol of the power of mythological explanation. The Temple of Apollo, with its huge pillars, lies below the stage of the Theatre. The Temple was the sanctuary of the Oracle of Delphi, whose predictions influenced the decisions and actions of the mightiest men in the western world for 2000 years of legend and history. On the lintel above the portico was the most famous of Greek mottoes, 'Know Thyself'.*

BELOW *17 000 years ago, at Lascaux in south-west France, Cro-Magnon people left a message that they had minds like ours. They decorated the walls of the caves with magnificent paintings of the animals that they hunted (left). But in a tiny crevice, deep in the caves is the only image of a human being, attacked by an injured bison (right). The man is a cryptic stick figure, a mere symbol of humanity. Even to the Cro-Magnon mind, the human species was already special.*

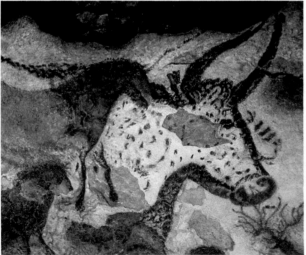

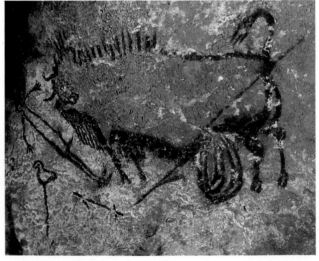

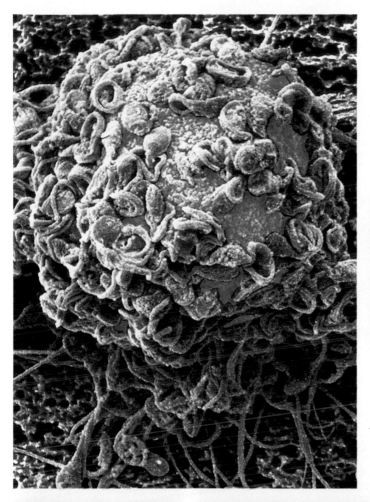

Sperm, their heads packed with DNA, smother the surface of a human ovum (*left*). Fertilisation is the first step in the creation of a new mind. Ovum and sperm each contribute twenty-three chromosomes to make up the full set of forty-six (*below*). These chromosomes contain the genes (perhaps as few as 50 000 of them) which are the inherited blueprint of a new human being – body and brain.

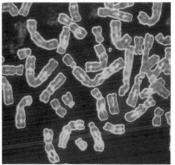

BELOW *In very simple animals many of the neurons are so distinctive and regular in arrangement that exactly the same cell can be identified from one individual to another. One neuron in the middle of the thorax of a grasshopper has been injected with a yellow fluorescent dye (far left), showing the full pattern of its dendrites and branching axon. During the early development of this cell, the tip of its axon, covered with fine, twitching hairs (left) grows across a scaffold of glial cells and makes contact with another bundle of nerve fibres, sticking to them and creeping along them, to find its correct target.*

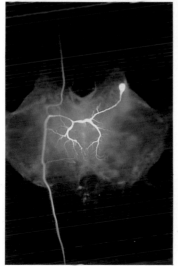

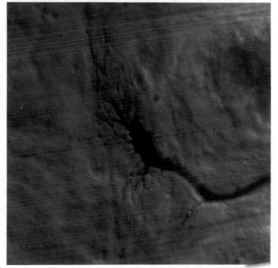

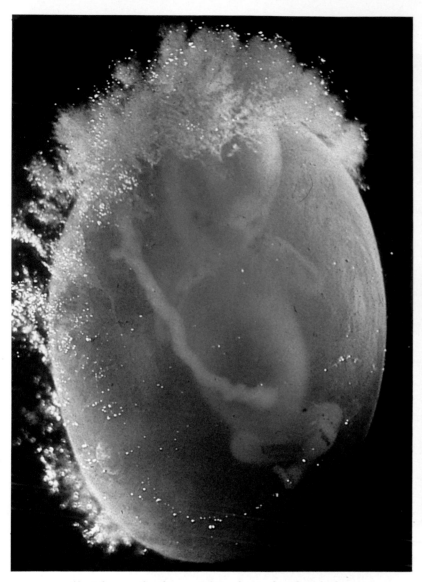

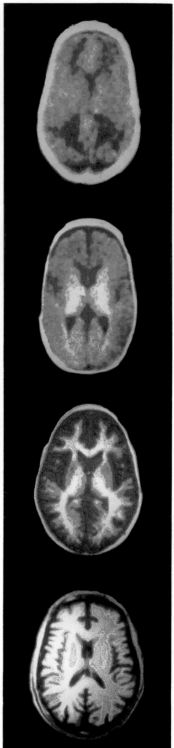

About three months after conception, a human fetus floats in the warm amniotic fluid. Its brain is reaching the end of the period of multiplication and migration of nerve cells, during which it is vulnerable to the effects of radiation and alcohol.

After birth, few if any new neurons are created, but the existing cells grow and connections between them continue to form. Nuclear Magnetic Resonance imaging, one of the new non-invasive methods of seeing inside the living brain, provides pictures of horizontal slices through the head, at birth, six months, five years and in an adult (right: from top to bottom). In each image, the forehead is at the top. The outer layer of cortex, covering the cerebral hemispheres, increases in thickness and area, and becomes progressively more infolded. The nerve fibres underneath, which carry messages in and out of the cortex, become thickly covered with myelin, a fatty sheath (shown as white in these scans) that helps them conduct impulses more quickly.

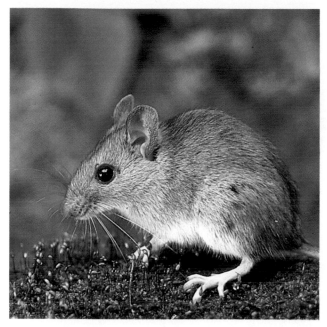

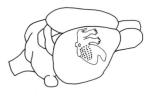

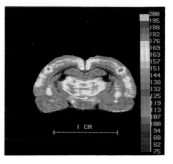

The large whiskers on the upper lip of a mouse (left) are very important sense organs. Huge numbers of nerve fibres carry information from the thirty-three whiskers on each side of the face through a pathway of connections to the opposite cerebral hemisphere, where the body surface is represented in the somatic cortex (above centre). A large area within this body 'map' is devoted to sensory information from the whiskers. The incoming nerve fibres arrive in the middle layer of the cortex. A microscopic section cut through this layer, parallel to the surface, shows the individual nerve cells as tiny blue dots (left, upper part). They form thirty-three rings, called 'barrels', each about 0.3 mm across, arranged in a pattern very similar to that of the whiskers on the face. The nerve fibres terminating in the middle of each barrel carry information from a single whisker. If a mouse is injected with a radioactive glucose derivative and just one whisker on each side of the face is gently vibrated, the radioactivity becomes concentrated in the activated nerve cells in the corresponding barrel on each side of the brain. The vertical section through the brain (above right) shows these activated barrels as red dots in the cortex.

The barrels form themselves during the first few days of life in response to the presence and activity of the incoming sensory fibres. If one row of whiskers is plucked out in a mouse less than about five days old, the corresponding row of barrels fails to form (left, lower part). The asterisk marks the missing row.

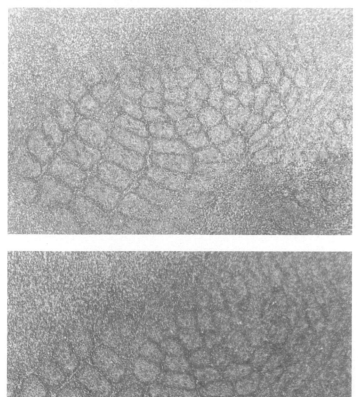

The attempt to assign particular functions to particular parts of the brain began in earnest with the pseudo-science of phrenology. Memory was said to be localised directly behind the eyes. Although phrenology was soon discredited in scientific circles, it was popularised (right) for more than 100 years.

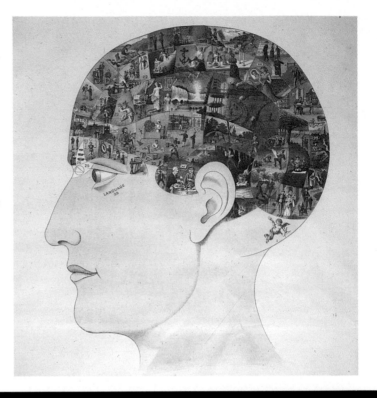

The human brain (below), sliced through the middle from front to back, reveals its major parts. The huge, convoluted cerebral hemispheres, where conscious memories are probably permanently stored, cover the top of the brain (frontal lobe to the left). The corpus callosum, appearing as a yellow horizontal band within the cerebral hemispheres, contains millions of fibres joining the two hemispheres together. Below is the brainstem, which runs down to join the spinal cord. The feathery organ on the back of the brainstem is the cerebellum, which is probably the site of the memory of motor skills.

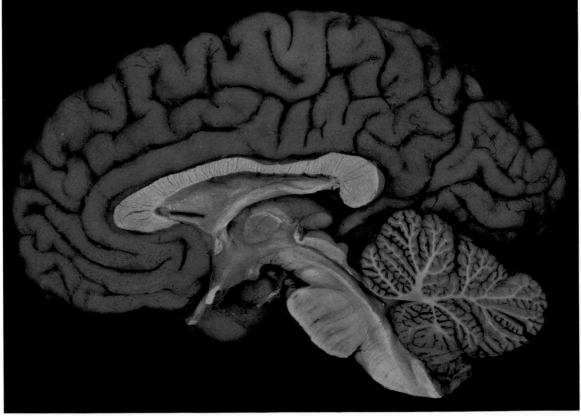

A honey bee (right) dances to demonstrate her memory of the whereabouts of a food source. The direction and length of the dance indicate the direction and distance of the food.

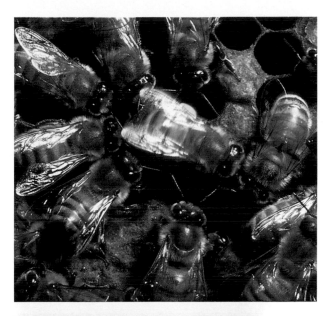

Eric Kandel holds a sea snail, Aplysia *(below left). This creature has a very small nervous system, but it can learn to change its behaviour. By recording electrical activity from individual nerve cells and fibres in this animal (below right), Kandel and his colleagues have tracked down the site of the underlying memories. For several sorts of learning, the change takes the form of the strengthening or weakening of individual synaptic connections between nerve cells. Rapid learning seems to depend on changes in the amount of chemical transmitter substance released from existing nerve terminals, but long-term learning probably involves actual growth or retraction of terminals.*

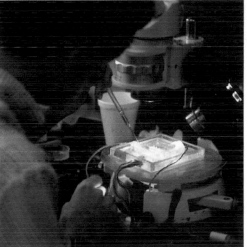

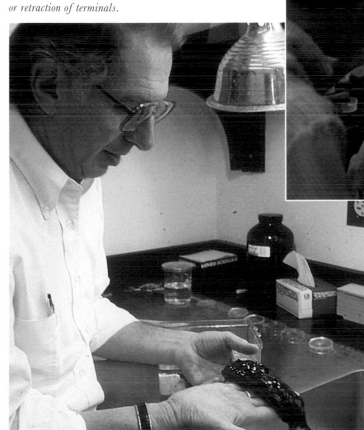

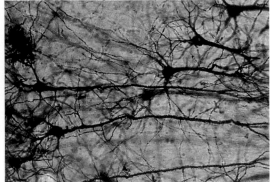

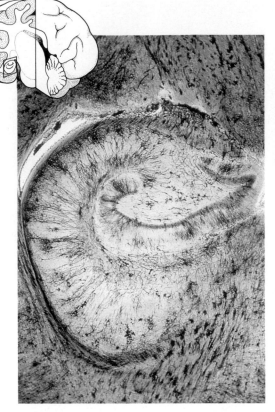

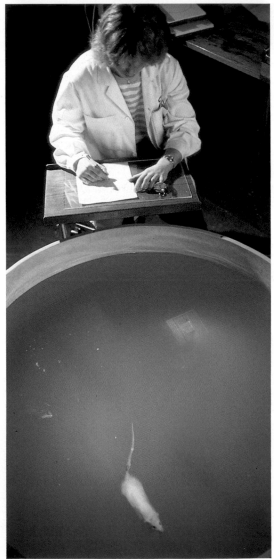

*Imagine the brain of a monkey viewed from behind, with
the rear half of the left hemisphere removed (top left).
The cross-section exposed reveals the hippocampus, out-
lined in red, rolled up within the temporal lobe. This
region is enlarged in a microscopic section (above), prepared by the Golgi technique, which stains only about
one nerve cell in fifty. A high-power view (above right)
shows some of the individual, large 'pyramidal cells', with
their many dendrites, where the terminals of incoming
fibres form synapses. A short burst of impulses arriving
along those incoming fibres causes 'long-term potentiation'
of the synapses, increasing their strength for several
weeks. This kind of change may underlie the initial
storage of information as consciously accessible 'declarative' memories in human beings.*

*The memory of a rat can be tested by training it to swim
in a pool of milky water to find a platform hidden under
the surface (right). A normal rat learns very quickly but
if the hippocampus is damaged, new learning is almost
impossible. The drug APV, which prevents long-term
potentiation, also interferes with this kind of learning.*

development of the corpus callosum, the huge cable of millions of fibres that connects together the hemispheres of the brain. In rodents, cats, monkeys and human beings, the corpus callosum contains a vast excess of nerve fibres in the fetus, joining together parts of the two cerebral hemispheres that do not remain connected in the normal adult.

All this attrition of cells and axons is far from the wastage that it seems to be. It is a clever trick that Nature has devised to sculpt the perfect neuronal machine from an over-abundance of cells and an excess of interconnection.

• LIFE BEYOND BIRTH •

Birth is the emergence of a baby from the dark constancy of the womb into a different universe, a world of sensory experience, which William James described as 'a blooming, buzzing confusion'. Lambs, colts and calves run and walk soon after they are born. Kittens and puppies are independent of their mothers within a few weeks. Even monkeys can look after themselves less than a year after birth. But human babies seem totally parasitic on their parents for years. No other species invests so much time in the rearing of its offspring; no other species takes so long to learn to be an individual. But this 'long childhood', as Jacob Bronowski called it, is no biological mistake, no waste of time. It is a period of maturation of brain and mind that goes far beyond anything that occurs or is needed in the rest of the animal kingdom. If any single characteristic of human beings makes them unique, separate from the beasts, it is surely the enormously protracted development of their brains.

But is a newborn baby truly helpless? Was the behavioural psychologist J. D. Watson correct when he said, 'All we have to start with in building a human being is a lively bit of squirming flesh'? To judge a baby by adult standards is as foolish as to assess the intelligence of a snail by comparison with a dog. The actions of babies are exquisitely adapted for their immediate purposes, not for their future lives. Until a few years ago, developmental psychologists, who are interested in the way that children gain understanding of the world around them, virtually ignored the first year or two of life. But increasingly they are exploring the mind of the speechless child.

Just a few minutes old, a baby will turn its head towards an object that touches its cheek, will work the object into its mouth and start sucking. The co-ordinated movements of head and neck, in response to sensory information, combined with appropriate reactions of breathing, sucking and swallowing, are all done without mistake the very first time. The urge to seek and suck is, of course, a programmed reaction – a reflex – designed to help the baby find the nipple. What the newborn child suckles from its mother for the first three days is colostrum, a deep yellow milk, rich in proteins, some of which help to give the baby early immunity. But the benefits go both ways. The sucking of the baby stimulates the release of a hormone, oxytocin, in the mother's body, which makes the uterus contract and hence helps to expel the afterbirth. And this immediate urge to suckle may help to promote the early emotional bonding between mother and baby. Indeed, many of the things that young babies do in response to signals from the environment can be interpreted in terms of the strengthening or modification of the relationship between the infant and its parents.

When do these behavioural programmes of survival first emerge in the growing fetus? Cecilia McCarton at the Neonatal Intensive Care Unit at Albert Einstein Hospital in the Bronx is studying babies who survive when born as much as fifteen weeks prematurely. Amazing technical advances in intensive care have made it possible for such immature infants to live, giving the psychologist a window on the state of development of such a fetus, only two-thirds prepared for birth. Even after just twenty-eight weeks of gestation, ten weeks before normal birth, a premature baby reacts to sound and light. It can turn to locate a sound; it can track a moving toy with its eyes (though whether it is using its cerebral cortex to do these things is not clear). A premature baby has made its entry on the stage of life a little early, but its brain is already prepared to deal with at least some of the blooming, buzzing confusion.

• INTO THE MIND OF A CHILD •

Most of what we know of the perceptions, thoughts and feelings of other human beings comes from what they *tell* us. Just because a young baby cannot *say* what it sees, or speak its thoughts, doesn't mean that it cannot think or perceive. But how are we to learn what a baby knows? Much of the progress of developmental psychology in the last few years has been based on the invention of ingenious methods of communicating with babies who cannot yet speak.

Of course, speech is not the only channel by which a mind can escape from the confines of its brain. The *actions* of animals write volumes about the nature of their sensations, their memories and their thoughts. The great advance in developmental psychology has come through finding and interpreting actions that babies *can* perform. One thing that babies do very well is to suckle, and they regulate the force with which they suck, depending on the apparent pleasure or novelty of the situation that they are in. A loud harsh voice will stop a baby sucking, while a soft and familiar voice will make it suck faster and harder.

William Fifer of Columbia Presbyterian Hospital in New York measures how strongly a baby sucks on an artificial nipple while it listens to tape recordings of voices. His research shows that, as soon as it is born, a baby not only sucks harder for the voice of a woman than for that of a man, but actually prefers its own mother's voice to that of other women. When a tiny microphone is placed inside the uterus of a pregnant woman, it picks up the mother's voice, though somewhat muffled by the layers of tissue through which the sound has to pass. It seems quite clear that the fetus not only *hears* inside the uterus but *learns* to recognise the distorted voice that it hears most. Indeed, a *newborn* baby actually prefers a recording of its own mother's voice electronically filtered to produce the same kind of distortion, rather than the pure sound alone. By about three weeks after birth, the baby learns to prefer the unmuffled version of its mother's voice!

The newborn baby also has a well-developed, though simple capacity to see. Jan Atkinson and Oliver Braddick at the University of Cambridge, and many other research workers around the world, study the visual worlds of babies. It turns out that even a newborn child has natural preferences. Confronted with two targets projected on a blank screen, the baby will turn its gaze towards the one with more *pattern*, more edges and lines. If one target is a set of black and white lines and the other is simply a grey patch of the same average brightness, the baby will look at the stripes. Making the stripes smaller, until suddenly the baby no longer prefers to look at them, provides a way of measuring the visual acuity of very young infants long before they can read an optician's test chart. The visual acuity of a newborn baby measured this way is worse than that of an adult rat, and fifty times lower than that of an adult human being. But even such poor vision gives the baby the capacity that it needs to deal with its own tiny world – the microcosm of existence that lies between its eyes and its mother's face as the baby is cradled in her arms. There is even some evidence that very young babies prefer to look at cartoon drawings of faces rather than scrambled-up versions of exactly the same shapes. The instinctive gazing at faces may further serve the vital function of bonding the parent to the child.

But a baby is not simply biologically programmed to elicit reactions from its parent; it is equipped with an inquisitive brain, constructed to discover new things in the world around it. Eric Courchesne of the Children's Hospital Research Center in San Diego, California, records brainwaves with electrodes pasted to the scalps of babies, in an attempt to understand the way that the baby's brain recognises new things in the world around it. Even the restful world of a contented baby is full of changing shapes and sounds. Courchesne simplifies that world by projecting a sequence of pictures in front of the baby's eyes while recording the evoked potential that each picture generates – the series of brainwaves that indicate the sequence of events in the brain as it processes the incoming sensory message.

The picture is a human face: it flashes on again and again, identical every time. Then, suddenly a new face is shown – something that would be seen as startlingly different by an adult. Certain components of the evoked potential, occurring about one third of a second after the stimulus is flashed on, also change dramatically in an adult human if a different picture like this is shown after a series of identical images. The same tell-tale change in brainwaves – an indication of the recognition of novelty – occurs in children as young as three months old. But, before that, there is little hint that the brain can distinguish between one face and another. By three months of age the cerebral cortex has just finished the most rapid phase in the formation of synaptic connections between nerve cells. The brain is now using the circuitry that it has constructed in order to learn about the nature of the world. Learning would be impossible without the ability to detect difference and change.

The new capacities of the baby's brain that appear at around two to three months of age are revealed in its behaviour too. Leslie Cohen of the Children's Research Laboratory at the University of Texas in Austin records a baby's sucking reactions while he projects patterns in front of the baby's eyes. He is interested in how babies recognise and categorise the simplest components of shapes – pairs of straight lines. If any pattern is shown again and again, without change, the baby appears to become bored; it sucks less and less strongly. Whenever the pattern changes, and that change can be recognised by the baby, interest is aroused and there is a new burst of sucking. Cohen flashes on a pair of lines forming a simple acute angle – a V shape. Time after time the lines are flashed and the baby 'habituates' and stops sucking. Now, a new stimulus is shown, either the same V angle but *rotated* to point in a different direction, or exactly the same two lines simply joined together to make an *obtuse* angle rather than an acute one. The latter stimulus is a completely different *angle* but it consists of the same two *lines*. A six-week-old baby does not notice the change from the acute angle to the obtuse one and does not increase its sucking. It is as if the baby has no concept of an angle and sees only the individual lines. By three months of age, the baby reacts strongly for the change from acute angle to obtuse but remains bored if the V is simply rotated. Apparently, by three months of age, babies have gained the concept of an angle, which may be a crucial step in understanding the objects that they see.

Psychologists used to think that human beings classify the things that they see by using *language* to group things together: a square is different from a diamond simply because it has a different *name*. Leslie Cohen thinks that his experiments, and those of many other psychologists who have studied 'categorisation' in both infants and animals, clearly establish that language is not necessary for this kind of classification. Cohen asks us to imagine a three-month-old infant who, because it has not mastered language, could not form simple concepts and categories through which to understand the nature of the world: 'Every time that infant saw a different person from a different point of view, it would be totally different. That baby would not survive in this world. The world would be totally chaotic.'

We know little about how the brain reorganises itself as it goes through each of the neurological milestones of development, but it is very likely that the signals coming in along the nerves from the sense organs help the brain to reconstruct and refine its circuits, so as to develop mechanisms for recognising the habitual conjunctions of simple shapes and sounds. The world is not composed of disembodied lines; it consists of lines joined together to form angles, which are the boundaries of real objects in space. Perhaps it is the constant appearance of lines arranged in angles in the image on the retina that allows the baby, by the third month of life, to build the machinery in its brain needed to categorise angles as angles, and not just as independent lines. The recognition of common combinations of stimuli in the world may form the basis of all sorts of sophisticated classification, of the sort that allows us to distinguish a dog from a cat or one person from another.

• A LESSON FROM •
THE WHISKERS OF A MOUSE

Hendrik Van der Loos, at the Institute of Anatomy in Lausanne, studies the whiskers of mice and the region of the cerebral hemispheres that is dedicated to these important sensory structures. Van der Loos views the whiskers as a 'sixth sense'. The nerve from the muzzle of a mouse, which carries the sensory messages from the whiskers, is several times thicker than the optic nerve itself! As a mouse explores its environment, it uses its whiskers, like constantly twitching fingers, to investigate the objects around it. No surprise to discover, then, that a large part of the cerebral cortex is devoted to the analysis of signals from the whiskers.

A normal mouse has thirty-three large whiskers on each side of its face and there is a remarkable correspondence between the *structure* of the whisker area of the brain in an adult mouse and the pattern of whiskers on its upper lip. When Van der Loos and his colleagues looked at microscopic sections through the middle layers of the cerebral cortex, where the sensory fibres bringing messages into the cortex terminate, they found an amazing pattern of nerve cells, packed together to form rings, or, more accurately, structures that looked like 'barrels'. While the neurons of the cortex form the walls of the barrels, the interiors are filled with nerve fibres carrying messages from the whiskers. The correspondence between barrels and whiskers was clear to see: there were thirty-three barrels on each side of

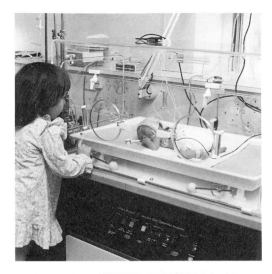

Advances in pre-natal care now make it possible for babies born as much as fifteen weeks premature to survive (left). These human fetuses, released before their time into the outside world, have provided insight into the early development of movement and sensation.

Psychologists have recently developed a variety of techniques for defining and measuring the abilities of babies before they can speak. One of the most useful is the 'preferential looking technique' (below left), in which a baby views two screens with projected patterns that differ in some respect. In this case, one consists of stripes and the other is blank. Even newborn babies have a natural tendency to look at the more complicated of two visual patterns, such as the stripes in this example. By observing the baby's eyes as thinner and thinner stripes are projected, it is possible to discover how narrow the stripes must be before the baby no longer prefers to look at them; this is taken as a measure of the baby's 'visual acuity'.

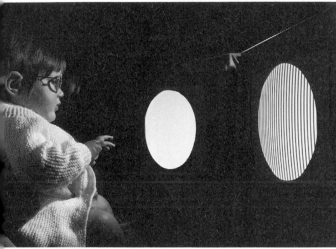

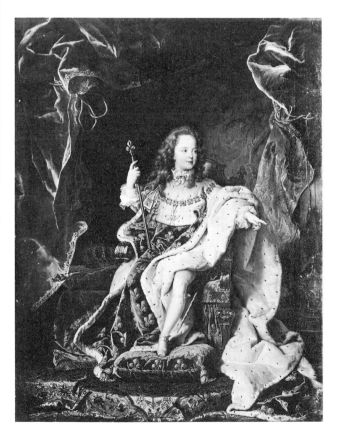

RIGHT Louis XV *by H. Rigaud. Louis was crowned King of France at the age of five, long before the stage of cognitive development at which a child would normally be ready for independent life. His weakness and indecision discredited the Crown and provoked the dissatisfaction that led eventually to the French Revolution.*

the brain, laid out in a pattern corresponding exactly to the array of whiskers on the opposite side of the face. Subsequently, neurophysiologists, using tiny microelectrodes to record activity from this region of the brain, confirmed that the cells clustered in the walls of a single barrel receive information from just one of the whiskers.

How is this extraordinary correspondence between the structure of the brain and the structure of the sense organs produced? Both anatomical structures – the whiskers and the barrels – could, of course, be predetermined by instructions in the genetic code. But, alternatively, the nerve fibres growing into the cortex, carrying signals from the whiskers, might somehow *induce* the formation of barrels in the cortex. When Van der Loos looked at the brain of a newborn mouse he could see no barrels; they first appear a few days after birth. In a crucial experiment, he removed a single row of whiskers on one side of the face in a newborn mouse and then waited until the cortex had gone through the phase of barrel formation. When he looked subsequently at microscopic sections through the cortex, he saw that one row of barrels, corresponding to the plucked whiskers, had totally failed to develop.

More recently, Van der Loos has been looking at the brains of inbred, mutant mice, with one or more extra whiskers on the face. In every case, the pattern of barrels in the brain matches the number and pattern of whiskers. It is inconceivable that a single genetic mutation could make *both* an extra whisker and an extra barrel. The conclusion is obvious: somehow, the nerves carrying activity from each whisker must cause the cerebral cortex to rearrange its nerve cells to make a barrel to deal with the incoming messages.

This is a very particular example of the way in which the sense organs and the messages that they generate influence the developing brain. But it is very likely that the brains of babies, especially during the first few months of life, are being moulded and modified in a variety of ways by the sensory signals that the brain is receiving. Experience writes a diary in the shifting circuits of nerve cells in the brain of the young child.

• CYCLES OF SENSITIVITY •

In Hendrik Van der Loos's experiments, the barrels in the brain fail to develop only if the corresponding whiskers are removed during the first few days after birth. Plucking the whiskers in an older mouse has no effect. This is just one example of a specific *sensitive* period in brain development. The effects of alcohol and radiation on the eight-week-old human fetus provide another striking example of sensitivity of the brain confined to a particular stage of development. Again and again, the growing, developing brain passes through brief episodes of sensitivity during which it must be exposed to the correct chemical signals or the appropriate experience if the programme of maturation is to unfold normally.

During these sensitive periods, the brain is particularly vulnerable to disturbances of the signals from the sense organs. The visual area of the cerebral cortex of a growing kitten or baby monkey passes through such a sensitive period during the first few weeks of life. Several weeks before a monkey's birth, axons that have grown out of cells of the lateral geniculate nucleus start to invade the partly formed region of cerebral cortex at the back of the hemispheres, which is destined to become the visual cortex. These fibres, which will carry messages to the cortex from the eyes, are still arriving at, and after, the time of birth. The activity reaching the brain from the two eyes seems to be used in some way to control the formation of connections. Normally, with equal visual stimulation of the two eyes, the left-eye and right-eye nerve fibres arrange themselves into a beautiful pattern, each eye's fibres laying down their connections in an array of dense bands about 0.3 mm across, making an alternating pattern of right-eye and left-eye terminals that runs across the whole of the visual cortex and provides a perfectly balanced input to the brain from the two eyes.

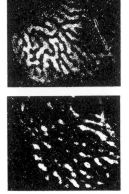

Sections cut parallel to the surface of a monkey's visual cortex reveal the incoming nerve fibres carrying signals from one of the eyes, which have been radioactively labelled and appear white. In a normal monkey (top), the nerve terminals form an array of stripes, each about 0.3 mm across. The gaps in between are filled with terminals from the other eye. If one eye is deprived of vision for as little as two or three days, during a sensitive period early in life, its nerve terminals fail to make normal connections and occupy only small patches (bottom).

Just as for the whisker barrels of a mouse, any disturbance of the sensory input during this crucial phase disrupts the pattern and leads to a highly abnormal arrangement of stripes. For instance, if a cat or a monkey has one eye covered, even for a short time, during the first few weeks of life, the fibres carrying messages from that eye fail to form normal bands of termination and end up occupying small, patchy islands in a sea of input from the other, normal eye. Thus, the actual connection of eye to brain is determined by the activity of the eyes early in life.

It is very likely that much the same kind of process takes place in the visual cortex of a human baby during the first few months of life. If a child suffers some imbalance between the two eyes at this early stage, for instance because of a cloudy cataract in the lens of one eye or a drooping eyelid on one side, the child will subsequently have very poor vision through that eye, even if the initial problem is entirely cured.

A baby's individual visual experiences, early in its postnatal life, influence the formation of nerve connections in its brain, which in turn affect the way that its brain can process visual information. The ability of the brain to modify itself, on the basis of its own experiences, liberates the individual from the chains of its own DNA; the minds of different people might otherwise be as similar as their muscles or their stomachs.

The concept of periods of sensitivity, which grew out of simple experiments on the structure and function of the growing brain, has had a strong impact in the field of developmental psychology. Human beings, even for many years after birth, pass through periods of 'cognitive sensitivity', when the state of maturation of the brain allows the child to form new mental abilities and concepts. Take language, for example. There seems little doubt that every normal human baby is born with the innate capacity to learn a spoken language – *any* language. Somehow a general capacity must become transformed into a very specific skill. Janet Werker of the University of British Columbia works among the Indians of northern Canada, discovering the way in which their babies learn their local dialect – the Thompson or Inslachetin language. For a baby to learn a language the first requirement is that it should recognise the characteristic sounds of that tongue. But not all languages use the same set of basic building blocks of sound. What Janet Werker has found is that babies lose their potential to recognise *all* possible sounds in languages as they begin to master a single dialect.

The Thompson language has a set of consonants that are not used in English and which adult English speakers cannot distinguish, such as the first syllables in 'Kachrem' (frying) and 'Kacherem' (to secure). Werker teaches the baby that whenever a sound *changes*, a group of toys will be shown to the child. The baby likes to look at the toys and turns its head whenever it expects them to appear. The head-turning response is, then, an indication that the child has recognised a change in the sounds being presented. Werker plays tape recordings of sounds from the Thompson language to see whether babies can spot a shift from one sound to another (such as the 'ka' of 'kachrem' to that of 'kacherem'), which is unrecognisable as a change to an adult English speaker. An eight-month-old baby, of whatever nationality, immediately detects the change, and looks expectantly towards the toys. But by a year of age, a baby that has not been exposed regularly to the Thompson language can no longer recognise the subtle shift of sound. As Janet Werker says: 'The young infant is born ready to learn any human language. And experience then functions to narrow that universal set of abilities ... to the particular language that the baby is learning.'

It seems so obvious that babies and children go through well-defined stages of mental development, but this is a relatively new idea. Around 1900, the American experimental psychologist, G. Stanley Hall, began to investigate the attitudes, knowledge, memory and thoughts of young children, by presenting them with questionnaires, asking such simple things as 'What happens to the sun when it sets?' In their time, the results of Hall's investigations were astonishing. He found that children simply do not understand many of the concepts that adults take for granted. By making comparisons between children of different ages, Hall began to formulate ideas about their perception of the world.

The name most associated with the study of the major phases of childhood development is Jean Piaget (1896-1980), the eminent Swiss psychologist who explored the cognitive world of the child through formal interviews and puzzles. One of his best-known tests involves pouring water from a short fat glass into a tall thin glass and asking the child which vessel contains more water. Young children will always say that the tall glass has more, even when they see the water literally being transferred from one to the other.

Piaget divided the development of a child into four stages. From birth until two years is the Sensori-Motor Stage during which the infant understands the world only in terms of its own immediate sensations. Show it a toy and it will track it with its eyes and attempt to reach for it until it disappears from view. Then the baby will react as if the toy no longer exists. According to Piaget the next stage, the Pre-Operational Stage, lasts from about two to seven. The child at this stage has a grasp of language and symbols but cannot yet think logically and cannot understand that another person can have a different point of view. Two toddlers at this stage, playing together in a room, do not play *with* each other; they play with their own toys and conduct their own monologues. According to Piaget, a child at this stage has an egocentric view of the universe.

From about seven to eleven years of age is the Stage of Concrete Operations, when the child will no longer be fooled by liquid being poured from one container into another of a different shape. The child starts to develop a natural concept of statistics, learning to judge the world in terms of the *possibility* or *probability* of things happening, rather than thinking in terms of *certainties*. By about eleven years, the Age of Formal Operations begins and the child has all the mental tools needed for adult life. From this point on, further development is simply a matter of the acquisition of knowledge.

Although details of Piaget's rather dogmatic views, especially concerning the timing of these stages, have been challenged by many developmental psychologists, the idea that there are major milestones of cognitive development is now firmly established. It is tempting to think that they represent stages of sensitivity in the brain, as circuits of nerve cells undergo crucial modification and refinement.

• THE EMERGENCE OF MIND •

Can we see any hint in the behaviour of a baby to indicate the onset of the concept of self? Does consciousness – the sense of awareness of the world, of intentions and of oneself – appear slowly and gradually, perhaps starting even in the uterus? Or is there a critical period for the development of conscious awareness, just as much as for the construction of barrels in the mouse brain or of connections from the two eyes in the visual cortex? Jerome Kagan of the Department of Psychology at Harvard University believes that there is a fairly precise stage, between eighteen and twenty-four months after birth, when normal children first become aware that they have intentions, that they have feelings, that they can act. This 'ah-ha' experience, as he calls it, 'requires interaction of the brain … with people. But all the interactions in the world won't lead to the sense of self until you're in the middle of the second year, because the brain is not yet mature.'

Put a spot of rouge on the nose of a three-month-old baby. Place the baby in front of a mirror and it will look at its reflection but won't touch its nose, because it does not recognise that the face in the mirror is its own. Even at nine or ten months of age a child cannot realise the meaning of the image in a mirror. But by eighteen or twenty months, perhaps because the sense of self has matured, a child with a dab of rouge on its nose will reach up and touch it as it looks at itself in a mirror.

Jerome Kagan sees many other signs of the growing sense of self around this age: the child first begins to use words of self-identity, such as 'I' and 'me' and 'my'. Laura Petito at McGill University in Montreal has discovered that even the deaf children of deaf parents, who learn to communicate by sign language, start to use the sign meaning 'I' at the same age that hearing children speak the same word (the very age at which they wipe the rouge from their noses).

Around the same time another distinctly human quality is emerging. According to Kagan, the child is developing a *moral* sense. At twelve months of age no baby will show concern when it sees a broken doll, a damaged toy car or peeling paintwork. But a little later it recognises these wrongs in the world. Such things are called 'broken', 'dirty', or 'bad'. Kagan interprets this to mean that 'the child now has a primitive understanding that there is integrity to objects, and that if the integrity is violated, somebody, some living thing, has done something *wrong*'.

There is no doubt that the awareness of self and the sense of right and wrong are fundamental in human life. Their emergence in the development of a baby should be viewed as an accomplishment no less profound than learning to speak or to work. The 'terrible twos' should not be thought of as a time of incomprehensible frustration and aggression, but as the phase when a child is trying to establish for itself what is right and what is wrong – to learn the rules by which we live.

Nineteenth-century and early twentieth-century theorists of the mind, most notably Sigmund Freud, thought that the development of primitive emotions formed the basis for the maturation of understanding and morality. For Freud, the id came first and then the ego. But the present-day view is quite different and it sees the earliest stages of a baby's life as a struggle for *cognitive* competence.

The well-known fear of strangers, which all babies develop at around eight to twelve months of age, could not appear unless the child were mature enough both to *recognise* different faces and to *remember* the past.

The *anxiety* associated with a stranger's face depends on advances in the perceptual and cognitive capacities of the baby. Before eight months of age, babies smile frequently at any face. This powerful reaction cannot be taken to indicate any recognition, nor perhaps any emotion in the child, but is more likely to be yet another automatic, reflex trick placed in the child by nature to encourage bonding and protective reactions from the adults around it. But, towards the end of the first year, as recognition and stranger-anxiety emerge, smiling changes from an unconscious demand for protection to a genuine indication of the child's emotional feelings. Perhaps the first smile of true pleasure marks the very birth of a new mind.

When a child starts to walk, a new world of opportunities to explore and to discover opens up; and the brain is now ready for these interactions. The child gains skill in walking, then in talking. Memory and learning improve and the child adapts readily to new situations, new demands. Between two and six years of age the restricted horizons of a baby's world fall away. Vocabulary explodes. Knowledge increases. A social sense blossoms. It is no surprise that all cultures have taken this period as the time to start discovering the child's real potential – to begin the process of formal education. The child is developing the ability to put concepts together, to relate the concept of self to the concept of events in the outside world. It becomes possible for the child to imagine abstract things. Four-year-olds are afraid of straightforward experiences that they might meet in their everyday worlds – darkness, burglars, spiders, big dogs. After the age of six, fears and worries sometimes focus on abstract, distant or mysterious things. For the first time, children will tell their mothers that they are afraid of nuclear war, of being kidnapped or of having cancer.

From fertilised egg to growing embryo; from the creation and migration of neurons to the development of personality: the changes are universal. Slowly, inevitably, in stages that are common to every society and culture, the child's mind emerges. From the cocoon of the womb, from the protection of the family, into the outside world. As Jerome Kagan puts it: 'Human beings are built to seek new information, to learn from it, to consolidate that knowledge and move on.'

REMEMBERING

O<small>N</small> 22 N<small>OVEMBER</small>, 1963, I was a medical student at Cambridge. It should have been like any other day, but it branded itself into the structure of my brain. If you were more than ten years old at the time, do you remember where you were that day? Let me put it another way. Do you remember where you were when John F. Kennedy was shot? That question has become a classic one in the armoury of tests that psychologists use to explore the memories of their patients.

I can see the stone of the steps to the dining hall of the college at which I studied, worn smooth by the shoes of generations of students. I can see the black formal gowns of the undergraduates ahead of me, as we shuffled up the stairs. I can even remember snatches of our conversation. Then the Master of the college, Sir Frank Lee, told us the dreadful news, that Kennedy had been shot and was feared to be mortally wounded. Within minutes, a man (I can still see his face so clearly) came into the hall and whispered to Sir Frank, who rose again to say that Kennedy was dead.

It is the vivid clarity of such *special* recollections that reminds us how little we remember of our everyday experience. Yet without the capacity to remember and to learn, it is difficult to imagine what life would be like, whether it could be called living at all. Without memory we would be servants of the moment, with nothing but our innate reflexes to help us to deal with the world. There could be no language, no art, no science, no culture. Civilisation itself is the distillation of human memory.

Robert Frost wrote:

But as I said it, swift there passed me by
On noiseless wing a bewildered butterfly,
Seeking with memories grown dim o'er night
Some resting flower of yesterday's delight.

Without memories, life would be continuous bewilderment. But animals *do* remember what they need to. A honey bee, home from a foraging expedition to a particularly rich patch of flowers, can *communicate* its whereabouts to her sisters by means of an extraordinary 'waggle dance', first described by Karl von Frisch. As they cluster around her on the wall of the hive, she does a rumba, pointing with her wriggling body in the direction of the source of nectar, using the vertical reference of gravity to *represent* the position of the sun. More astonishing is the fact that she can update her memory, as the hours pass, to take account of the movement of the sun across the sky. If she arrives at the hive late in the afternoon and dances her abstract map next morning, she anticipates the *new* position of the sun as she symbolically represents the source of food.

Memory is virtually ubiquitous in the animal kingdom. To remember things and change behaviour appropriately are almost defining characteristics of animal life.

In the broadest sense, learning is the acquisition of knowledge; and memory is the storage of an internal representation of that knowledge. Every organism is created with an inbuilt repertoire of understanding of the world, acquired through natural selection and represented, symbolically, in the genes responsible for constructing circuits of nerve cells that control the behaviour that expresses that knowledge. This inherent wisdom, the distant memory of the experiences of ancestors, consists of a battery of reflexes – adaptive reactions produced automatically in response to stereotyped events in the outside world. Contraction of the pupil of the eye in bright light, the snatching of a hand from a flame, salivation in response to the taste or smell of food; these are primitive reflexes, unconditioned reflexes as Ivan Pavlov called them. They are gifts of knowledge to each animal from its predecessors – a minimum kit of understanding about the world. But if an animal had no more than this small repertoire of behaviour, how impoverished its life would be.

The evolution of a mechanism for storing new information in the brain of an individual animal, during its lifetime, must have been a simply transcendent step in evolution. The ability to learn allows an animal to escape from the confines of knowledge of its own DNA. Yet that very ability must itself be inherited. Our genes give us both a basic repertoire of inbuilt behaviour *and* a capacity to capture new information about the world. Animals are organisms of prediction: they benefit from experience and gain the power to anticipate the future.

To our conscious mind, the recollection of past events can be a joy.

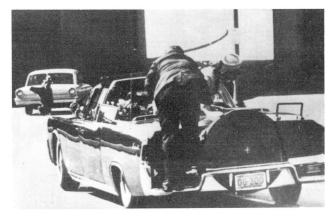

ABOVE *The assassination of John F. Kennedy in Dallas on 22 November 1963. Why do the memories of important and emotional events stamp themselves with such clarity on our minds?*

RIGHT *The founder of phrenology, Franz Joseph Gall (1758–1828), believed that the 'organ of memory' was localised in the brain directly behind the eyes. The cerebral cortex may indeed play a part in the storage of long-term memories, but Gall's observations were merely anecdotal and his specific ideas were soon discredited.*

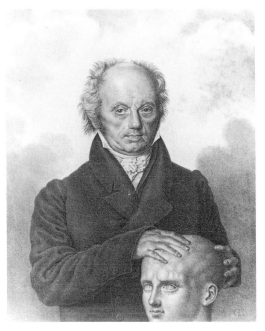

BELOW *Ivan Pavlov (1849–1936) is best known for his discovery of 'classical conditioning' in which a stimulus, such as a bell, can be associated with a reflex response, such as salivation for food. If bell and food are presented together a few times, a dog will soon salivate for the sound of a bell alone. This kind of simple learning may well involve the cerebellum and probably underlies a good deal of animal and human behaviour.*

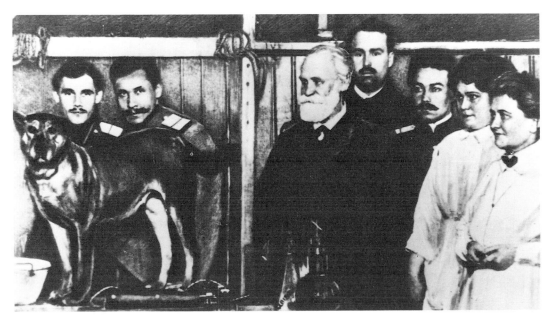

In his novel, *Remembrance of Things Past*, Marcel Proust described the hypnotic quality of a distant memory brought to mind by the taste of a little cake called a *petite madeleine*, dipped in lime tea. It reminded him of teatime as a child, at his Aunt Leonie's house in Combray: 'the town from morning to night and in all weathers, the square where I used to be sent for lunch, the streets along which I used to run errands, the country roads we took when it was fine ... the whole of Combray and its surroundings, taking shape and solidity, sprang into being, town and gardens alike, from my cup of tea.' But the biological advantage of remembering is surely not that it permits its owner to reminisce but that it allows him to predict, to anticipate, to plan.

• THE FRUITLESS SEARCH • FOR THE ENGRAM

Over the centuries there has been no shortage of analogies for the way in which the brain stores information. Remembrances have been likened to scratches in a wax tablet, holes in a linen cloth, exposure of a photographic emulsion or a holographic plate, and storage in a computer memory. All of these metaphors are concerned with the way in which individual fragments of experience can be held in the brain. But it is important to note that we use the word 'memory' in two ways – to describe both the stored records (we speak of having pleasant memories of the past) *and* the machinery for making them (we might say, for instance, that someone has a good memory). If past memories were books in a library, the memory that made them would be a printing press. To explain the process of remembering we must identify both the press and the books in the brain. But long before science tackled directly the question of *what* memory might be it started to think about *where* it lives in the brain.

During the nineteenth century a battle raged back and forth across Europe: an intellectual debate, between anatomists, neurologists, physiologists and a newly emerging breed of scientists, behavioural psychologists. The issue that they were contesting was whether function is specifically localised in the brain, especially in the cerebral cortex.

The Viennese anatomist Franz Joseph Gall astonished the scientific world in the first decades of the last century by his 'discovery' that the character and even the intellectual and moral characteristics of human beings are revealed by the pattern of bumps on their heads, each area of the skull reflecting the size of an innate 'organ', dedicated to a particular faculty, in the brain below. His methods of observation founded a noble tradition in brain research – an attempt to correlate the structure and function of parts of the nervous system. However, with no proper experiments and no knowledge of statistics to guide him, his procedures seem pitifully inadequate by modern standards. His evidence was anecdote rather than systematic observation.

For instance, Gall claimed in 1812 that, when he was a young boy, he had noticed that friends and acquaintances who had large protruding eyes also had especially good memories; he concluded that the 'organ' of remembering must be located in the brain immediately behind the eyes.

The pseudo-science of phrenology was popular with the general public for more than a hundred years. Gall was by no means a charlatan: he made a substantial contribution to the study of the anatomy of the brain and, for a short time, even enjoyed the applause of his scientific colleagues. Before long, though, suspicion fell on the nature and validity of his observations. The French physiologist Marie-Jean-Pierre Flourens was one of phrenology's most bitter opponents. Clinical neurologists were, at that time, starting the painstaking task of analysing the results of damage to the human brain and Flourens decided to use the same approach, in a much more controlled fashion, in animals. He chose birds as the subjects for his work and examined the effects of damage to the forebrain. 'Animals deprived of their cerebral lobes,' he wrote, 'have neither perception, nor judgement, nor memory, nor will. The cerebral lobes are therefore the exclusive seat of all the perceptions and all the intellectual faculties.'

In contrast to the phrenologists, though, Flourens argued that these various functions, including memory, are simply spread across the fore-brain structures. He could find no evidence that specific skills depended on particular parts of the brain (though it must be said that his surgical techniques were rather crude and that the forebrain of a bird is quite different from the cerebral hemispheres of a mammal).

Despite the reaction against phrenology, the march of genuine evidence in favour of localisation of function was inexorable. By the end of the last century, vision, hearing, speech and movement had all staked their claims to circumscribed pieces of cortical territory. But what of memory? Flourens's results suggest that the forebrain is needed for memories to be stored (or retrieved), but that neither the storing device nor the stored traces are strictly located in one part of the brain.

The German physiologist Friedrich Goltz came to much the same conclusions. He toured Europe demonstrating dogs whose cerebral cortex had been surgically damaged. In 1892, Goltz wrote: 'They do not learn from past experience. They do not *have* experiences, for only he who has memories can have experiences. The decerebrated dog is essentially nothing but a child of the moment.' Again, the remembrances seemed to be in the cortex; but *where*?

Karl Lashley, a psychologist working at Harvard University in the first half of this century, spent much of his career searching for what he called the *Engram*, the individual neural record of remembered events.

The participants in his experiments were laboratory rats and he borrowed the techniques of the American school of behaviourism to train them to run simple mazes, with pellets of food as the reward. When each animal had learnt the task, Lashley would surgically damage some region of the cerebral hemispheres, and then test the rat to see how well it could remember the maze. Far from finding that injury in one specific place had a particular effect on learning, Lashley discovered that the magnitude of the loss of memory seemed to be roughly proportional to the area of damaged cortex, *wherever* the injury was actually made. He coined the term 'mass action' to describe the way in which the cerebral hemispheres seemed to be involved in the storage of information. So frustrated was Lashley in his search for the Engram that he wrote, in 1950, 'I sometimes feel, in reviewing the evidence on the localisation of the memory trace, that the necessary conclusion is that learning is just not possible.'

Learning *is* possible, of course, and Lashley's experiments amply demonstrated that the record of past successes and failures involves the cerebral cortex. But he failed to discover a single, specific library of the brain in which the volumes of experience are stored.

• CIRCUITS AND SYNAPSES •

As Lashley himself became increasingly frustrated in his search for individual memory traces, one of his students, Donald Hebb, was conceiving an entirely new approach to the question of storage of information in the brain – an approach that was ahead of its time. Shortly before his death in 1985, Hebb, who lived in an old house outside Halifax, Nova Scotia, reminisced about his time in Lashley's laboratory:

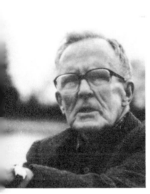

Donald Hebb, who died in 1985, was the first to suggest that memories might be stored in circuits of nerve cells, which he called 'cell assemblies'. This view has its modern echo in the current interest in the efficiency of storage of information in parallel networks, both in the brain and in computers. Hebb was also the first to propose that the changes underlying the storage of memories take place at the individual synaptic connections between nerve cells.

All the theories that I knew made the brain out to be completely controlled by the things that were going on around it, by the sensory events that the brain was exposed to. But it occurred to me about 1945 that the brain might be functioning independently of the messages it is getting from the outside. I came up with the idea that brain activity is actually the activity of a number of separate systems that I call *cell assemblies*. Thanks to these cell assemblies, activity can go on in the brain without any external stimulation at all.

In his influential book, *The Organisation of Behaviour*, Hebb put down his new theory. Every individual activity of the brain, he argued, requires a circuit of nerve cells, each exciting the next, forming a closed loop in which impulses can run round and round, escaping through side branches to influence other parts of the brain or to cause a movement or some other action. Just as the resonant ring of a bell is a kind of memory of the hammer that struck it, so the traffic of nerve impulses around a cell assembly could be used to store in the brain a record of a previously experienced event. This, Hebb suggested, could be the basis of immediate memory of past experience.

Hebb knew quite well, however, that impulse activity in the nerve cells of the brain could not be the basis of lifelong memories. For one thing, a concussive blow to the head, which presumably disrupts millions of nerve circuits, can lead to amnesia for the events of the preceding few hours or minutes leading up to the accident, but it does not obliterate much earlier memories. Equally, if an animal is trained to remember something, such as how to run a maze, is then quickly cooled down to a temperature that stops all nerve impulses in the brain, and subsequently warmed up again, it cannot remember the task, though it performs perfectly well on other tests that it learned days or weeks before.

This all implies that there are two sorts of memory trace. The first, usually called short-term memory, holds a record for minutes or perhaps hours after a particular experience, which depends on the electrical activity of the brain. Then, a more permanent record, called long-term memory, takes over, in which information is represented in the *structure* of the brain and no longer depends on the ability of nerve cells to transmit impulses. In fact, there may well be several different sorts of short-term and long-term memory, with different durations and different locations in the brain. One view is that short-term memories become converted or consolidated into long-term ones, but the two processes might go on completely independently of each other.

Hebb's cell assemblies, those reverberating circuits of firing nerve cells, could function as short-term but not long-term memories, because they require electrical activity. Hebb therefore went on to postulate that the repetitive patterns of firing in circuits of neurons might, gradually, modify the synapses – the *connections* between those cells – in such a way that each junction becomes more efficient. If the synapses become stronger, it is more likely that the whole assembly of neurons will be triggered off by some small signal coming into one of the cells in the assembly. This synaptic modification, he suggested, might be permanent; it could be the way in which the memories of a lifetime are stored.

Not everything that we remember for a brief period becomes permanently stored. Think of the thousands upon thousands of people, places, telephone numbers and addresses that you deal with for a few minutes and keep in your mind as you do so, but which you may never need to remember again. Vast amounts of information roll through the temporary storage of short-term memory – doodles on the sketch-pad of experience. The remarkably efficient filter of forgetting throws out the ephemeral dross of everyday memories but keeps the masterpieces of experience that deserve to be saved for ever. According to Hebb, the forgetting of short-term memories before long-term ones are established could be due to the running down of activity in the circuit of neurons. But once the synapses between the cells are adequately strengthened, only extensive damage to the circuit might obliterate the memory.

The way in which memories are chosen for the privilege of permanence remains a mystery. It might depend on a signal (perhaps a chemical signal) transmitted from some other part of the brain, which facilitates the strengthening of any synapses that are active at the time. Such a signal might be turned on whenever the animal finds itself in a situation of great danger, of great pleasure, or of significance in some other way.

We all live in fear of forgetfulness, that archetypal symptom of senility; but what would life be like *without* the ability to forget? Every trivial experience, every number, every face would clutter your mind, hiding the wood of wisdom with the trees of triviality. Alexander Luria, the eminent Russian neuropsychologist, described a patient with exactly that problem in his book *The Mind of a Mnemonist*. The man in question, called simply 'S' by Luria, worked as a reporter for a newspaper in Moscow, in the early 1920s. His astounding ability to produce reports rich in the minutest factual detail, without ever taking a note, so amazed the editor that he sent him for a psychological evaluation.

S was examined by Luria, who had for years been studying human memory and the amnesia caused by various forms of disease. But Luria had never encountered anyone like S. He wrote: 'It appeared that there was no limit either to the capacity of S's memory or to the durability of the traces he retained.' He could commit to memory, in a few minutes, long lists of numbers, and recall them in perfect detail hours, days or weeks later. Luria tested him thirty *years* after they first met and S could still remember quite perfectly the tables of numbers that he had first learned!

S seemed, quite spontaneously, to have developed mnemonic tricks to help him remember such detail; he would, for instance, associate, in his mind's eye, lists of objects that he wished to remember with familiar features of a street or some other place that was well known to him. He would mentally place each object in some spot in the scene, so that all that he had to do to remember the list was to recall a mental image of the scene and look around it for each object on display. He would imagine himself walking along a street in Moscow looking in each hiding place for the object that he had left there! 'Sometimes I put a word in a dark place and have trouble seeing it as I go by,' S wrote.

This trick of associating numbers, words or objects with familiar scenes is one that has been used for millennia by professional mnemonists. Committing vast tracts of factual information to memory is a skill that seems to have been virtually lost in the modern world, but past civilisations relied on traditional oral history, poetry and story-telling for the transmission of culture. The Roman orator Cicero tells the story of a poet, Simonides, who was invited to recite a poem at a banquet in the honour of a nobleman, Scopas. Simonides left the room after his performance, just before the roof of the hall collapsed, killing and mutilating beyond recognition Scopas and his many guests. Because of the extraordinary richness of his memory, Simonides was able to help the relatives to identify the dead, by recalling precisely where everyone had been seated. Cicero gave an account of the mnemonic method that Simonides had used and it was remarkably similar to the tricks of Luria's S. 'Persons desiring to train this faculty of memory', Cicero wrote, 'must select places and form mental images of the things they wish to remember and store those images in places, so that the order of the places will preserve the order of the things, and the images of the things will denote the things themselves.'

Trevor Emmott, a British mnemonist, remembers lists of thirty-six digits at a time by linking the numbers with letters and then converting those letters into words. He demonstrates his skills with a pristine list of numbers generated randomly by a computer. Emmott first divides the list into six groups of six numbers each and concentrates on finding a word-picture code for each six-digit number. From the innocent number 351639, he came up with an image of a chimpanzee hitting a lantern with a mallet!

First, he had to remember that this particular sequence of numbers was the fourth group of six in the whole list. Emmott uses a conversion table that he has memorised to translate each number into a consonant or other non-vowel sound: 4 translates into the letter R. So, he remembers that this is the fourth row by thinking of the letter R. To make it easier to remember, he adds 'ay' to the R, to make the word Ray. He thinks of a ray of light and therefore of a lantern. The first three digits of the sequence, 351, convert to the letters MLT. Emmott adds some vowels to come up with the word 'mallet'. The other three numbers, 639, translate into ChMP. With the addition of 'i', this becomes 'chimp'. So the whole of the fourth sequence of six digits becomes, in the mind of Trevor Emmott, an *image* of a chimpanzee hitting a lantern with a mallet.

Almost all techniques for improving memory involve the linking of symbols (numbers, letters, words, names, etc.) to imagined places or events. Surely this must imply that scenes and events are somehow easier to remember than numbers and names. Perhaps it is the conversion of something that is essentially nonsense (a string of unrelated words or digits) into something that has *meaning* and can be visualised and understood, that makes this form of mnemonic trick so effective. After all, the brain was designed to remember things about the natural world, not lists of random numbers! When we normally recall places that we have visited, people whom we have met or things that we have done, we bring our knowledge of the world and our expectations about it to bear on the reconstruction of the particular memory. If you try to recall a room that you have visited, you won't need to remember that it had a door and windows, because most rooms have those things. Equally, in trying to conjure up the image of someone's face you could start with the *assumption* that he or she had a nose, two eyes and a mouth. Our memories of everyday events are a synthesis of genuine factual recall and assumption based on our knowledge of the real world.

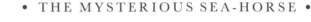

• THE MYSTERIOUS SEA-HORSE •

Several decades after his time in Karl Lashley's laboratory, Donald Hebb collaborated, in Montreal, with another pioneer in the science of memory, Wilder Penfield. Penfield was a leading neurosurgeon who pioneered techniques for treating epilepsy. The fits that epileptics suffer are due to explosive spasms of electrical activity that start from one diseased spot in the brain – the focus of the seizure. Penfield devised various ways of detecting the position of the focus, so that he could cut it out. One of his methods involved stimulating the surface of the patient's cerebral hemispheres with a mild electric current delivered through a needle. The patient was fully conscious, the operation to reveal the brain having been done under local anaesthetic. (Surprisingly, the tissue of the brain itself is completely insensitive to pain.) Penfield hoped to find a place on the surface of the brain where electrical stimulation would produce strange feelings, hallucinations or sensations typical of the 'aura' that normally preceded the onset of a fit. If the aura was, as most neurologists thought, the result of rhythmic activity building up in the focus, before the onset of a full fit, the spot at which electrical stimulation produced such an aura would surely be the tissue to remove. The technique worked and Penfield gained an international reputation for his success in treating epileptic patients. But the method also gave him the chance to explore the workings of the brain of fully conscious human beings, rather like an electrical engineer probing a circuit board with pulses and monitoring equipment to try to discover how it works.

When Penfield stimulated the motor cortex, a narrow strip running down the side of each cerebral hemisphere, parts of the patient's body would twitch briefly and uncontrollably. High up, at the top of the strip, stimulation caused the patient's toes or feet to jerk; lower down, the thumb, fingers or hand would quiver with each electric shock; and at the very bottom of the strip, the muscles of the face would twitch. Thus, Penfield was able to prove in a few minutes what neurologists had speculated about for a century – that the muscles of the body are represented in a systematic fashion along the motor strip, almost as if the body were painted as a strange, distorted picture across the surface of the cortex.

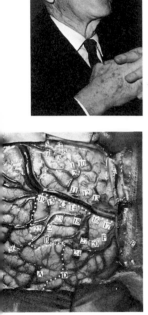

Canadian neurosurgeon Wilder Penfield (1891–1976) exposed the surface of the cerebral hemispheres (bottom) under local anaesthetic, while the patient was fully conscious, and electrically stimulated at the positions indicated by the numbers. Stimulation of the temporal lobe often evoked vivid impressions of sounds or complex visual scenes, some of which seemed familiar.

Penfield went on, exploring every readily accessible crag and crevice of the strange landscape of the cerebral hemispheres. Stimulation in the visual cortex, at the back of the brain, made the patient see brief sparks of light or moving coloured shapes in front of his eyes. Stimulation of the auditory cortex produced weird buzzing noises. And when the electrode was placed on the somatic sensory strip, which lies directly behind the motor cortex, it produced strange tingling sensations felt by the patient in some part of the skin of the body: here too was a 'map', lined up with that in the neighbouring motor strip.

These results were amazing enough, but it was the temporal lobe, the huge mass of cortex on each side of the head, that was Penfield's main continent of adventure. For here, the experiences that were unleashed by the touch of the stimulating electrode were not mere involuntary twitches or atoms of sensation; they were whole remembrances or experiences, imaginary hallucinations or vividly real recollections. Often, patients found themselves, as if in a dream, transported to a scene from the past.

Penfield really believed that he had achieved what Lashley had spent a lifetime of research failing to do. He thought that he had tracked down the elusive Engram and that its lair was the temporal lobe. Penfield imagined that all our remembered experiences are packed together there in a kind of neural library. But that conclusion was probably too hasty and too simplistic. For one thing, as Donald Hebb has pointed out, many of the hallucinations reported by Penfield's patients were bizarre, dream-like experiences, and few of them said that they portrayed familiar incidents from their own past. Perhaps Penfield's electrode did little more than provoke a jumble of signals on which the astonishing interpretive mechanisms of the brain then got to work, constructing a convincing account of the neural nonsense.

There remains another interpretation. The current from Penfield's electrodes might have spread *through* the temporal lobe to a part of the cerebral hemispheres tucked underneath. Penfield may indeed have located a brain structure critical in the process of memory, not on the outside of the temporal lobe but within it.

Folded in on the undersurface of the temporal lobe is an ancient part of the cerebral hemispheres, one of the first structures to appear in the evolutionary development of the cerebral cortex, called the hippocampus, Latin for a sea-horse, because a cross-section through it has that shape. It is a huge structure in a human brain, laid out in a simple and regular pattern of cells and interconnections repeated a millionfold along its length. At its front end it touches the amygdala, a nucleus, the size of a grape. Both hippocampus and amygdala have rich and complex inter-connections with many parts of the brain; but, most significantly, they gather information from areas of the cerebral cortex that are thought to be involved in processing sensory information. In turn, they communicate back to vast areas of the cerebral cortex, as well as to an array of other structures deep in the engine of the brain that are involved in emotions and appetites. In other words, both hippocampus and amygdala seem perfectly placed, in the midst of the stream of information through the brain, to play a part in the machinery of memory.

The first and still the most dramatic evidence that this hidden part of the brain plays a crucial role in memory came not from careful anatomical studies, not from painstaking experimentation in animals or human beings, but from the blade of a well-meaning surgeon. In 1953, a young man, who had suffered epileptic fits of devastating frequency since the age of sixteen, was sent by his local doctors to a hospital in Hartford, Connecticut. Nothing that they had tried, none of the drugs that they had prescribed, had relieved him of the convulsions that consumed his life. All the neurological evidence pointed to a region within the temporal lobe as the focus of his epileptic fits, and both sides of the brain seemed to be equally affected. So this man, known by his initials HM, became the subject of a surgical operation that had never been tried before, an operation that miraculously cured his fits but at a terrible cost. The region under the temporal lobes was removed on both sides by the neurosurgeon, William Scoville. The seizures stopped and elation spread through the hospital team until, within the first few hours after surgery, it became clear that HM had a new disease. He could not recognise the medical staff; he could not find his bedroom in the hospital; in short, he seemed entirely unable to remember any new fact or event.

HM now lives in Boston, supported by the Massachusetts General Hospital, but his life is tragically different from normal human experience. Brenda Milner of the Neurological Institute in Montreal, has known HM for a quarter of a century, yet she is a stranger to him every time they meet. She wrote of HM:

> His intelligence as measured by standard tests is actually a little higher now than before the operation yet the remarkable memory defect persists, and it is clear that HM can remember little of the experiences of the last years. HM is still unsure of his present address ... [He will] read the same magazines over and over again without finding their contents familiar.

The very fact that HM can speak shows that he has not forgotten language; in fact, he has good recall for his life up until a few years before the operation. But new events, faces, telephone numbers, places now settle in his mind for just a few seconds or minutes before they slip, like water through a sieve, and are lost from his consciousness.

Is, then, the hippocampus (which was certainly damaged on both sides of HM's brain) the site of Karl Lashley's elusive Engram? Probably not. The current view is that the hippocampus is essential for the process of storage of new long-term memories but is not the place where the messages are permanently stored. In the metaphor of the library, the hippocampus may be a printing press, not the final printed page.

Clive Wearing used to be chorus master of the London Sinfonietta, a world expert on Renaissance music and a producer for BBC Radio. In March 1985 he suffered a rare infection of the brain by the cold sore virus, *Herpes simplex*. It started with just a headache but six days later he was admitted to St Mary's Hospital, London, in a state of semi-consciousness. Clive's physical life was saved by an antiviral drug but the virus, which has a predilection for the hippocampus, had already destroyed that crucial region, as well as other parts of the cerebral cortex. Clive, like HM, now lives in a snapshot of time, constantly believing that he has *just* awoken from years of unconsciousness. As Clive's wife Deborah enters his hospital room for the third time in a single morning, he embraces her as if they had been parted for years. 'I'm conscious for the first time,' he says. 'It's the first time I've seen anybody at all.' Deborah says, 'Clive's world now consists of a moment, with no past to anchor it and no future to look ahead to. It's a blinkered moment.'

At first, Clive's confusion was total and very frightening to him. Deborah remembers him holding a chocolate in the palm of one hand and covering it with the other for just a few seconds, until the image of it disappeared from the fading snapshot of his memory. When he uncovered it, it was, to him, as if he had performed a magic trick, conjuring up the chocolate from nowhere. He repeated it again and again, with total astonishment and growing fear as the chocolate appeared anew each time.

Clive now lives a sort of life, constantly playing patience and obsessionally keeping a diary; every few minutes he makes a note that he has *just* woken for the first time, scoring out the previous entry as he does so. He still has much of his previous *general* knowledge of the world. He can still speak and walk; indeed he can still read music, play the organ and conduct. Moreover, Clive, HM and other amnesic patients can still *learn* new skills, benefiting from their experience, in a variety of puzzles and tests of recognition, motor co-ordination and so on. For instance, such patients can be taught to mirror-read – recognising words printed in mirror reversal. Over the course of a few days of testing, the speed of reading such words doubles, and the task can be done just as well three months later; yet, to the patient, the test is a new one every time. Other skills show the same unconscious improvement – recognising complicated pictures; drawing while viewing through a mirror; logical puzzle tasks.

This all suggests that there are two main kinds of long-term memory; the kind of unconscious, 'non-declarative' memory needed to learn such new skills, and 'declarative' memory, which can be consciously brought to mind. Declarative memory, which seems to depend on the hippocampus,

Clive Wearing (below), before the viral infection that damaged his brain and robbed him of the ability to lay down new conscious memories. His diary (right) reveals the horror of this constant sense of awakening, as well as his persistent thoughts of his wife, Deborah, and his dependence on the card game of patience.

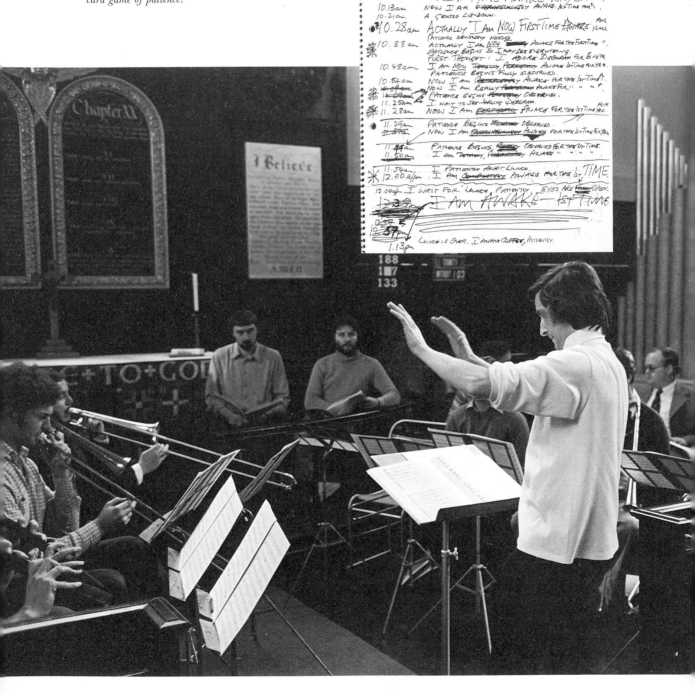

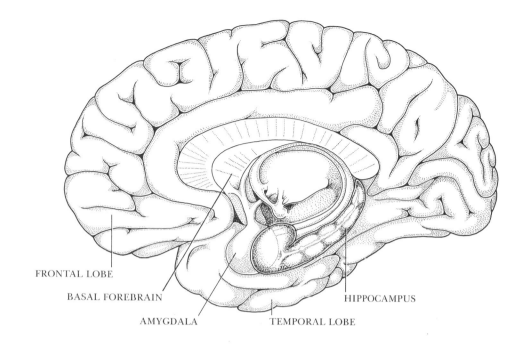

FRONTAL LOBE

BASAL FOREBRAIN

AMYGDALA

TEMPORAL LOBE

HIPPOCAMPUS

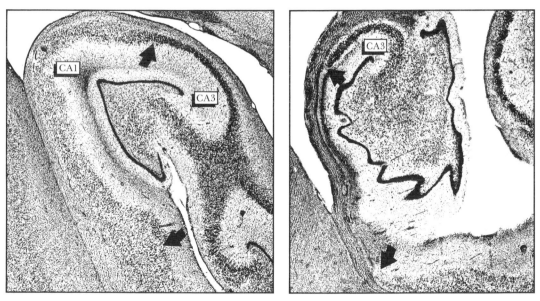

The diagram (top) shows the right hemisphere of a human brain, viewed from inside, after the brain has been split lengthways down the middle. The hippocampus, which is rolled up inside the temporal lobe, has been extensively damaged in Clive's case. Injury to the frontal lobe, the temporal lobe or the basal forebrain, can also produce amnesia. The microscopic sections show the normal human hippocampus (above left) and the hippocampus of a man, 'RB' (above right), who suffered from amnesia after a surgical operation. In his case, virtually the only part of the brain that was damaged was the region between the two arrows (the so-called CA1 region) throughout the whole length of the hippocampus.

is further subdivided by psychologists into semantic memory (general knowledge) and episodic memory (of particular places, people and personal experience).

The extraordinary thing about deeply amnesic patients is that their lives are, effectively, ruined because of their lack of *conscious* recollection, even though their brains retain the ability to learn. As Deborah says of Clive, 'without consciousness he's in many senses dead'. The distinction between these various kinds of memory may explain why most normal human beings are quite unable to recall specific episodes from their very early childhood, even though they are obviously learning all sorts of skills – walking, language, perception – during those early years. Perhaps episodic memory does not function properly until a child is a few years old – indeed, until the child is aware of its own independent existence in relation to the world around it.

The unconscious forms of memory may well reside in the cerebellum, the tightly wrinkled structure, the size of an orange, that protrudes from the brainstem, beneath the skull above the back of the neck. The human hippocampus, it seems, is needed for the imprinting of individual experiences. It may have taken over this job from a rather different role in simpler animals. John O'Keefe from University College London has recorded the impulses of individual neurons in the hippocampus of rats, as they go about their ratty business. As the rat moves from place to place in a large open cage, any individual nerve cell in its hippocampus waits silently until the rat reaches a particular region in its little world, and then the cell fires vigorously. As the rat moves away from that spot, the nerve cell stops firing, but if it returns, the cell starts to respond again. Different cells, scattered through the hippocampus, fire off their messages in different particular regions of the cage, and O'Keefe has suggested that they constitute a kind of short-term working 'map' of the immediate environment, which the animal keeps in its head. Thus, in simpler animals, the hippocampus may store information about where the animal has already been, which helps it to plan the future exploration of its world. Indeed, if the hippocampus is damaged in a rat, its ability to search around a complex maze for several hidden pieces of food is severely disrupted.

• THE SYNAPTIC SWITCH •

What we have so far is little more than an anatomy of memory. The hippocampus seems to be needed for long-term storage of general knowledge and personal experience but the cerebral cortex is probably the ultimate home of those persistent records, each of them spread out in some way over the cortex, quite unlike the orderly arrangement of books on a shelf.

If we want to know *how* memories are formed, we have to peer into the brain with sharper eyes, at the synaptic connections between nerve cells. In view of the fact that long-term memories can survive after the total cessation of impulse activity in the brain, they must take the form of structural modification, almost certainly changes in the strength of connections between nerve cells. Ivan Pavlov's dogs told him that some simple forms of learning involve the formation of new connections in the brain. A hungry dog dribbles at the sight of tasty food: presumably the interconnected pathway of nerves responsible for *that* response is constructed innately. But now, ring a bell before the food is presented a few times and the dog will drool when the bell alone rings (just as you and I do when we hear the clatter of plates in the kitchen). This new reflex, a *conditioned* reflex as Pavlov called it, must surely be due to the linking together of the nerve cells in the brain that are activated by the bell and those switched on by the sight of food, in such a way that either food or bell can now cause salivation.

Most researchers in the field of memory believe that a method for the rapid modification of connections between nerve cells must have appeared at a very early stage in evolution, allowing simple, mindless creatures to learn from their successes and mistakes – even animals as simple minded as a sea snail. Eric Kandel from Columbia University in New York, a psychiatrist by training, has devoted many years to the analysis of learning in the Californian sea snail, *Aplysia*. Let's be honest. *Aplysia* is neither beautiful nor bright. Its entire nervous system consists of some 18 000 neurons and it does little more than eat and have sex of a snaily sort. However, remarkably, *Aplysia* can learn. The animal has a gill, like a fish's gill, which it pushes out into the water to breathe. But if the gill is touched, an innate reflex (like a dog's salivation to food) makes it pull back. This gill withdrawal reflex is controlled by one tiny cluster of nerve cells containing six motor neurons (whose fibres run out to the muscles) and twenty-four sensory cells (which receive information from receptive endings around the gill and elsewhere). Touching the gill activates the sensory neurons, which send impulses along their fibres to end in synaptic contacts on to the motor neurons, which in turn send impulses out to the muscles to make them contract.

If the gill is touched lightly, time after time, the sea snail gradually stops withdrawing it. This kind of successive reduction in response, called habituation, is generally accepted as a simple sort of learning. Kandel chose *Aplysia* as the subject of his research because of the simplicity of its nervous system and the huge size of the nerve cells, which makes them relatively easy to study electrically and chemically. The site of habituation was narrowed down to the synaptic junction between the sensory nerve cell and the motor cell. Kandel showed that successive impulses arriving along the sensory fibre, set off by the series of touches to the area of the gill, caused progressively less and less chemical transmitter substance to be squirted out from the nerve ending. This reduction in transmitter release explained the reduced motor response.

Now, when the little animal has grown accustomed to the tickling of its gill, if a different part of the body is prodded the gill reflex *returns* in all its former strength and glory. Here is another form of simple learning, called sensitisation. Again, Kandel has shown that the return of the reflex is due to a change in the amount of substance released at that same synaptic junction – a change that is itself triggered by a different chemical transmitter substance released by other sensory nerve fibres transmitting news about the stimulation of some other part of the body.

Aplysia can even learn associations between one thing and another, rather like Pavlov's dogs, and that sort of conditioning depends on changes in the strength of synaptic connections through a mechanism not too different from that originally proposed by Donald Hebb.

Many people are surprised, even amused, that an eminent scientist and a large team of research workers have dedicated two decades to the study of such trivial forms of learning in an animal that looks revolting and has little more intelligence than a stone. But the work of Kandel and many others who search for the secret of memory in the nervous systems of the simplest animals is of fundamental importance for our understanding of ourselves as more than 'children of the moment'. If the magic power of memory was discovered very early in the history of life on Earth, it would not be far-fetched to think that the mechanisms in our brains use chemical machinery not too different from that of the humble sea snail.

In fact, there is a bridge between the beautifully simple biology of *Aplysia* and the complex results of brain damage in man. A tiny slice taken from the hippocampus of a rat or other animal can survive for some hours in a suitable oxygenated fluid, providing the experimental physiologist with an opportunity to do the kinds of experiments on a mammalian brain that Eric Kandel performs on the sea snail. Tim Bliss of the Medical Research Council's National Institute for Medical Research in London was one of the first to show that synaptic contacts in the hippocampus can be changed, rapidly and dramatically, depending on the traffic of nerve impulses through them. A burst of nerve impulses, caused by electrical stimulation of the nerve fibres that carry information into the hippocampus from sensory areas of the cerebral cortex, causes a progressive *increase* in the electrical response of cells in the hippocampus to each successive incoming impulse. Once induced these changes can last for days or even weeks.

At the University of Edinburgh, Richard Morris uses a swimming pool to test the ability of rats to learn. Hidden just below the surface at some point in the pool is a platform on to which the rat can clamber. Rats normally learn quickly to swim to the platform, from wherever they are put into the water. But they have great difficulty in learning if the hippocampus is damaged or even if they are given a drug called APV, which specifically prevents the changes of synaptic strength in the hippocampus.

Just as in *Aplysia*, the crucial process in the hippocampus seems to take place at the individual synaptic contacts. The increased response of each nerve cell seems to be caused by changes in the reaction of the cell itself to the chemical transmitter substance released at the synapses on to it, as well as an increase in the amount of transmitter squirted out for each impulse. Gary Lynch and his colleagues at the University of California at Irvine have shown that just a brief burst of nerve impulses passing through the synapses of the hippocampus can, within hours, cause changes in the shapes and sizes of synaptic contacts, and even the number of synapses, visible in the electronic microscope. Recent results from Kandel's laboratory show that long-term learning can also change the number and size of individual synapses in *Aplysia*.

Cells of the cerebral cortex also have the ability to change the strength of their responses to incoming signals, using cellular mechanisms similar to those of the hippocampus. It seems possible, then, that short-term conscious memory depends on reverberating activity in cortical circuits, that the transfer of signals to the hippocampus starts the process of long-term storage and that signals sent back to the cortex from the hippocampus result in a permanent change in a distributed network of cortical cells.

To remember is to alter the brain. Yet the brain changes spontaneously and constantly throughout life, like all parts of the body, as molecules break down and are replaced. Gary Lynch describes this paradox:

> We have been faced with a phenomenon which seems beyond the possible. For instance, you are sitting here right now, registering an incredibly modest signal – a word. Somehow that word, which stays in your head as an electric signal for no more than a few seconds, can, if you wish, leave a trace that will last for years. Your brain is literally tearing itself apart; the cells and the proteins that constitute cell membranes in your brain are being broken down and replaced. And yet the traces that you stored are still there.

Looking back, the prescience of Donald Hebb seems quite extraordinary. Hebb defined what the differences between short-term and long-term memory must mean in terms of the mechanisms of the brain; Hebb first saw that the world must be represented, piece by piece, in the activity of small assemblies of nerve cells; Hebb speculated about the way in which those internal representations could be stamped in through the strengthening of individual connections between nerve cells.

It was Hebb, too, who conceived of the brain as a vast, intermingled, parallel network of circuits or assemblies of cells. In just the last few years, ideas very much like these have seized the world of computer science and promise to revolutionise the efficiency with which computers can do the things that our brains do so well.

A new generation of computer scientists, with one eye on the brain, is exploring the extraordinary computing power possessed by simple networks of components, connected in parallel, with junctions that can change their strength depending on the signals that have passed through them. These are early days to judge the profundity of this new movement, even in a subject that races ahead as quickly as computer science. But astounding claims have been made for this new style of parallel computation, with its uncanny resemblance to Hebb's image of the brain. Simple networks of imagined nerves and modifiable synapses, all collaborating in *each* memory, can store vast amounts of information. The memories can survive local damage to the network, with merely a general reduction in the clarity of recall (much like the blurred and muddled memories of brain-damaged people).

Memory is a central problem that must be solved if we are to explain more general mysteries, such as the nature of perception and thought. 'All that we are is the result of what we have thought,' a Buddhist text, the Dhammapada, says. Just as the unravelling of the structure of DNA, the medium of memory from generation to generation, has allowed molecular biology to march on at such a furious pace, so the unlocking of the door of remembering will let us through into a new world of understanding. The most coveted reward that the unravelling of memory offers is the clue that it will bring to the nature of conscious human experience.

RHYTHMS
OF LIFE

WE LIVE IN a restless world. From the vibrations of molecules to the endless cyclical wanderings of comets, the universe is a vast, swinging, revolving, throbbing clock. The sun rises and sets; the tides ebb and flow; the moon waxes and wanes; the seasons come and go. These rhythms have profound effects on the environment and animals have evolved to be part of this natural order. For an animal with eyes, what event could be more cataclysmic than the loss of the sun? Yet it happens every night, without fail. For animals that forage for plant food, what could be more disastrous than the death of vegetation and its covering with snow that comes with every winter? For a warm-blooded animal, which must maintain its body temperature, or a cold-blooded one, whose ability to move at all is dictated by the temperature of the environment, the changing seasons present a tremendous physiological challenge. To survive in the rhythmic universe, living things must fall in step with its tempo; their behaviour must resonate with the shifting state of the physical world around them. The brain itself must be a rhythmic organ.

It is the dawn of a new day. Birds are singing. Flowers turn towards the rising sun; their petals open. Many animals emerge from their nests; other, nocturnal species are hurrying home to sleep.

It is the spring. Many species of birds that fled south for the winter are on their way back; winter visitors are leaving for the north. The leaves are bursting open; shoots push through the soil; hibernating species emerge from their winter's sleep. The urge to mate is everywhere; to reproduce and give the next generation the advantage of the summer months.

The cycles of nature are reflected in these and many other ways in

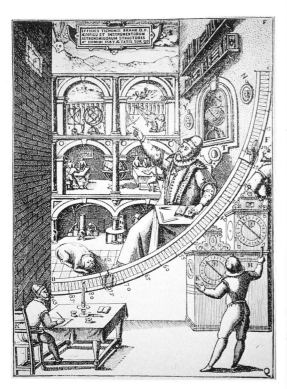

ABOVE LEFT *The Danish nobleman turned astronomer, Tycho Brahe (1546–1601), built this 'mural quadrant' at Uraniborg. It was a pre-telescope device for siting planets and stars, measuring their elevations accurately and defining the rhythms of the universe.*

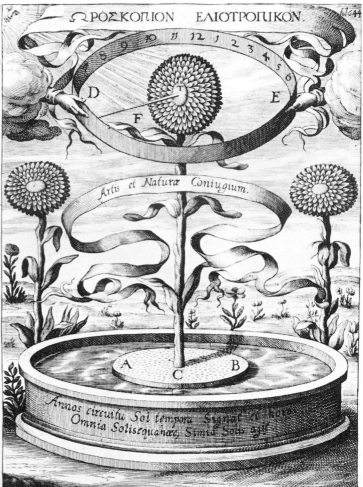

ABOVE RIGHT *The ability of plants to respond to the seasons and the motion of the sun has intrigued scientists for centuries. In this illustration by Athanasius Kircher, published in 1643, the movements of the sunflower are attributed to a 'magnetic' attraction from the sun.*

the actions of living things. Animals and plants seem to be slaves to their environments. But surely human beings are different. We think that we are in control, that the pattern of human life depends on our *voluntary* reactions to the world around us. We eat, sleep and make love when we want to. We may, for convenience, match our actions to the state of the world around us, but the choice is ours. That is how things seem to be, but when we look closely we find that many of the cycles of our lives, like those of the animals around us, are beyond our control. We too are slaves to the rhythms of life.

Our animal past is most apparent when we look deep into the human brain. Imagine that we peel away the cerebral hemispheres that have evolved so rapidly in the past 50 million years: we are left with a brain about the size of that of a cat. Now strip away the rest of the forebrain, and we are left with something comparable to the brain of a giant lizard. It is here, at the level of the reptile beneath the man, that the brain dances to the beat of nature.

• DARK TIMES •

The clocks of our brain normally tick away quietly and reliably. Most of us hardly notice them; but others hear nothing else. Pat Moore, from The Plains, Virginia in the United States, suffered severe depression for several years before she noticed that the onset of a depressive period often coincided with the start of winter, and that her melancholy would lift with the arrival of spring. Her condition has been properly recognised by the medical world only recently – a condition called Seasonal Affective Disorder (with the appropriate acronym SAD).

In the winter, Pat Moore slept up to twelve hours a day. She lacked energy and enthusiasm, and life had no pleasure in it. For many animals, winter is a time of inactivity and a period that tests the powers of survival. Perhaps it is not surprising that as summer slips into autumn and autumn fades into winter most people too feel less energetic and perhaps a little less enthusiastic for life. Many cities in Scandinavia, near or above the Arctic Circle, have a higher suicide rate in the winter than in the summer.

For most of us, seasonal changes in mood are subtle. But for Pat Moore, swings of emotion are so severe that they interfere with her ability to function. They may well be triggered by the same mechanisms in the brain that cause seasonal changes of behaviour in animals. What signals could the brain use from the environment to detect the onset of winter? Detecting variations in the daily temperature would be unreliable, but the length of daylight changes inexorably through the year; any animal that could follow the variation in day-length could know the time of year and predict the coming season. Many animals are indeed able to sense the shifting length of the day and they use this information to trigger seasonal changes in their behaviour.

Seasonal Affective Disorder has been the subject of intensive research at the National Institute of Mental Health in Bethesda, Maryland. Thomas Wehr and his colleagues reasoned that if the decline of depression in people like Pat Moore coincided with the longer days of springtime, then such patients might be lifted out of their winter gloom by a procedure as simple as showing them extra, artificial sunlight during the darkness of night. Pat Moore became the subject of a curious experiment. Every morning in winter, she set her alarm clock and struggled out of bed a few hours before sunrise. She then sat, with her radio for company, in front of her artificial sun – a bank of full-spectrum fluorescent lamps, which bathed her in bright white light. This ridiculously simple experiment paid off. Within just a couple of days she began to emerge from her depression and to experience the energy and good feelings that were, for her, typical of the spring. This simple procedure has had a dramatic impact on the treatment of SAD sufferers, many of whom now find relief in winter from a prescription of lights rather than pills.

• THE CLOCKS WITHIN •

It takes a case like that of Pat Moore to remind us how closely we are linked with the animal world. Clocks and watches, newspapers, holidays, schedules of work, mealtimes, vacations; all these man-made features of our life remind us of the passage of time. It is easy to forget that we may be tied in a much more primitive way to the rhythms of the physical world. What would happen if we were to *remove* all the external cues to the nature of time, even the ones that nature provides? In a world without alarm clocks and meal breaks, without day and night, could our bodies still have their own rhythmic existence? What would happen without the *Zeitgeber* – the 'time-givers' of the world around us?

In the early 1960s these questions assumed great scientific importance, partly because of the political as well as scientific interest in the prospects of space travel. Michel Siffre, a young French cave explorer, was one of a number of intrepid volunteers who agreed to isolate themselves from the *Zeitgeber* of the normal world, living underground with no cues to the time of day. In 1972 Siffre spent seven months, deep in a cave in Texas, entirely alone. He had a stockpile of food and water, books to read and equipment on which to exercise. But his was a world of constant temperature and artificial light, without a clock in sight. His only contact with the outside world was via a telephone line, permanently manned, and through a computer and video camera link-up to scientists on the

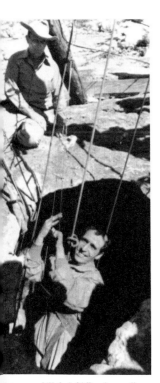

Michel Siffre descending into the cave near Del Rio, Texas, in 1972.

surface, who monitored his activities, his physiological functions and his comments about his states of mind.

In some ways, the results of this bizarre experiment were not surprising. Siffre organised his life into a fairly normal pattern of alternating periods of activity and sleep. His 'day' was punctuated with the normal pattern of meals. But what was remarkable about this self-made universe was that the day he chose to live by lasted twenty-five hours rather than twenty-four. Every real day that passed, Siffre rose an hour later, as if he were living by a clock that was running a little slow. He was! That clock was in his brain.

For all the advances of modern society, we cannot afford to ignore the rhythms of the animal brain within us, any more than we can neglect our need to breathe or eat. Without the biological clocks in our brains, our lives would be chaotic, our actions disorganised. The brain has internalised the rhythms of nature, but can tick on for months without sight of the sun. But how can a piece of brain – a wet, living tangle of cells – act like a mechanical timepiece?

In 1729 Jean Jacques Dortous de Mairan reported a surprising observation, in the *Proceedings of the Royal Academy of Sciences of Paris*.

> The sunflower reacts to sunlight and the day: its leaves and stems contract and close towards sunset. [But] sunlight and air are not necessary for this phenomenon to take place ... the reaction is only slightly less pronounced if the plant is kept in complete darkness. It continues to open very distinctly at sunrise, closes again in the evening, and remains closed the whole night. The sunflower therefore responds to the sun without being exposed to it in any way.

Despite de Mairan's encouragement to scientists to continue his work, the science of chronobiology (the study of biological time) did not blossom until the middle of this century. Interest soon shifted from plants to animals and evidence grew rapidly that most animal species, from single-celled organisms upwards, exhibit circadian rhythms (from the Latin *circa*, meaning 'about' and *dies*, 'day') – alternating patterns of rest and activity, in time with the twenty-four hour clock. Many species continue to maintain rhythmic behaviour, in a circadian pattern, even if they are kept in total darkness. A rat, like a human being, has an inherent rhythm of about twenty-five hours, which dominates its cycle of sleep and activity as soon as it is put in the dark. Despite the fact that this internal clock is slightly out of step with nature, it is, nevertheless, as reliable and regular as most man-made clocks; the rhythm does not deviate by more than a few minutes over several months. There is obviously an internal rhythm-generator that is normally reset each day to the cycle of the real world. Subsequent research showed that a brief exposure to light in the early morning, as little as a single flash in some species, is sufficient to synchronise the animal's activity to the twenty-four hour cycle.

In 1972, Fred Stephan and Irving Zucker of the University of California at Berkeley, narrowed the search for the clock down to a tiny cluster of nerve cells, the suprachiasmatic nucleus in the hypothalamus. If this region is damaged in rats, the circadian rhythm of rest and activity, which is normally maintained even in constant darkness, disappears completely. The animal's movements, its periods of rest and of eating and drinking become randomly distributed through the whole day. This tiny nucleus, smaller than a pinhead in a rat, seems to be the clock itself, or at least a vital part of it.

Since then the evidence has grown that the few hundred or thousand nerve cells of the suprachiasmatic nucleus constitute a timing mechanism used by the brain to regulate many of its rhythms. When neurophysiologists placed tiny microelectrodes in the nucleus, to pick up impulses from the cells as a rat went about its business, they found that the neurons in this part of the brain fire off in a remarkably regular pattern, almost like the ticking of a clock. Moreover, the rate of nerve ticking varies systematically through the day; the cells fire slightly faster when the rat is active (during the night) than when it is resting (during the day). If the suprachiasmatic nucleus is isolated from the rest of the brain by cutting the bundles of fibres running in and out of it, the nerve cells in the nucleus continue to tick in their regular pattern and to vary their frequency of firing through the day. Even if this minute structure is removed completely from the brain and maintained alive in an oxygenated dish of fluid, the nerve cells still persist in their fantastically regular, clock-like rhythm of firing.

Most timing devices invented by man contain some kind of regular oscillator, such as a swinging pendulum or a vibrating crystal. But to register the passage of time, something more is needed; there must be an integrator (such as the hands of a conventional clock) or a counter (such as the numbers on a digital watch) to keep track of the number of ticks or oscillations that have passed. We do not yet know how this component of the brain's clock operates and it may use a principle quite different from that of man-made timepieces. There is certainly no evidence of a counting mechanism in the brain; the slow variation in the frequency of firing of nerve cells in the suprachiasmatic nucleus suggests that the oscillator in this biological clock is giving a *direct* indication of the time of day, rather like a clock with a pendulum that swings faster at some periods in the day and slower at others.

But if the suprachiasmatic nucleus is the home of the brain's own, slightly slow, clock, how is it reset each day by the natural cycle of light and dark? The *position* of this little mass of nerve cells is the clue: it lies directly above the optic chiasma – the junction of the two optic nerves on their way from the eyes to the brain. A tuft of thin nerve fibres branches off from the main optic nerves and penetrates the hypothalamus above, forming synaptic connections on to cells in the suprachiasmatic nucleus. This anatomically insignificant pathway is the link between the outside world and the brain's own clock. This may be the route by which bright lights in the early morning can wipe away the winter blues of patients such as Pat Moore.

Until very recently the idea of transplanting pieces of the brain from one individual to another lay in the realm of science fiction; but nowadays neural transplantation is a reality. Several research groups around the world have been attempting to restore the circadian rhythms of rodents, after destruction of the suprachiasmatic nucleus, by transplanting into the brain a fragment of the hypothalamus of another animal.

In 1987, Michael Lehman, Rae Silver, Eric Bittman and their colleagues from New York and from the University of Massachusetts at Amherst, reported dramatic results from such experiments. They made tiny areas of damage in the region of the suprachiasmatic nucleus in normal adult golden hamsters and confirmed that such animals immediately lose their cyclical pattern of activity and rest, whether they are kept continuously in the dark or in a twenty-four hour pattern of dark and light. Then, they took fragments of immature brain tissue from the appropriate region of the hypothalamus of fetal hamsters, shortly before the normal time of birth. Using a tiny needle, they injected these clusters of embryonic cells into the brains of the rhythmless adult hamsters. Within a few days the animals began to show rhythmic circadian patterns of activity, which were maintained over weeks or months in total darkness. The cyclical activity had a rhythm of a little more than twenty-four hours, just as in completely normal hamsters kept in the dark. When they subsequently examined the brains of these animals, they found that the grafted tissue had connected itself to the hypothalamus of the adult animal and that within it were groups of nerve cells characteristic of the normal suprachiasmatic nucleus, containing peptide substances thought to be involved in chemical communication between the suprachiasmatic nucleus and other parts of the brain.

In those cases in which the graft had attached itself close to the optic chiasma, nerve fibres from the eye were seen penetrating the graft. However, such animals did not adopt a twenty-four hour rhythm if they were exposed to a normal cycle of light and dark, so the new connections between eye and graft may not have been fully functional. More remarkable was the finding that even if the graft attached itself to some completely different part of the brain, a natural circadian rhythm of activity was restored. This all suggests that these tiny morsels of brain from fetal animals, which have never experienced the rhythms of day and night, can, nevertheless, generate cyclical patterns of activity, which can be

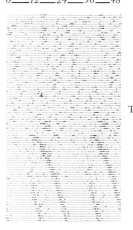

HOURS
0——12——24——36——48

ABOVE *This record illustrates the remarkable experiments of Michael Lehman and his colleagues. It shows the pattern of activity of a hamster over six months, the lines representing successive forty-eight hour periods. The thickened regions on each trace indicate times when the hamster was highly active. A normal hamster would be active during the night but not during the day, but the tiny suprachiasmatic nucleus in the hypothalamus of this animal had been destroyed, causing it to lose its normal daily cycle of activity. At the time indicated by the 'T', it was given a transplant of tissue from the suprachiasmatic nucleus of a fetal hamster. About a month later, a clear, cyclical pattern of activity appeared, roughly once a day but slightly longer than twenty-four hours.*

used by the host brain to control activity and rest. These remarkable experiments bring us closer to understanding the nature of the biological clock and even the chemical messages by which it communicates with the rest of the brain.

• RESETTING THE CLOCKS •

Nathaniel Kleitman and Bruce Richardson, two sleep researchers at the University of Chicago, did a simple experiment in 1938 to try to discover how readily the brain's clocks can be reset. They spent thirty-two days deep in Mammoth Cave in Kentucky, not living by their internal clocks alone but trying to adapt to a twenty-eight hour day – nineteen hours of artificial light for waking and 9 of darkness for sleep. They forced themselves to try to sleep, wake and have their meals according to this curious schedule. It turned out that Bruce Richardson adapted well to this rhythm, but Kleitman could not and his sleepiness and body temperature followed a cycle much closer to twenty-four hours.

Human beings are, by nature, nomadic. Curiosity, territoriality and greed have driven people to move on and out, beyond the patch of land that would serve the immediate purpose of survival alone. For the first few million years of hominid evolution, travel was so slow that it could not disrupt the inbuilt sense of time. But the aeroplane brought with it an unprecedented physiological problem. Imagine that our internal clocks were set exactly and unalterably to a twenty-four hour cycle: each of us would be shackled, by our brain, to a single spot on earth. We have to thank the fact that our internal clocks are reset every day for our ability to adjust to the patterns of time in other parts of the world. However, the internal clock does not allow itself to be shifted without a struggle. Fatigue, insomnia and disorientation often ruin the first few days of a holiday or a business trip abroad. Knowledge of the characteristics of the biological clock makes it easy to understand one apparently curious feature of jet lag – the fact that most people suffer much less when journeying in a westerly direction than when travelling from west to east. When going westward, chasing the sun, the day is temporarily lengthened. Since the *natural* cycling time of the biological clock is about twenty-five hours for most people, an increase in day-length is much easier to deal with than a decrease. Indeed, the ideal way to travel would be to go always from east to west, in short hops of one time zone each day, making each day of the journey precisely equal to the body's natural twenty-five hour rhythm.

Although the root cause of jet lag is quite clear, we still do not fully understand how the cycles of the biological clock become transformed into physiological states, such as needing to sleep. The finger of suspicion, though, points at melatonin, a hormone produced by the enigmatic pineal gland, a tiny organ that sits on top of the brainstem. The secretion of this hormone varies with the time of day, reaching a maximum during the night. It turns out that the cyclical production of melatonin by the pineal gland is regulated in some way by the suprachiasmatic nucleus, the tiny structure in the hypothalamus that listens in on signals from the eye. Somehow, the activity of nerve cells in the suprachiasmatic nucleus inhibits the production of melatonin by the pineal gland during the daytime.

Now, after a long jet flight, the cyclical release of melatonin stays locked to the pattern of day and night of the home country for some days. Josephine Arendt and her colleagues at the University of Surrey think that the surge of melatonin that normally occurs at night may play a part in triggering fatigue and sleep. The cyclical production of melatonin in a pattern inappropriate for the destination at which a jet traveller arrives might cause the fatigue experienced during the day and the insomnia at night. They therefore administered melatonin to jet-lagged volunteers during the evening, when they ought to be feeling sleepy. Far fewer of the volunteers who received injections of melatonin reported feeling the ill effects of jet lag than did a group of control volunteers who received only a placebo injection, without melatonin. The pineal gland may play a role of enormous significance, co-ordinating the rhythms of the body by relaying cyclical signals from the brain.

Except for airline pilots and cabin staff, most people have to worry about jet lag only once or twice a year. But as industry strives for greater and greater production, as more and more industrial and commercial processes require round-the-clock human supervision, the demand has grown for people to work at times when Nature tells them to sleep. The lives of shift workers can be disturbed just as much as those of international travellers: they suffer from insomnia, digestive problems, irritability, fatigue and even depression. Workers who rotate shifts each week also have more accidents on the job and their productivity is low.

Preston Richey, plant manager of the Great Salt Lake Minerals & Chemicals Corporation, on the salt flats of Utah, read a newspaper article about Charles Czeisler, who studies biological rhythms at Harvard University, and invited him to help them. The plant had 130 shift workers, who were constantly complaining of insomnia and a variety of other problems. They worked a weekly schedule: first a week on day shift, then a week on night shift, then a week on evening shift, and so on. This is one of the most common shift schedules used in industry, but it seems almost deliberately designed to present the worst possible challenge to the rhythms of the body. The shift rotation essentially has the workers toiling in New York one week, Paris the next, Tokyo the third and so on – travelling constantly from west to east and never quite overcoming their jet lag. Laboratory studies show that animals placed on this kind of rotating schedule of light and dark suffer from increased incidence of heart disease and have shorter life spans.

All the experimental evidence suggests that the normal cycling time of the clocks in the brains of most animals and of human beings is set *longer* than a twenty-four hour day. Yet the workers in Utah were being forced to rotate their clocks *backwards* by eight hours each week. Czeisler recommended, first, that the shifts should rotate forwards in time (taking advantage of the natural preference of the body) and, second, that each shift should last for three weeks (because most people take more than a week to adjust completely to a new time zone).

The effects were rapid and remarkable. The workers liked the new schedules, their health was better and they were able to make fuller use of their leisure time. The managers were pleased too, because productivity dramatically improved by as much as 22 per cent. Charles Czeisler and his team did more than simply change the work schedule. They taught the men and the management something of how the body works, about the timing mechanisms in the brain, in order that they could all understand the problems that they faced and could learn how best to deal with them. Most of the workers now try to plan their periods of sleep to ease the move to the next shift period: they go to bed a little later each week, so that they are, in effect, shifting their clocks in small steps every few days.

• THE PARADOX OF SLEEP •

Our planet is a dangerous place; there is ruthless competition for limited resources; only the fittest survive. And yet all the most advanced animals, normally alert, shrewd, watchful, drop their defences to sleep. Even human beings, the most spectacularly successful species, spend one-third of their lives more or less paralysed and senseless. If sleep is so risky it must bestow a huge benefit on animals that indulge in it, or it would have been eliminated by the powerful forces of natural selection. Animals that did not need to sleep would surely have evolved and prevailed over their sleepy competitors. With only this prejudice in mind – that sleep must surely be valuable – let us examine this strange altered state of mind.

Speculation about the causes and significance of sleep gave way to scientific enquiry at the turn of this century. The breakthrough that propelled this area of research was the discovery that the brain has electrical activity – brainwaves – that can be recorded through the skull and the scalp of a living animal. In the 1870s, Richard Caton, an amateur scientist and sometime mayor of Liverpool, battling with incredibly primitive electrical recording equipment, discovered that tiny fluctuations in voltage could be detected through electrodes placed on the surface of the brain or on the skulls of rabbits and monkeys. But it was a German psychiatrist, Hans Berger, who first recorded such an electroencephalogram (EEG) from the human brain. In his spare time, after his day's work in the clinic in Jena, he followed an unusual experimental interest – in the supernatural. When he was a young man, at the end of the last century, Berger was serving in the German army; one day his horse stumbled and he fell, narrowly escaping injury. That same evening he received from his father a telegram, prompted by a premonition that his sister had had, enquiring about his state of health.

Largely as a result of that curious event, Berger switched from astronomy to psychiatry in his studies at the University of Jena. He became fascinated with the possibility that electrical discharges from the human brain might be correlated with conscious experience and might even be responsible for the transmission of thoughts. In 1924, his long and unsuccessful series of experiments began to pay off: he picked up tiny electrical signals from wires stuck into the skin of the scalp of his young son Klaus. Berger had hoped to see bursts of electrical activity radiating from his son's head whenever the boy concentrated on some deep thought, but whenever Klaus opened his eyes, spoke or tackled mental arithmetic, the electrical recording went virtually flat. And when the boy relaxed completely, closed his eyes and tried to think of nothing, a regular, rhythmic pattern of electrical waves began to grow, beating out a thought-less message ten times every second.

Hans Berger's discovery was either ignored or rejected by most of his psychiatric colleagues. It was Edgar Adrian, Professor of Physiology at the University of Cambridge, who brought his findings to the attention of the scientific world. Adrian repeated and confirmed Berger's observations, and recognised the potential importance of the EEG in studying the state and activity of the human brain. But what of that odd fact, that the waves of the brain become huge rolling breakers when the mind is empty and settle to a calm ocean of tiny ripples when consciousness wells up and active thought takes over? To understand this we have to ask about the state of activity of the millions of individual nerve cells in the cortex under the skull, whose massed electrical responses somehow generate the single signal of the EEG. To produce a clear, steady, slow oscillation of the type that Berger saw when Klaus's mind was resting, those vast populations of nerve cells must all fire in unison, in a mindless synchronised chant of impulses. But when the brain is occupied, when the mind is busy, the nerve cells of the cortex go about their own individual business, each one bursting or pausing as it plays its part in the chatter of neural communication that underlies a thought. No wonder, then, that the wires in Klaus's scalp picked up nothing more than a tiny, rapidly changing, *desynchronised* signal whenever he was alert.

When neurophysiologists recorded from individual nerve cells in the brains of freely moving animals, they fully confirmed this speculation. When an animal is awake and active, the cells of its cortex fire their impulses in irregular bursts, each following its own pattern, depending on the part that that cell is playing in the computing task in hand. But when the animal becomes relaxed, even drowsy, the cells of the cortex pick up a common theme, the whole vast mantle of the cortex drumming out a regular pattern of impulses, singing in time with the throbbing rhythm of an ancient conductor, deep in the brain.

Through the 1930s the techniques of electroencephalography improved rapidly and it played its part in medical diagnosis, particularly in the study of epilepsy and coma. As methods improved, research workers began to detect minor differences in the form of the EEG waves during different states of consciousness. In particular, their interest turned to sleep. In a restful state of drowsiness, just before the onset of sleep, Hans Berger's alpha rhythm – the ten per second waves that he first described – wells up and dominates the EEG. Eyelids droop; consciousness flags; perception fades. As the person slips into the arms of Hypnos, the waves of the EEG beat more slowly – small in amplitude at first but gradually growing in size, as the neurons chant their lullaby with a slower and firmer beat.

Is sleep the natural state of the brain, interrupted only when sensory stimulation, hunger or thirst rouses the nervous system from its rhythmic idyll? Or is alertness the normal state, interrupted by some powerful signal from the blood or the brain, forcing the cortex into slumber? The debate has raged since the turn of the century. Frederic Bremer, a Belgian neurophysiologist, operated on the brains of animals, interrupting the pathways carrying messages from the senses into the brain. Such animals fall into comatose sleep, their EEG consisting of a constant pattern of slow, sleep-like waves. This seems strong evidence in favour of the *passive* theory, suggesting that sleep is indeed the natural state of the brain. But through the following decades, experiment after experiment demonstrated that sleep is far from a passive process; it is actively organised, in all of its complex stages, by a network of neural engines deep in the brain.

In 1948, Giuseppe Moruzzi, recently appointed as Professor of Physiology at the University of Pisa in Italy, who had studied ten years earlier with Bremer in Brussels, went to work for a year in the laboratory of Horace Magoun at Northwestern University in Evanston, Illinois. Moruzzi, who died in 1986, described this period in the United States as one of the most fruitful in his life. In their pioneering experiments, Moruzzi and Magoun demonstrated that there is a tangled network of nerve cells – the reticular formation – that runs through the centre of the brainstem and seems to be responsible for both actively turning the brain on during the waking state and deliberately switching it off during sleep.

It turns out that nerves from the sense organs, as well as providing direct information to the cortex about the nature of the outside world, also send branches into the reticular formation, where the activity from the senses is mixed together. From groups of nerve cells in the reticular formation, small but vital systems of nerve fibres pass up to higher parts of the brain, including the cerebral cortex, to provide a constant indication of the degree of sensory stimulation. Direct electrical stimulation, with minute currents, in this upper part of the reticular formation would arouse a sleeping animal, mimicking precisely the natural pattern of waking. But, more surprisingly, if the stimulating electrodes were moved to the lower parts of the reticular formation, deeper in the brainstem, repetitive stimulation would make the animal stretch, curl up, close its eyes and fall into apparently normal sleep! Indeed, Walter Hess, a physiologist working at the University of Zurich, found that sleep could be *actively* produced by electrical stimulation in many parts of the brain, including the hypothalamus and regions of the forebrain directly above.

• PERCHANCE TO DREAM •

By the early 1950s, neurophysiologists had a delightfully simple and satisfying view of the steering of the cycles of sleeping and waking. Two rival systems, both in the reticular formation, appeared to run the engines of the brain; one monitoring constantly the level of sensory stimulation and arousing the brain in relation to it; the other actively pulling back the throttle and sending the brain into sleep. The cycle of life was thought to be simply the swinging of the pendulum of power between these two commanders of the brain. But research work on humans, in the laboratory of Nathaniel Kleitman in Chicago, added an enigmatic complication to this simple story.

In 1952, Kleitman suggested to one of his graduate students, Eugene Aserinsky, that he should study the rolling movements of the eyes that occur early in sleep. Aserinsky taped an extra pair of electrodes on to the volunteers who came to sleep in Kleitman's laboratory. These electrodes, one on each temple, picked up signals each time the eyes moved. As the volunteers became drowsy, the electrodes detected the slow rolling eye movements that could easily be seen through their lids. Aserinsky continued to watch the pen recorders as the subject fell deeper into sleep. The eyes became still and it looked as if the experiment was over. But, to the great surprise of Eugene Aserinsky, an hour or so after the start of sleep, the eyes suddenly began to move again, not just swinging slowly from side to side but darting rapidly back and forth. Bursts of these rapid eye movements continued over the next few minutes until, once again, the eyes came to rest.

Kleitman was, at first, sceptical about this extraordinary observation but he and another student, Bill Dement, went on not only to confirm Aserinsky's strange finding but also to show that the phases of rapid eye movements, occurring every ninety minutes or so throughout the night, represent a distinct and vitally important stage of sleep. I went to visit Bill Dement, now the director of a well-known sleep laboratory, at Stanford University in California.

With a tangle of wires stuck to my face and scalp, tethered by the plaited cable to a panel above my head, I fell asleep quickly in one of Bill Dement's special bedrooms. The cable of wires, eavesdropping on my brain and eyes, emerged in the neighbouring room, a laboratory lined with racks of electronic equipment, where a dozen pens scribbled out the story of my slumber on a recording machine.

Down I went, through the classical stages of sleep, with the deepening, slowing pattern of waves punctuated by occasional 'complexes' and 'spindles', which Bill Dement subsequently interpreted. And there, suddenly, was the predicted event: furious twitching of my eyes behind the closed lids. And, with it, a characteristic but strange change in the EEG, the huge slow waves of normal deep sleep being replaced by a higher-frequency pattern, closer to the brainwaves of the waking state. But I was far from awake: indeed, this stage, called rapid eye-movement sleep, is also sometimes known as paradoxical sleep, because the sleeper is actually more difficult to awaken, even though the EEG suggests that the brain is active. Indeed, most of the muscles of the body are quite literally paralysed, cut off from the restless activity of the brain by inhibitory signals descending from a tiny region deep in the brainstem. Just a few overt responses of the body indicate the frenzied activity taking place in the brain. The eye movements are one. Sometimes the fingers twitch or the teeth grind together; in males, the penis erects.

And then the shock. Just after the burst of paradoxical sleep, one of Bill Dement's assistants woke me! 'Have you been dreaming?' I had; a bizarre dream about earthquakes and aeroplanes, full of twisted versions of the events of the past day. Bill Dement was the first to wake sleepers during paradoxical sleep, and he discovered that they were much more likely to say that they were having a vivid dream than if they were woken at other times during sleep. If he selectively deprived people of paradoxical sleep by waking them each time the pen recorder showed the signs of an impending phase of eye movements, they would, next day, show many more of the signs of a sleepless night than if Dement had woken them the same number of times but during other stages of sleep. And the next night they would spend more time than normal in paradoxical sleep, as if they needed to catch up on the dreams that they had lost.

Soon, the paradoxical stage of sleep was identified in animals; the same rapid eye movements, irregular breathing and heartbeat, the same signs of limp bodies but busy brains. And this discovery in turn led to the identification of yet more regions, in the reticular formation of the brainstem, that might control this specific phase of sleep.

During the normal waking state, the EEG consists of small, rapidly fluct-uating waves and the lower trace registers the movements of the eyes as I look around the room.

Awake, but very relaxed, my EEG shows 'alpha rhythm' – very regular waves at a rate of about ten per second.

The arrow marks the onset of sleep – a transition to slightly slower EEG activity.

In the early stages of sleep, the waves of the EEG begin to deepen and become lower in frequency. The eyes roll slowly from side to side.

After several minutes, I reach the deeper stages of 'slow-wave sleep', in which large slow-waves dominate the EEG.

Every ninety minutes or so during sleep there is a period of 'paradoxical sleep' in which the EEG returns to something closer to the waking state, while the eyes jerk rapidly back and forth. Vivid dreams occur during these REM episodes.

EEG

EYES

These signals were picked up with electrodes stuck to my scalp and face, while I slept in Bill Dement's laboratory in California. In each case the upper trace (labelled 'EEG') shows the electroencephalogram, which reflects the activity in the cerebral cortex, while the trace below shows the movements of the eyes.

The Swiss artist Henry Fuseli (1741–1825) specialised in the por-trayal of grotesque subjects, par-ticularly nightmares. He was a friend of William Blake and a teacher of Landseer and Constable.

During the 1960s, the growing interest in the *chemistry* of the brain had its impact on sleep research. Pharmacologists realised that a wide variety of different transmitter substances were used by nerve cells to communicate with each other. New methods were developed, mainly by Swedish neuroanatomists, to make visible under the microscope different classes of nerve cells that use different transmitter substances for their communication. The reticular formation, previously seen as a more or less homogeneous mass of nerve cells and fibres, was revealed by these new techniques as a set of chemical plants – groups of neurons specialising in the use of one transmitter substance or another, distributing their fibres through the brain, to dump their chemical product over vast areas of the nervous system whenever the cells are active. One chemically distinct region in the lower brainstem, the raphe nucleus, contains the transmitter substance serotonin. This is the structure that Moruzzi had shown is essential for normal sleep. Nearby, on each side of the brainstem, was another tiny structure with a distinct chemical signature, the locus coeruleus, whose cells are rich in the transmitter substance nor-adrenaline. Although there are only a few hundred or a few thousand cells in this little nucleus, their axons spread to almost every corner of the brain, including the whole of the cerebral cortex.

Could each major phase of sleeping and waking be understood in simple chemical terms, one transmitter system for each aspect of consciousness and sleep? Michel Jouvet, working in Lyon, France, combined the advances in anatomical and pharmacological understanding into the beginnings of such a grand chemical theory during the 1960s. Ordinary, slow-wave sleep, he argued, might be due to the release of serotonin, throughout the brain, from the terminals of nerve cells in the raphe nuclei. The paradoxical phase of sleep might be caused by a sudden spasm of activity in the locus coeruleus, distributing nor-adrenaline. This elegantly simple theory has had some elements of confirmation but a number of contradictions. The involvement of serotonin in slow-wave sleep is broadly accepted, but direct recordings from the cells of the locus coeruleus showed that, far from increasing their activity during paradoxical sleep, they actually subside to near-silence. Attention has focused on other, nearby groups of nerve cells, and on other neurotransmitter substances, including acetyl choline and a number of different peptides (small protein fragments).

The notion that sleep is triggered by a chemical produced by the brain – or the body – was by no means new. Even Aristotle suggested that sleeping eliminates warm, sleep-inducing vapours that rise from the stomach. Early this century the French physiologist Henri Pieron speculated that the irresistible need for sleep that builds up after many hours awake might well be due to the generation of a natural 'poison'. 'Our studies', he wrote, 'have established that the accumulation of the hypnotoxin produces an increasing need for sleep.'

The last few years have seen a flurry of interest in the possibility that a particular substance produced in the body or the brain first triggers the onset of sleep. Pieron himself had reported that transfusion of liquid (the cerebrospinal fluid) from the cavities of the brain of a sleepy dog into a normal dog caused the latter to fall asleep. John Pappenheimer of Harvard Medical School in the 1970s showed that the sleepiness of goats could actually be transferred to rats and rabbits into which the extracted cerebrospinal fluid was injected. Pappenheimer concluded that the fluid must contain a sleep-producing substance – 'Factor S', as he called it. He and his colleagues tried to isolate the elusive Factor S, which they knew must be present in minute quantities in the fluid of the brain. Fortunately, they soon discovered that this substance is quite stable, chemically, so they argued that it must finally be eliminated from the body, in its unaltered form, in the urine. Starting with 3000 litres of human urine, they demonstrated that the sleep substance was indeed present, and then went on to isolate 7 millionths of a gram of Factor S from the urine and to analyse it. It turned out to be a tiny peptide, consisting of only five amino acids. To date, research groups as far afield as Japan, Mexico and Romania have all reported different peptide substances that appear to be produced by the brain and to trigger different stages of sleep. Some of these substances are amazingly potent: one report suggests that just 600 molecules of the peptide arginine vasotocin can trigger normal sleep in a cat! This kind of experimental work offers hope of the development of new and completely natural substances for the treatment of insomnia.

• THE STUFF OF DREAMS •

Poets, artists, not to mention psychoanalysts, have been obsessed with the fantastical quality of dreams. But when I read through Sigmund Freud's descriptions of his patients' elaborate and bizarre dreams, I ask myself why mine (when I can recall them, which is not often) are usually mundane, incoherent and quite boring. Huge and careful studies of the reports of people about their dreams confirm that very few contain the extraordinary elements that the surrealist writers and artists would have us believe are typical. In two American studies of 1650 people, two-thirds of the dreams they reported simply involved the dreamer standing still – speaking, listening or looking – or moving around in some conventional fashion. There did, though, tend to be one strong theme. The majority of dreams involved some sort of failure, defeat or unhappiness, and feelings of fear or anxiety were much more common than happiness.

Bill Dement's discovery that rapid eye-movement sleep is particularly rich in dreams gave a new twist and a sudden scientific respectability to the study of dreaming. As it happens, dreams most certainly do not occur *only* in paradoxical sleep. If a sleeper is awakened during the first hour of sleep, before the first episode of rapid eye movements has occurred, he or she often reports a dream. However, it does seem that the most vivid and striking elements of dreams occur during the rapid eye-movement stage. Moreover, the dreams that take place seem to occupy the entire period of active EEG and jerking eye movements.

The relationship between these paradoxical stages of sleep and the occurrence of dreams made it possible for scientists to look back (to the young baby) and down (to animals) for evidence of the origins of dreams. To those who believe that dreams are metaphorical and symbolic accounts of the unresolved problems of childhood sexuality, it must be disturbing to discover that newborn rats spend three-quarters of their sleep in the rapid eye movement phase! Virtually all vertebrate animals, at least down to the level of fish, spend some part of the day in a phase that resembles sleep. And nearly all mammals and birds, when asleep, have clearly recognisable phases that resemble human paradoxical sleep. There is even evidence that animals do indeed experience something comparable to the hallucinations of dreams. Michel Jouvet destroyed the tiny region of the brainstem in cats that is responsible for the paralysis of body muscles during the rapid eye-movement stage. Paradoxical sleep still occurred; but far from collapsing, with little more than a twitch of the tail to indicate the storm in their brains, these cats raised themselves, leaped up and acted out what must surely have been their dream experiences, stalking and attacking imaginary mice or retreating, fur erect, from an invisible dog.

The universal and primitive nature of the dream stage of sleep became even more apparent when researchers studied the sleep of normal human infants, of premature babies and even of the fetus in the womb. Newborn babies sleep, of course, for an enormous fraction of the day, and approximately *half* their sleep is of the rapid eye movement type. Indeed, the fraction of paradoxical sleep within the total time of sleeping decreases throughout life. Premature babies sleep almost constantly, and much of their time is spent in a very exaggerated version of paradoxical sleep, with constant twitching of the eyes and parts of the body. The ultrasound imaging techniques that can now be used to give such a clear view of the fetus, long before birth, reveal that the eyes move constantly, as if the unborn baby were dreaming for much of the time.

What, then, are dreams for? Current scientific opinion divides, basically, into two diametrically opposed viewpoints. The first suggests that dreams are the useful rehearsal of activity in the brain, perhaps allowing nerve circuits to be strengthened, memories to be stamped in, or difficult mental problems to be solved. The other suggests that dreams are the elimination of unwanted nonsense, the tossing out of bugs in the neural programmes of the brain.

The unexpected champion of the second viewpoint is Francis Crick, who won the Nobel Prize for his discovery of the structure of DNA, but who now enjoys theorising about the workings of the brain at the Salk Institute in California. In 1983, together with Graeme Mitchison, from the University of Cambridge, Crick proposed that we dream in order to *forget*. Learning, they argued, is a process that must involve constant modification of the circuits of the brain. Whatever rule is used by the brain to guide the strengthening or weakening of synaptic connections, it must surely make mistakes. Odd backwaters of neural circuitry are bound to develop 'parasitic' modes of strengthened excitation, little unwanted pieces of modified circuitry that would disturb the progress of normal learning, if left unpruned. Crick and Mitchison suggested that dreams are, quite literally, a kind of shock therapy, in which the cortex is bombarded by barrages of impulses from the brainstem below, while a different mode of synaptic modification ensures that the unwanted elements of each circuit are unlearned. The perceptual content of dreams would, then, correspond to the internally generated patterns of activity set up in the cerebral cortex as a result of the barrage from below. The fact that the narrative of a dream, though sometimes bizarre, is at least coherent (the dream tells some sort of story) must surely reflect interpretive processes, at higher levels of the brain, probably in the frontal lobes, trying to impose order and plausibility on the chaos of activity in the sensory areas of the cortex. In the terminology of Freud, 'dream work' is being done, weaving together the tangle of represented ideas and sensations, to make a coherent story from the whole.

John Hopfield at the California Institute of Technology in Pasadena, who has been a pioneer in the development of parallel computing techniques, based loosely on the structure and mechanisms of the brain, showed that a learning computer that has been given superfluous information consolidates the correct memories more efficiently if it is put through a period of 'reverse learning' like that proposed by Crick and Mitchison.

Then what would happen to an animal that could not dream? Its cortex would fill up rapidly with the unwanted junk of unrepresentative experience. In order to survive *without* dreams, an animal would have to have a much larger cerebral cortex. There are, in fact, two well-known examples of higher mammals that seem to have no rapid eye-movement sleep – the spiny ant-eater (an Australian marsupial) and the dolphin. These animals do indeed have an abnormally large cerebral cortex for their size and evolutionary development. Crick postulates, then, that these two species might need oversized brains to accommodate all their useless memories because they have little or no ability to unlearn them.

What would be the consequences, for us, of a failure to rid our brains of the detritus of experience? Perhaps an inability to unlearn would cause the mind to become fixated on repetitive or unreal states – in short to hallucinate. A virtually universal feature of the accounts of volunteers who have taken part in sleep deprivation experiments is that, after three nights without sleep, disturbances of perception and thought frequently occur. Solid objects seem to tremble; faces appear from nowhere; the floor or walls may seem to be covered with cobwebs, insects or sticky particles. The sleep-deprived subject often hears voices, apparently talking about him or her.

Auditory hallucinations of this sort, are, of course, one of the classic symptoms of schizophrenia. On the other hand, the opposite pole of psychotic disease, depression, has been successfully treated by deliberate deprivation of sleep (and therefore of dreams). As many as 40 per cent of depressed patients respond to this odd form of treatment and their depression lifts, for a day or so at least. To Sigmund Freud, dreams were a window on the unconscious mind, a potent clue to the nature of neurotic disease. Now, we begin to see that the apparently esoteric study of sleep and dreaming may give profound new insights into the crippling psychotic diseases of schizophrenia and depression.

• THE CLOCK OF SEX •

Sleeping, eating, drinking; they all have their own cyclical patterns, their own clocks in the core of the brain. The hypothalamus is the centre of the most biologically crucial urge of all – the drive to reproduce.

The cycles of the universe show themselves most obviously in the seasonal reproductive patterns seen in the vast majority of animals. Courtship, breeding, nest-building, gestation, birth, caring for the young; all of these complex behaviours are locked to the seasons of nature, to optimise the chances of survival of the offspring. Even the apparently ceaseless sexuality of human beings contains subtle seasonal variations, reflected in an annual variation in the birth rate. But there are other, more powerful rhythms that lie at the heart of the sexual behaviour of human beings. The body of a woman cycles in time with the moon: one of her ova (all of which are present in her ovaries at the start of puberty) is released every twenty-eight days. The cycle of maturation and release of the egg, its journey from the ovary to the uterus, the preparation of the wall of the womb to receive the implanting embryo and the shedding of that wall if the ovum goes unfertilised – this whole astonishing pattern is controlled by a cocktail of hormones. The start of the cycle is a monthly stirring of activity in the hypothalamus. The first ingredient in the mixture of hormones, gonadotrophin-releasing hormone (GRH), is squirted out by specialised nerve cells in a region very close to the suprachiasmatic nucleus. The GRH runs down through the network of tiny blood vessels that link the hypothalamus with the pituitary gland, which hangs from this part of the brain. In response to GRH, the pituitary produces and releases two further hormones for the cocktail, which in turn flow through the bloodstream of the body to encourage the ovary to prepare and release one of its precious eggs. The ovary responds with its own addition to the cocktail, the hormone oestrogen, which circulates back to the pituitary to control the further outflow of its hormones. Two weeks into the cycle and the egg is launched. The ovary then adds the final component of the recipe, progesterone, the hormone that not only prepares the wall of the uterus but also acts back on the pituitary gland to reset the balance of its hormones.

We still do not understand how the monthly cycle, so astonishingly precise in most women, is timed and controlled. But in many animals, the female cycle is certainly influenced by light, just like the circadian patterns of activity and sleep. A female hamster, for instance, ovulates every ninety-six hours under normal circumstances, but every one hundred hours when kept in constant very dim light, which also causes the internal activity rhythm of more than twenty-four hours to appear. So, the cycles of sleeping, waking and ovulation may be linked together, sharing part of the brain's clockwork.

Although it is now a familiar concept that the brain is as much a chemical as an electrical machine, the close similarity of hormones (the chemical messengers that travel in the blood of the body) and neuro-transmitters (the chemicals used to communicate between nerve cells) is a relatively recent discovery. It was Geoffrey Harris, working at Cambridge, London and then Oxford, who laid the foundations of our understanding of the brain as a hormone-producing organ. He demonstrated that the hypothalamus (part of the brain) influences the pituitary (a classical hormone gland) by means of chemical substances produced by nerve cells and distributed in the blood from hypothalamus to pituitary. The credit for the identification of GRH goes to Andrew Schally of Tulane University in New Orleans and a Frenchman, Roger Guillemin of the Salk Institute in California, who won the Nobel Prize for their work in 1977. But even these crucial discoveries, of the pathway between brain and pituitary, and of the exact chemical nature of the hormone, did not provide a complete description of this chemical trigger. The experiences of Mitch Heller, an engineer from Stow, in Massachusetts, help us to find the missing piece of the jigsaw.

Mitch is an amateur hockey player, a sports enthusiast, a red-blooded American male. He married at the age of twenty-two and was looking forward to the children that he and his wife, Debbie, planned to have. Then, in August of 1978, Mitch was involved in a car accident. He suffered no more than a minor blow to the head, but about a month after the accident Mitch realised that his desire for sex was decreasing. Gradually he began to lose the hair of his body and face. As Mitch said: 'I was both horrified and concerned. I knew something was going on inside my body and I didn't know what.'

Mitch's local physician suspected trouble in his hypothalamus and he referred Mitch to William Crowley, an expert on hypothalamic function at Massachusetts General Hospital in Boston, who diagnosed a specific defect in the hypothalamic secretion of GRH. In males, the GRH produced by the hypothalamus causes the release of further sex hormones from the pituitary, just as in women. These hormones in turn influence the male testes, making them produce sperm, and also encouraging them to secrete their own hormone, testosterone, which circulates to the rest of the body and the brain, stimulating many typically male characteristics – not just the growth of facial hair but also the urge for sex. In Mitch, this intricate chemical cascade had been interrupted at its very source.

Recent research had made it possible to produce GRH, which could be injected into Mitch to substitute for the natural function of his hypothalamus. But Crowley knew that straightforward administration of GRH, either continuously or as a series of occasional injections, would not be successful in restoring pituitary function and hence the secretion of the pituitary hormones essential for normal function of the testes. A research group working under Ernst Knobil at the University of Pittsburgh had discovered in studies on monkeys that the hypothalamus normally releases its hormones rhythmically, in short bursts. Crowley incorporated this rhythmic feature into a simple device that he made to treat Mitch. A tiny pump and automated syringe were strapped to Mitch's belt and a tube from the syringe led to a needle that was inserted under the skin of Mitch's abdomen. Crowley fitted a timing device that made the pump deliver an injection at intervals, every two hours, round the clock. 'Only by administering the hypothalamic message in a pulsatile fashion', Crowley explained, 'could the normal physiology and normal endocrine conversation of the hypothalamus, pituitary and gonads be mimicked.'

For the first few days Mitch hated the regular injections but by the end of a week he hardly noticed them. His libido reblossomed, and so did the hair on his chest. More slowly, his sperm count rose too, and, five and a half months into the treatment, his wife, Debbie, became pregnant. Mitch grew a beard, perhaps the final self-assurance of masculinity, in time for the birth of the Hellers' daughter Tovah. To Mitch and Debbie Tovah was a miracle baby, but to an objective observer she was the product of decades of painstaking research to understand not only the complex chemical signals that link brain and body together but also the nature of the rhythmic pacemakers whose beating within our brains is as essential to normal life as the heartbeat itself.

No area of brain research does more than the study of its inherent rhythms to tell us that people, despite all their intellectual sophistication, are, at root, children of the animal world. Despite the veneer of mental liberation, on which we pride ourselves, our brains still listen to the sun, the moon and the seasons. The rhythms of life reveal our kinship to the animals with which we share this restless world.

PRISONERS OF PLEASURE

Human existence is a tapestry of ambitions. We are driven by needs that seem to have little to do with the natural order of animal survival. Yet those very impulses, to create, to discover, to consume and to gratify, have driven mankind to extraordinary cultural achievements.

The more that we learn of the lives of animals, the richer, more intelligent and creative they seem to be. Nevertheless, however wonderful the behaviour of even a troop of chimpanzees, it is still easy to see, hidden just beneath the veneer of social behaviour, the obvious and brutal demands of life. To eat, to drink, to create other individuals of the same species carrying forward the genes that will build a brain to do the same thing; these are the natural needs of life on earth. Of course, these primitive urges are as vital to a human being as they are to a worm: some of our social behaviour is little more than an intricate, highly refined and decorative showcase for swallowing and sex. But somehow the human brain has channelled the powerful and primitive urges of survival and procreation into education, work, religion, charity, science, art – activities and achievements that are distantly removed from crude necessity.

The capacity to link habits to deep biological needs is vital for the survival of animals and human beings. But the cycle of need, action and satisfaction, which has been embellished to generate all human culture, can be subverted by chemicals and perverted by self-deception. Addiction is the dead-end of human drive. In the brain of an addict the elegant machinery of satisfaction has been short-circuited: gratification has become an end in itself. The junkie, dying in an alley; the housewife seeking solace in gin; the child lying to buy cigarettes: we can all learn from them about our needs and pleasures. Without addiction of a sort, none of us could survive.

• AN EXPERIMENT ON THE STREETS •

All human societies live with addictions, with behaviours that are repeated over and over again, for the sake of pleasure or to avoid the pain of stopping. Alcohol and tobacco are used throughout the world. They can kill, but they are not against the law, so they are freely available; powerful drugs that attack body and brain. And behind the glamorous and socially acceptable exterior of every big city is a world of addiction in which pleasure becomes a disease: a world of smack and crack, and a growing catalogue of other chemicals that subvert the systems of need and reward in our brains.

The revolution in trade and transport that has brought tropical fruits to London in mid winter has carried with it drugs of addiction from every corner of the globe. In the back streets of Manhattan, of Tokyo, of London, the intoxicating distillations and concoctions from the plant products of distant countries are also on sale. Mind-altering substances that local societies have learned to live with over centuries of use are suddenly available for a ruthless, efficient and competitive international market.

As soon as people could write down their ideas, they wrote about their drugs and the pleasures they gave. About 5000 BC, the Sumerians used an ideogram translated as HUL, meaning 'joy' or 'rejoicing', to represent opium; an Egyptian papyrus of about 3500 BC is the earliest historical record of the production of alcohol, in an Egyptian brewery; by 2500 BC, the lake dwellers of Switzerland were eating poppy seeds. And as early as 2000 BC, an Egyptian priest wrote to a pupil, 'I, thy superior, forbid thee to go to the taverns. Thou art degraded like the beasts.'

Though it is likely that alcohol had already been used for millennia as a sedative and an analgesic, the intertwining of medicine and addiction began in earnest at the start of the sixteenth century when Paracelsus introduced laudanum, or tincture of opium, into medical practice. That relationship has had a long and tortuous history, a dilemma of benefit and abuse that continues to the present day. The realisation that pure, natural organic chemicals extracted from plants could have powerful effects (some of them indubitably beneficial) on body and brain stimulated the science of pharmacology. The search for other natural plant products that might be of benefit to man was soon joined by a quest, in the laboratories of Europe and America, to improve on Nature – to purify and modify natural substances and even to invent entirely new ones. In 1844 cocaine was isolated in its pure form; in 1864 came the first barbiturate; in 1898, heroin, a potent derivative of the opium alkaloid morphine; in 1938, LSD, the first of a growing catalogue of artificial substances that take the mind into a world of dreams and nightmares.

The attitude of western society to its drugs has always been equivocal; it rests on a constantly shifting mixture of legislation, taxation, supply, scientific opinion, fashion and prejudice. Between 1839 and 1860, Britain fought two wars against China to force the Chinese government to accept the importation of opium from India. In 1868, Dr George Wood, author of a major textbook, *Treatise on Therapeutics*, wrote of opium: 'The intellectual and imaginative faculties are raised to the highest point compatible with individual capacity.... It seems to make the individual, for the time, a better and greater man.' In 1909 the United States prohibited the importation of opium and three years later the first international Opium Convention, meeting in The Hague, recommended drastic measures for the control of the international trade in opium.

Between 1870 and 1915, the tax on alcoholic liquor provided between one-half and two-thirds of the entire tax revenue of the United States. Attitudes changed rapidly, however, during the first two decades of this century. In 1917, the president of the American Medical Association endorsed the prohibition of alcohol, and the association passed a resolution resolving that it opposed 'the use of alcohol as a beverage' and 'that the use of alcohol as a therapeutic agent should be discouraged'. In 1918, the Anti-Saloon League called the trade in alcohol 'un-American, pro-German, crime-producing, food-wasting, youth-corrupting, home-wrecking, treason'. The following year the Eighteenth Amendment to the US constitution was passed, prohibiting the social use of alcohol. By 1928, the medical profession in the United States was earning an estimated 40 million dollars a year by writing prescriptions for whiskey, and the illicit supply of liquor grew to massive and ludicrous levels. The Eighteenth Amendment was repealed in 1933. By 1970, the consumption of alcohol in the United States had risen to the highest value in the world – equivalent to almost 7 gallons of pure alcohol per adult per year in Washington, DC.

Following Columbus's discovery of the American continent in 1493, the habit of smoking tobacco leaves, essential to the religious and social rituals of North American Indians, quickly took hold in Europe and was to spread like wildfire around the world. The growth of opposition was equally rapid and widespread. James I and VI at the turn of the sixteenth century, condemned tobacco as unhealthy and immoral; but even his elevation of the duty on tobacco by 4000 per cent did little more than stimulate the smuggling trade. Sultan Murad IV of the Ottoman Empire 'was fond of surprising men in the act of smoking, when he would punish them by beheading, hanging, quartering or crushing their hands and feet.... Nevertheless ... the passion of smoking still persisted.' In 1967, when the American tobacco industry spent an estimated 250 million dollars on advertising, Senator Robert F. Kennedy, of New York, speaking at the first world conference on smoking and health, said 'Every year cigarettes kill more Americans than were killed in World War 1, the Korean War and Vietnam combined.' The next year, Americans smoked 544 billion cigarettes. The consumption of tobacco in many Third World countries has more than doubled in the past decade.

• DRUGS OF DELIGHT •

In a sixth-century grave in Peru, there were, in addition to the usual collection of utensils, food and other accoutrements for the afterlife, several bags of cocaine. Could the man in question not tolerate the thought of eternal life without his source of eternal joy? During the sixteenth century, the conquistadors brought back reports to Europe of the invigorating properties of the leaves of the coca plant. About 1750, they were being imported and by the middle of the last century coca was being promoted as an invigorating, health-giving tonic with universal powers. Elixirs and syrups of coca were hawked for everything from headaches to hysteria. In 1885, John Pemberton, a resourceful pharmacist anxious to capitalise on the craze for coca, formulated a product which he called 'French Wine of Coca, Ideal Tonic'. A year later, enhanced by the addition of the kola nut and extra syrup, it was launched as Coca-Cola, the 'brain tonic', aimed principally at the temperance market.

The medical respectability that cocaine briefly enjoyed was partly due to the enthusiasm (and addiction) of Sigmund Freud, who first took cocaine in 1884: he called his reports of his use of this drug 'a song of praise to this magnificent substance'. He recognised its aphrodisiac qualities and persuaded his fiancée Martha Bernays to share cocaine with him. An article by W. H. Bentley in the *Therapeutic Gazette* of 1880 had proposed the use of cocaine in the treatment of opium and alcohol addiction so, when Freud's close friend Ernst von Fleischl-Marxow fell victim to morphine addiction after the amputation of a badly infected finger, Freud persuaded him to take cocaine to 'cure' him of the addiction. Fleischl's lust for morphine decreased, but his desire for cocaine simply grew in proportion. He hallucinated 'white snakes' sliding over his body. His death in 1891 shocked Freud into disenchantment with the drug whose administration he had previously called an 'offering' rather than a dose.

By the turn of the century, cocaine's miraculous image was tarnished, its reputation much affected by the autobiographical account *Eight Years in Cocaine Hell*, written by a Chicago woman, Annie Meyers, and published in 1902. The following year caffeine was substituted for cocaine in Coca-Cola. But cocaine kept its hold on the western world and it will never go away. Two generations after its public disgrace, cocaine has made an insidious come-back, assisted by new and more potent methods of deliv-

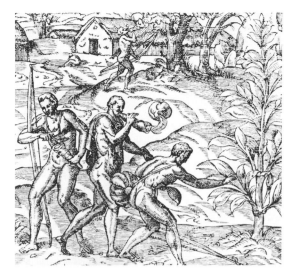

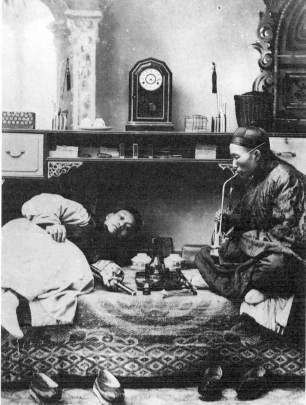

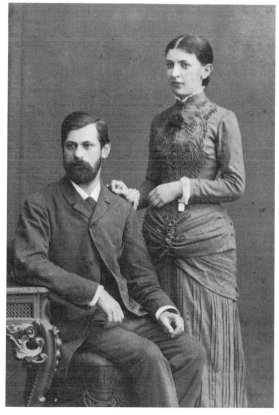

ABOVE LEFT *The first known printed illustration of the use of tobacco, from the* Cosmographie Universelle *of Thevet, 1575.*

ABOVE *The Opium Wars, fought by Britain in China, forced the Chinese to import Indian opium, so as to encourage the opium-smoking habit, which caused immense social problems in China.*

LEFT *Sigmund Freud and his fiancée, Martha Bernays, experimented with cocaine together.*

ering the drug to the brain. For 'freebasing', raw cocaine powder is purified by dissolving it in ether and drying it out, before it is smoked. 'Crack' is a form of freebase cocaine that crackles as it is smoked because baking soda is mixed with the drug.

Cocaine, now sweeping through Europe, seems to have replaced heroin as the main target of government publicity and law enforcement action in the United States. Yet all the objective evidence shows that cocaine, though powerfully addictive, is less harmful to the body as a whole than alcohol or tobacco.

For any drug that has been discovered by the international market, the same kind of story can be told, of alternating fashion and disfavour, of tolerance and crusading prohibition. Yet for all the campaigns against them, for all the efforts of drug squads and governments, no major drug has ever been entirely eradicated once it has infected a community. The brute force of prohibition and control will never prevail. To understand addiction, we must ask what these chemicals do to the brain; why some but not all people are magnetised by them; and what they provide, which life without these chemicals might otherwise give.

One of the great mysteries that emerge from the studies of drug-taking is that addiction is a process as special as falling in love: it lets a person walk away from some drugs, unimpressed and unscathed, but gives other drugs the power to invade every crevice of the thoughts and passions of the same person.

Five years ago, Jim Sloan from Philadelphia was a heavy cigarette smoker. He managed to break that habit but one day he tried freebasing:

> It was like every pain, every ache in my body was gone. And it was like having an orgasm with every nerve ending in my body at the same time. It was like the sexual act magnified. From that point on, I was a cocaine addict.... You are playing with death, you know. I have had sessions where I would fall on the floor; my heart would be palpitating and I would get very frightened that I was going to die. And while I was lying there, I would swear to myself and to God that once it was past I wouldn't do this again. And I'd get up right off the floor, and five or ten minutes later I would be getting high again.

Never again; always again. That is the liturgy of addiction.

• LEXINGTON DAYS •

A prison hospital in Lexington, Kentucky, was the unlikely birthplace of the 'biological' approach to psychiatry in the United States. Between 1935 and 1970, the Addiction Research Center in that remote prison hospital was the world focus for the study of drug addiction. Elsewhere in the world, governments were hesitant to acknowledge that they had a drug problem at all. In Britain, government reports were denying the growing crisis of addiction as late as the middle 1960s.

Conan Kornetsky, who was a graduate student at the University of Kentucky, came to the Addiction Research Center in Lexington in the late 1940s. Narcotic addiction, especially to heroin, was common amongst the prisoners, and Kornetsky and his colleagues observed and catalogued their ecstasies and agonies in the first truly scientific study of addiction and withdrawal. Volunteers among the prisoners agreed to be given drugs in varying doses while the scientists looked on. At the time, they believed that the key to the driving force of addiction was withdrawal, the torture that addicts suffer when denied their drug. Restlessness and spasms of pain are replaced by fever, sweating, vomiting and goose-flesh (hence the term 'cold turkey'). The involuntary twitching of the legs gave rise to the expression 'kicking the habit'; at their worst, these convulsions are much like an epileptic seizure.

Kornetsky was unhappy with the failure of the psychotherapeutic techniques used in the hospital to help these patients, but he was also alarmed by the virtually universal tendency of addicts to revert to their habit even after weeks of abstinence and the complete disappearance of withdrawal symptoms. He began to suspect that the key to the addictive progress might be the craving for the *high*, the magical rush that comes with each new shot of the drug.

The work at Lexington was revolutionary, the first real scientific study of the nature of addiction, but there were obviously ethical limits to what could be done and hence to what could be discovered. Drugs act on the brain; that was clear. But where, and how? Those were questions that could be answered only by a journey into the brain itself.

• THE PLEASURE PRINCIPLE •

The idea of emotion as a subject fit for scientific study is very young. True, Freud emphasised the significance of emotion in determining human behaviour but attempts to classify and study human emotion scientifically began only in the 1940s. Emotion was seen as a factor intervening between powerful stimuli in the outside world and the animal's behavioural response. The appearance of a competitor might produce the *sensation* of anger, followed by the action of attack. The sight of a predator produces fear and retreat. The discovery of food or an attractive partner produces pleasure, which stimulates eating or mating. Psychologists began to think that the *feelings* associated with emotion might play an important part in the control of learning, because they predict the outcome of the animal's behaviour and hence help it to plan its future actions. Animals will learn to avoid circumstances in which they have previously been afraid or to seek out situations in which they have had pleasure. Neurologists, using as their evidence the experiences of human patients who had suffered from local brain damage or from the stimulating effects of epilepsy, pointed to the frontal lobes of the cortex and the associated deep structures of the limbic system, below the forebrain, as the anatomical substrate of emotional reactions.

Techniques had already been developed for implanting electrodes deep in the brains of experimental animals and, in 1950, Robert Heath, in the Department of Psychiatry and Neurology at Tulane University in New Orleans, decided to implant stimulating electrodes in the brains of severely ill human patients in order to explore the basis of their emotional disturbances. Once the fine metal wires were in place, the patient could move freely, without pain, and they could be used either to record the brain's own electrical activity or to deliver minute electric shocks to stir into action the nerve cells at the tips of the implanted electrodes.

Heath's experiments, usually performed on mentally ill or severely epileptic patients, were, to say the least, controversial. For one patient, a chronically depressed, suicidal, homosexual drug addict, he provided a prostitute to participate in one such experiment. But if we can overlook the highly unorthodox nature of this research, some of Heath's observations are of great significance.

In his early work in the 1950s, Heath's attention focused on a region in the base of the forebrain, below the frontal lobes of the cerebral hemispheres. Heath and his colleagues had already shown that removal of this region, called the septum, could produce changes in an animal's emotional behaviour that 'resembled the impairment in psychological awareness and emotionality of the schizophrenic patient'; and in human patients, at the peak of orgasm, Heath had recorded convulsions of electrical activity in this same region of the basal forebrain. In 1952, he first described the effects of artificially stimulating this very region, through deep electrodes in the brains of twenty-six schizophrenic patients. The earlier work on the results of damage to the septum in animals suggested to Heath that this region may be underactive in the schizophrenic brain and he reasoned that stimulation there might be therapeutic. As the patient lay, fully conscious, Heath passed brief electrical pulses through the electrode whose tip lay in the septal area. The effects were remarkable; pleasure, even ecstasy, at the tip of a metal wire. The patient would recall pleasurable events, good feelings and, very often, specific sensations of sexual pleasure.

Quite independently of Bob Heath, two experimental psychologists were working on the same mysterious area, in the brain of the rat. Peter Milner, an engineer who enrolled at McGill University in Montreal as a research student in psychology, was especially interested in the new techniques for electrical stimulation through fine wires implanted into the brain that were being used by Walter Hess in Zurich. Milner was joined in the early 1950s by Jim Olds, a Harvard graduate, who had the foresight to see that these new methods might be capable of revealing mechanisms in the brain corresponding to the theories of learning that had been developed by the influential behaviourist school of psychology at Harvard.

Olds and Milner attended the seminars of the neurologist Wilder Penfield and the neurophysiologist Herbert Jasper at the Montreal Neurological Institute. Penfield and Jasper were full of the news of the discovery of a structure called the reticular formation, which runs through the core of the whole of the brainstem. They learned that damage to this region could cause an animal to become comatose and electrical stimulation of it could arouse a sleeping animal. Milner wondered whether stimulation of the reticular formation might enhance the ability of rats to learn mazes; but his own early experiments were entirely unsuccessful. In 1954, Jim Olds decided to try to implant electrodes in the same area but his inexperience in the surgical techniques led him to make a mistake – a mistake of enormous significance. Instead of penetrating the reticular formation, his electrodes entered the septal area. Olds delivered shocks through the electrode as the rat was running around an open arena. The animal abruptly turned and ran back to precisely the spot at which the shock had been given! It returned again and again if it was stimulated there each time. Fortunately, Olds had the insight to see that this was not just a failed experiment but a *new* experiment. He and Milner quickly constructed a Skinner box (named after the famous Harvard psychologist Burrhus F. Skinner), in which there was a small lever for the rat to press. They connected the lever to the rat's own electrode and found that, as soon as the rat discovered the effect of pushing the lever, it pressed it continuously, for hours on end.

Skinner had used his box to measure the strengths of animal desires in terms of the frequency with which an animal would press the lever in order to obtain a particular reward, food or liquid. A hungry rat will press the lever 100 times or even more per hour if it receives a tiny pellet of food each time, but only five or ten times an hour if no food is delivered. Skinner took this increase in the rate of bar-pressing as a measure of the rewarding effect of the food. To the amazement of Jim Olds and Peter Milner, their rats pressed the lever up to 5000 times an hour, just to be stimulated in the septal region of the brain. The reward of this self-stimulation seemed more potent than any genuine satisfaction of the animal's bodily needs. One hungry animal, given a choice between food and the magic lever, chose to ignore the food entirely and pressed the lever an average of 2000 times an hour continuously for twenty-four hours without sleep! Olds and Milner were certain that they had discovered an anatomical system at the base of the forebrain that was responsible for sensations of pleasure normally associated with eating, drinking and sex.

When Bob Heath in New Orleans then gave his patients buttons connected to the electrodes in their brains, these people, too, repeatedly pressed them in order to deliver shocks to the septal area. And depressed patients, in particular, found it improved their state of mind. Even the pain of terminal cancer was briefly relieved by a shock to the centre of pleasure.

• DRUGS AND THE • PATHWAYS OF PLEASURE

Only a year or two after Jim Olds discovered the power of self-stimulation, he began to think about the possibility that addictive drugs might tap the same system of insatiable desire. The clue to the relationship between self-stimulation and the euphoria of drugs is the overwhelming *strength* of the effects on behaviour. Another clue came from the suffering that animals would bear in order to secure the opportunity to stimulate the pleasure regions of their brains. Faced with the sight of the magic lever on the other side of its cage, a rat will run across an electrified grid giving a shock to its feet so unpleasant that a starving rat would not cross it to obtain food. The animal is willing to pay almost any price in order to stimulate that crucial part of its brain.

Jim Olds himself found that injection of a variety of different addictive drugs could alter the rate at which a rat would self-stimulate its brain. And in the mid 1970s, Conan Kornetsky devised a sensitive way of testing the effects of addictive drugs. He simply measured the minimum electric current that had to be applied through the electrodes in a rat's brain in order to encourage the animal to stimulate itself. He found that a well-defined level of electrical stimulation was needed, but that certain drugs could increase the sensitivity of the animal to brain stimulation, causing the threshold current to fall. As Kornetsky said, 'The fascinating thing was that we found in our laboratory that every single drug that increases sensitivity of the animal to brain stimulation was either an abuse substance or a substance that has potential for abuse.'

It looks as if most if not all of the drugs that give a strong sense of euphoria – opiates, cocaine, amphetamine, angel dust – have effects on the brain that are similar to those of electrical stimulation in the septal region. Indeed, drugs and electricity add together, so that a drugged animal needs less electricity to satisfy its needs. It was a short step (though it took many years of research) to develop methods for injecting a tiny drop of a drug directly into the same brain regions in which the tip of an electrode will cause self-stimulation. Animals, it turns out, will work

For thousands of years people have made timepieces, which override the biological clocks inside their heads and rule their lives.

BELOW *Stonehenge, built between about 2500 and 1500 BC, is a megalithic 'clock', predicting the solstices.*

RIGHT *An astronomical clock in Besançon, France.*

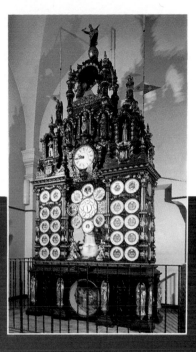

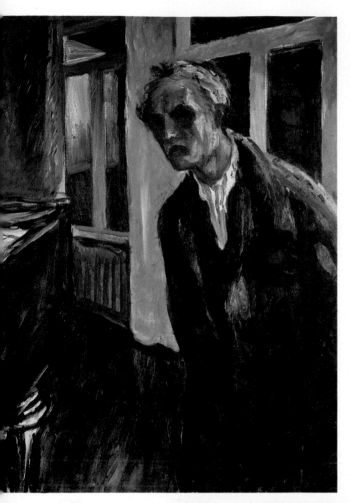

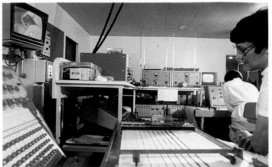

ABOVE *In Michel Jouvet's laboratory in Lyon, France, a scientist observes the* EEG *(brainwaves), muscle activity and eye movements recorded continuously through electrodes taped to the scalp and body of a volunteer, who is visible on the television screen, sleeping in a neighbouring room.*

LEFT Wanderer by Night: Self Portrait *by Edvard Munch (1863–1944). Insomnia, an enormous medical problem, is the focus of much current research.*

BELOW *Hypnos, the Greek god of sleep, and his brother Thanatos, god of death, carry dead Sarpendon, prince of Lycia and ally of the Trojans. Red-figured Attic vase (c. 515 BC).*

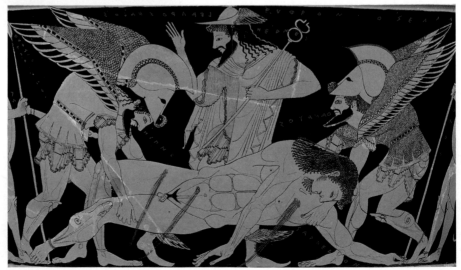

RIGHT A mouse rests contentedly on a small platform that stands in a shallow pool of water. But when its muscles relax completely during rapid eye movement (REM) sleep, it slips from the platform and wakes up. Michel Jouvet has studied the behavioural and pharmacological changes produced by selective deprivation of this stage of sleep. In human beings, vivid dreams occur during REM sleep and selective deprivation of this kind of sleep produces fatigue and inability to concentrate the following day. During the next sleep, more time than usual is spent in REM, as if catching up on the need to dream.

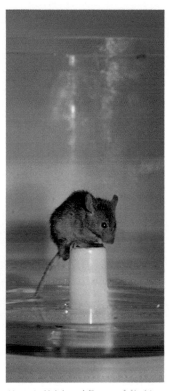

BELOW Mysterious Dream *by William Blake (1757–1827).*

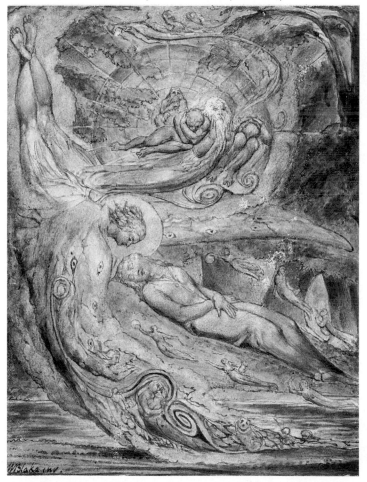

Francis Crick and Graeme Mitchison have suggested that REM sleep is needed for the efficient storage of memories in the cerebral cortex. The Australian spiny ant-eater (below), a primitive egg-laying mammal, seems not to indulge in REM sleep and it also has a surprisingly large cerebral cortex, perhaps to accommodate its inefficiently stored memories.

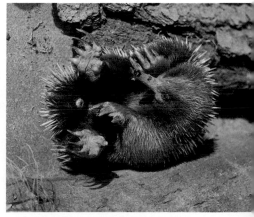

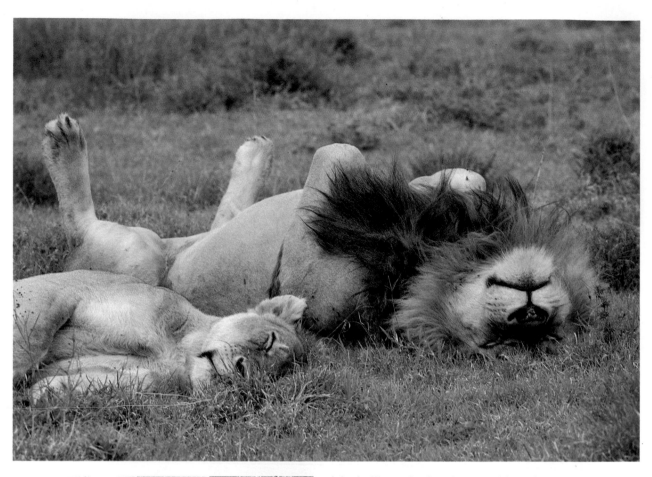

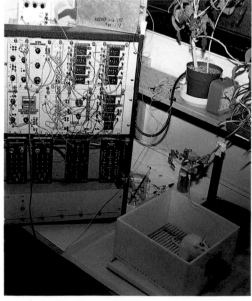

Animals, like people, show the outward signs of pleasure
(above). A rat pressing a lever to stimulate its nucleus
accumbens (left) may be exciting brain systems that are
normally active during the pleasure of eating or sex. Cocaine
turned on the same pathway in Jim Sloan's brain (below).

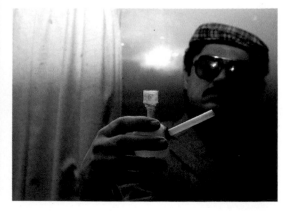

Conan Kornetsky (right) with the skyline of Boston. The pattern of drug use varies across the city – mainly heroin in the depressed Roxbury district, cocaine in fashionable Back Bay, and a variety of drugs in the mixed community of South End.

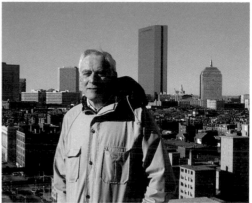

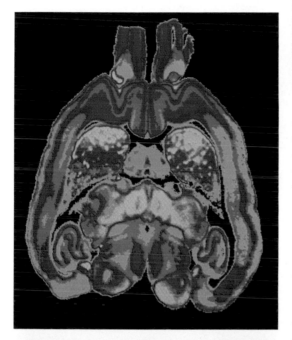

The enkephalins and other natural peptides in the brain, released from nerve terminals, act on specific receptors in the membranes of other neurons. These opiate receptors can be revealed by incubating brain slices with a solution of radioactive enkephalin and then measuring the distribution of radioactivity.

LEFT In this horizontal section through the rat brain (front of the brain at the top), a high density of receptors (yellow) is seen in parts of the forebrain and brainstem that are concerned with pleasure and pain. Morphine and the other opiate drugs act on these same receptors.

BELOW LEFT In this section of visual cortex from a monkey, high receptor density appears red, intermediate green, and low blue. The inset diagram shows a theoretical interpretation of the action of an enkephalin molecule (left side) and morphine (right side) on opiate receptors (the red shapes embedded in the blue nerve membrane). Both molecules fit into the receptor and trigger a response from the nerve cell.

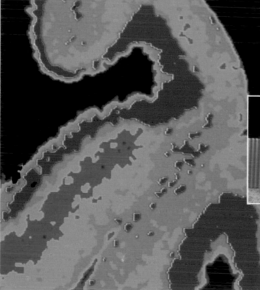

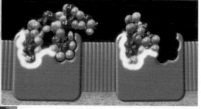

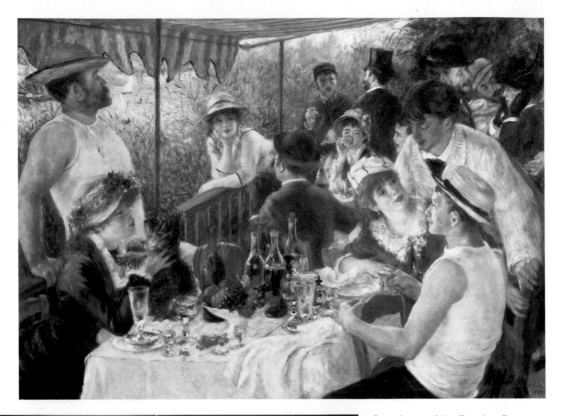

Luncheon of the Boating Party (*above*) *by Pierre Auguste Renoir* (*1841–1919*). *Socially acceptable indulgence in one of the most potentially harmful of addictive drugs – alcohol.*

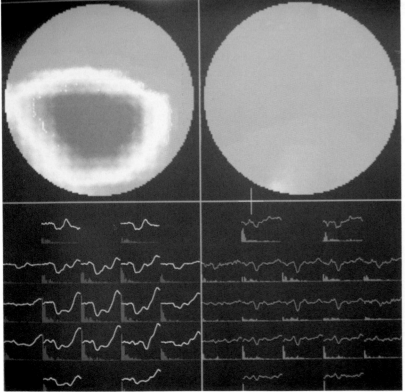

LEFT *Henri Begleiter uses brain-wave techniques to study alcoholics, abstinent alcoholics and the children of alcoholic parents. The television display shows responses recorded through electrodes in different places on the scalp. Above these records are reconstructions of the distribution of one wave – the P_3 wave – across the brain. This response is associated with the recognition of novel sensory events in the outside world. Each circle represents the head, with the forehead at the front. The records on the left came from a boy without alcoholic parents: there is strong P_3 activity (red area) over the back of the brain. Those on the right, with very little P_3 activity, came from the young son of a type 2 alcoholic.*

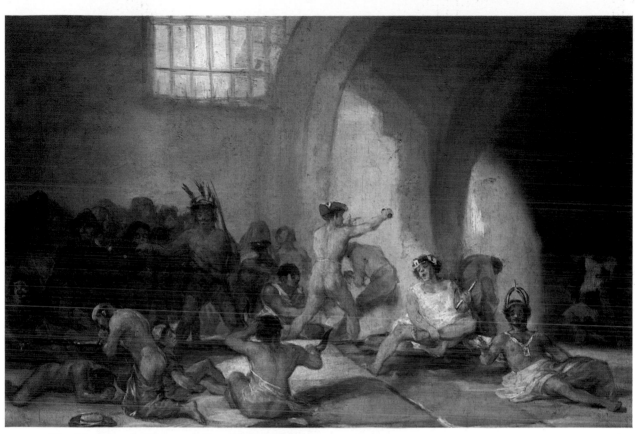

The Madhouse *by Francesco de Goya (1746–1828)*

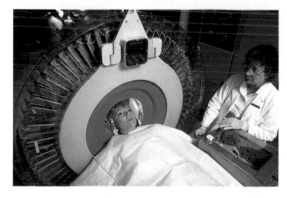

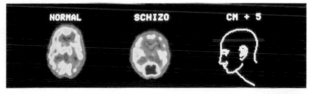

*Positron Emission Tomography (*PET *scanning) provides images, equivalent to thin slices, of the living brain. The patient's head lies within a ring of detectors, which measure positrons emitted as a result of the breakdown of radioactive isotopes injected in the bloodstream.* PET *scanning can be used to measure blood flow, oxygen utilisation and many other aspects of brain function. It is enormously valuable in the diagnosis of brain disease, but can also be used to study the function of the normal brain.*

A PET *scanner uses a computer which reconstructs a horizontal section of the brain, as shown in the diagram (above). The two scans show such sections, with the forehead at the top. In these cases a radioactive glucose derivative was injected and taken up by highly active nerve cells throughout the brain. The colour scale on the right indicates the level of glucose uptake: the most active regions appear red, the least active blue. These* PET *scans came from a normal volunteer and a schizophrenic patient, each lying quietly in the scanner. Interestingly, activity is relatively high in the visual areas at the back of the cerebral hemispheres in this schizophrenic patient, but is lower in the frontal lobes.*

The paintings and drawings of the mentally ill give us a special insight into their disturbed perceptions and thought processes.

RIGHT William Kurelek set out to depict his psychological state in The Maze, *painted in The Maudsley Hospital in 1953. He provided his own interpretation of the complex symbolism: 'The subject, seen as a whole, is of a man (representing me) lying on a barren plain before a wheatfield, with his head split open . . . the thoughts made in his head represented as a maze. . . . The white rat curled up in the central cavity represents my Spirit (I suppose). He is curled up with frustration from having run the passages so long without hope of escaping out of this maze of unhappy thoughts.'*

RIGHT The Fairy Feller's Master-Stroke, 1855–1864, *by Richard Dadd, the Victorian artist who was a patient at the Bethlem Royal Hospital from 1844–1864. Bethlem was originally founded as 'Bedlam' in 1247.*

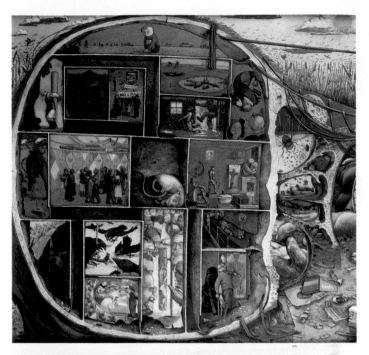

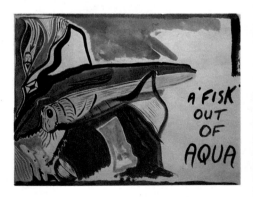

A 'Fisk' out of Aqua, *by an anonymous 'chronic paraphrenic patient'.*

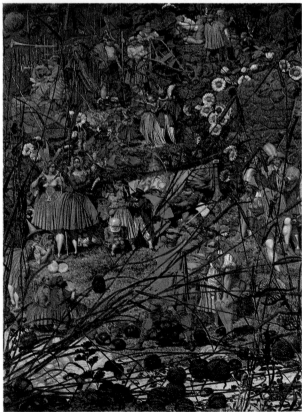

in just the same way to inject themselves with morphine, cocaine or amphetamine in this same general area of the brain.

During the 1960s, anatomists had been developing methods of selectively labelling nerve cells containing certain chemical substances that are released at the endings of axons, to convey the message across the synapse to the next cell in the chain. They discovered that nerve cells containing high concentrations of one transmitter substance called dopamine lie in distinct clusters in the upper part of the brainstem, just below the base of the forebrain. The pathway followed by the fibres of one of the main groups of dopamine nerve cells was precisely the same as the distribution of points that Olds and Milner had identified as being the best sites for electrical self-stimulation.

The crucial group of dopamine cells (called the A10 cell group) sends its fibres forwards and upwards through the septal area in a cable of axons called the medial forebrain bundle, and they terminate mainly on another small cluster of nerve cells, the nucleus accumbens. Some of the fibres run on into the cortex of the frontal lobe above. Electrodes placed in any of these areas will precipitate self-stimulation in the rat. Dopamine seems to be the crucial chemical in this pathway of pleasure. One view, popular at the moment, is that this pathway in the brain is normally active under conditions of incentive and reward, whenever the animal sets about the task of satisfying its natural needs.

The addictive drugs – heroin, morphine and the other opiates – act directly on the A10 neurons, chemically provoking them into activity. Cocaine and amphetamine have their influence at the other end of the pathway, increasing the amount of dopamine released from the terminals of the A10 neurons up in the nucleus accumbens. The high of these drugs is the pure essence of pleasure. They have broken into the natural cycle of need, action and satisfaction. It would be an over-simplification, however, to suggest that these drugs act on only a single circuit of nerve cells. The subjective quality of the experience is quite different for different drugs and each of them affects a variety of brain structures apart from this crucial reward system. Indeed, recent advances in imaging techniques for viewing the organisation and activity of the conscious human brain have shown that each drug sets up its own unique pattern of nervous activity. The PET scan (Positron Emission Tomography) shows that morphine shuts down the cerebral cortex but leaves the underlying structures of the emotional circuits of the brain still active. Cocaine seems to boost the excitement of the whole brain but especially stimulates not only the primitive centres of emotion but also the frontal lobes, which are thought to be involved in some of the highest of human mental functions.

Tony Phillips and Chris Fibiger at the University of Vancouver in Canada believe that the nucleus accumbens lies at a crucial crossroads within the pathways of the brain that are active when an animal *craves* –

for food, for water, for sex or for a drug. They have been using a new and sensitive technique for detecting the natural release of dopamine from nerve terminals in the living brain – a method called *in vivo* voltametry. A small electrode inserted into the brain is able to pick up signals relating to the release of chemical transmitters. When the tip of such an electrode lies in the nucleus accumbens, it detects a tiny surge of dopamine from the terminals of the incoming nerve fibres when a hungry rat sees food. Indeed, if the conditioning techniques invented by Ivan Pavlov are used to train a rat to anticipate food whenever a bell is rung, the sound of the bell alone is enough to set off the natural release of dopamine.

• THE BRAIN'S OWN MORPHINE •

A natural system within the brain for signalling incentive and reward is subverted by drugs of addiction: that is the conclusion of a detective story of research that began forty years ago. But how can substances extracted from plants exercise such power over neurons in the human brain? The answer to that question, the next step in this story, began with the Vietnam War.

War is never glorious, but as wars go, the one in Vietnam was singularly futile. By all accounts, it was wretched and humiliating, and a whole generation of clean-cut American boys, drafted to fight a battle that they didn't believe in, in a country they didn't understand, turned in massive numbers to opium and heroin, more cheaply and easily available than a cold beer and much more effective at shutting out the nonsense of war. In the small towns of America, mothers and fathers, ever fearful of telegrams announcing the death of their sons, began to fear their return – as drug addicts. America feared a wave of addiction of epidemic proportions following the return of its forces from Vietnam.

In 1971, four years before the withdrawal from Vietnam, the US government began to pour funds into research on addiction. The work of Heath, Olds, Kornetsky and so many others had pointed to the pathways of the chemical transmitter, dopamine. And new techniques were being developed for exploring the way that transmitters and other substances have their actions on nerve cells and terminals. Far away, in the University of Aberdeen, a German émigré, Hans Kosterlitz, received a little of the Vietnam money for his own research; but his work on morphine and his revolutionary idea about its action had started years before, in the early 1960s.

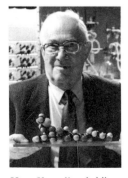

Hans Kosterlitz, holding a model of the enkephalin molecule.

Kosterlitz is a pharmacologist, interested in the way in which drugs act throughout the body. He knew that morphine, in addition to its pain-relieving qualities and the euphoria that it produces, has many other highly specific actions on organs other than the brain. In particular, the opiates slow down the contractions of the intestine, an effect that made morphine a favourite remedy for diarrhoea. Kosterlitz had been studying the effect of morphine on such contractions. Like many other pharmacologists around the world, Kosterlitz had realised that the powerful actions of the opiates depend on the *shape* of their molecules. Solomon Snyder and his student Candace Pert, working with support from the Vietnam addiction grant programme at Johns Hopkins University in Baltimore, had shown that morphine adheres selectively to the membranes of samples of tissue from the brain of a rat or the intestine of a guinea pig. By analogy with the hormone insulin (which was known to bind to particular, specialised receptor sites on cell membranes) opiates might have their own particular receptor mechanism too. In the early 1970s, Snyder in Baltimore, Eric Simon in New York and Lars Terenius in Uppsala, Sweden, raced to produce the definitive evidence for such a receptor system. They all published papers in 1973 claiming the discovery of the opiate receptor.

A crucial step in the understanding of how opiates work was the development of highly specific antagonists of the opiates, substances that block the action of morphine and heroin but do not mimic the euphoria or painkilling and other effects. As early as 1915, German pharmacologists, pursuing the relentless but futile search for a non-addictive opiate, found that a tiny molecular modification of codeine (another opiate) produced a substance that had no analgesic action of its own but that blocked the effects of codeine and other opiates. In 1940, Klaus Unna discovered another antagonist, a derivative of morphine called nalorphine. An animal at the point of death from morphine poisoning was revived miraculously by a tiny administration of this substance. The only possible conclusion was that the two substances, the drug and the antagonist, were competing with each other for a highly selective receptor mechanism scattered through the body and brain.

At first, these antagonist compounds were thought to be of no practical use, but in 1951 Abraham Wikler realised that they might be effective in treating narcotic poisoning in human addicts. He injected nalorphine into patients at the Addiction Research Center in Lexington and found that it immediately precipitated severe withdrawal symptoms, just as if the opiate drug had been instantly removed from their bloodstream. Wikler also gave nalorphine to non-addicted people and discovered, to his amazement, that they became extremely anxious and developed feelings of discomfort, which could even progress into near psychotic states with high enough doses.

In 1973, a new, extremely potent antagonist, naloxone, was synthesised. Solomon Snyder showed that if naloxone was applied to the membranes of cells from the brain or the intestine, morphine would no longer adhere strongly to those same membranes. The naloxone must have stuck to the opiate receptor molecules and prevented the morphine from doing so. It was Hans Kosterlitz, already more than seventy years old, who saw most clearly and most quickly the implications of all these discoveries. For many years, he had been studying the action of morphine on various tissues of the body, but in the early 1960s he had shared with a student his secret hunch:

> He asked me, 'Now, why do you do that; why are you interested in morphine?' I hesitated; I didn't want to say what I really thought. But this young man forced me, and I said 'Well you know, if you keep it to yourself and don't tell anybody, I have a suspicion that there may be a morphine-like substance in the brain.'

Hans Kosterlitz had pursued the argument of chemical logic to its inevitable conclusion. If opiates are effective because of their specific chemical shape and there are specific receptor molecules in the membranes of cells in the body and the brain, then Kosterlitz could see only one conclusion. Opiate receptors, sensitive to the extracts of a poppy, could not simply be a chance mistake of evolution. The brain itself must produce a substance that acts on its own opiate receptors, probably as part of a natural process of regulating pleasure and pain.

Kosterlitz sent his student John Hughes to the local abattoir early each morning to collect huge numbers of pig brains. They tested extracts from the brains on small pieces of muscle from the intestine and elsewhere. Kosterlitz recalls now that everyone else in the field thought that such an enterprise was crazy. But it was not. Hughes and Kosterlitz found that brain extracts could indeed stop the contractions of muscle, in exactly the same way as morphine. And the antagonist naloxone blocked this action just as effectively as it did for real opiates. The brain does produce its own natural morphine-like substance.

It then took two years, and the help of Howard Morris from the Laboratory for Molecular Biology at Cambridge, to concentrate an active factor and work out its structure. Two tiny peptide molecules, each a chain of merely five amino acids, were the active substances. Hughes and Kosterlitz called them enkephalins (from the Greek meaning 'in the head').

It is hard to exaggerate the general significance of Hans Kosterlitz's idea. For one thing it turned the attention of the chemists of the brain to that vast family of substances, the peptides. It was the first clear demonstration that nerve cells synthesise and release peptides as transmitter substances. That finding opened the pharmacological door to the discovery of a vast array of active peptides in many parts of the brain. Some of them, like the enkephalins, are probably involved in the regulation of pain. But others are concerned with the control of temperature, blood pressure and a variety of other crucial bodily functions. Others again seem to play a part in the control of growth and even the subtle regulation of the actions of many other non-peptide transmitters. Disturbances in peptide transmitter systems may play an important part in the psychotic diseases of depression and schizophrenia. In the past decade, we have come to see that peptides are among the most widespread and important transmitter chemicals in the brain.

• PAIN, PLEASURE AND TOLERANCE •

The discovery and isolation of opiate receptors and the enkephalin transmitters opened up new opportunities for mapping out the chemical organisation of the brain. Both enkephalin terminals and opiate receptors are densely concentrated in the ventral tegmental (A10) area, which contains the dopamine neurons whose axons make up the bundle of fibres that terminate in the nucleus accumbens. Enkephalin terminals and opiate receptors are also found in neighbouring regions of the hypothalamus (so much concerned with eating, drinking and sex) and the limbic system (a network of structures long thought to be involved in the regulation of emotion). But the enkephalins and their receptors are also found in a second major system within the spinal cord and brain, in the pathways relating to the sensation of *pain*. They are found in the spinal cord, at the point where sensory fibres from the skin terminate. They are also found in a number of other centres in the brainstem that are known to be involved in the regulation of information flowing through the pain pathway.

Thus, it appears that the two major actions of opiate drugs, their painkilling effect and the pleasurable high, are due to the fact that the drugs act parasitically on these two major systems in the brain for the regulation of pleasure and pain.

The discovery of the opiate receptor and the brain's natural morphine-like substances has taught us to see many of the strange phenomena of addiction in terms of the natural chemistry of the brain, in particular tolerance (the fact that opiates insidiously decrease in effectiveness, so that addicts need higher and higher doses to give them the same gratification). The attachment of enkephalin or an opiate drug to the opiate receptor triggers various chemical reactions inside the nerve cell. If the receptors are constantly exposed to morphine, there is a gradual change in the strength of the chemical response inside the cell, so that more and more morphine is needed to cause the same reaction.

Cocaine and amphetamine probably produce their highs by influencing the release of dopamine from nerve terminals right in the nucleus accumbens, so they do not trigger the mechanism for tolerance that is coupled to the opiate receptors on the nerve cell bodies. Cocaine is not needed in larger and larger doses, as heroin is, and the desire to take cocaine again and again, which is so overwhelmingly powerful for many people, has nothing to do with avoiding the pain of withdrawal. It is, as Conan Kornetsky had speculated, a result of the craving that the addict feels for the pleasure of the high itself.

Nicotine, too, almost certainly has some of its most important actions on the reward pathway. About 2000 people die every week in Britain as a result of smoking, yet more than 40 per cent of all adults continue to smoke. Within seven or eight seconds of the first puff of a cigarette, nicotine has been absorbed and has already reached the brain – faster than an intravenous injection of heroin. Its concentration in the brain peaks just as the cigarette is finished and within half an hour it has tailed off, the effects of withdrawal urging the smoker to reach for another cigarette. Though nicotine has many effects in the brain and the body, the pleasure that it produces is probably due to direct action on the dopamine neurons of the reward system.

• THE DOWNER DRUGS •

While the brain's pathway for pleasure and reward is the target of so many addictive drugs it is not the only system that can be invaded and captured by chemicals. A second major class of drugs is taken to calm and reduce anxiety rather than to achieve a euphoric high.

The age-old drug alcohol has complex effects, partly dependent on dose, but the most profound of these is relaxation, sedation and depression of the nervous system. It is hardly surprising that alcohol has a multitude of influences on the brain. Even the modest consumption of alcoholic drinks at a cocktail party is quite sufficient to raise the alcohol level in the brain to a concentration millions of times greater than the levels needed for other drugs to have their effects. Indeed, the blood alcohol level in a chronic drinker is so high that the fatty membranes of cells throughout the body are probably literally partially dissolved by it. However, John Littleton from King's College, London, believes that alcohol interferes selectively with the transmission of chemical signals between nerve cells and this property may produce its sought-after qualities and its addictive power.

Jeffrey Gray of the Institute of Psychiatry in London thinks that all the downer drugs have their main action on one particular system in the brain, anatomically very close to the reward pathway but functionally diametrically opposed to it. Gray calls it the punishment system and believes that it consists of the septum (through which the A10 dopamine fibres pass on their way to the nucleus accumbens) and the hippocampus, that long, curved organ that lies under the temporal lobe, and which is also thought to be involved in the formation of memories. Damage to this general area in animals produces a remarkable reduction in aggression, fear and anxiety. Alcohol may, then, specifically damp down this punishment pathway in some way. Significantly, that other major class of sedative drugs, the barbiturates, also seem to have selective action on the punishment system.

• SOMA WITH A •
TWIST IN ITS TAIL

The search for drugs of contentment has been a major enterprise of the drug industry. One that many thought to be near miraculous in its effects, close in its properties to soma, the perfect palliative of Aldous Huxley's *Brave New World*, was discovered by accident in 1955. Leo Sternbach, a Polish chemist, then working for the Roche Drug Company in Nutley, New Jersey, had spent years working on a group of chemicals that he had synthesised twenty years earlier at the University of Cracow. Roche had invested an enormous effort into the search for an anti-anxiety drug that would not cause drowsiness. Sternbach had searched through his full catalogue of compounds without success and didn't even bother to send the last substance in the batch for testing on animals. A year and a half later, as he was cleaning up his laboratory, Sternbach came across the last bottle. Rather than throwing it out, he decided to send it off for routine screening tests. The word came back; it was more active in reducing anxiety than any of the forty other substances that Sternbach had already developed. This was Librium, the first of a class of seemingly miraculous drugs called the benzodiazepines. By early 1960, Librium was on the market as an anti-anxiety drug and a number of other benzo-diazepines had already been manufactured. The most powerful of these, Valium, was released for clinical use in 1963. They did produce drowsiness, but were rarely lethal, even in massive doses. Soon after Librium and Valium were put on the market, a number of patients with suicidal tendencies consumed the entire contents of their bottles of pills, a hundred or more of them. But they simply slept for a couple of days and woke up not much the worse for wear.

Through the 1960s and 1970s, the demand for these apparently perfect tranquillisers grew and their safety record encouraged doctors to prescribe them freely. They were given for insomnia, for anxiety of all forms, as a pre-anaesthetic medication, for the symptoms of alcohol with-drawal, for epileptic seizures, for cerebral palsy, for tetanus, for backache. In 1975, 100 million prescriptions for Valium and related drugs were filled in the United States alone. In 1981, about one in ten of all men and

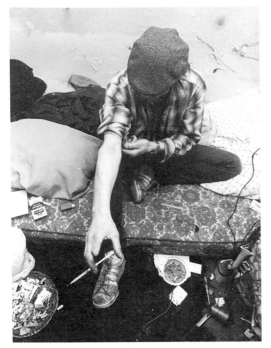

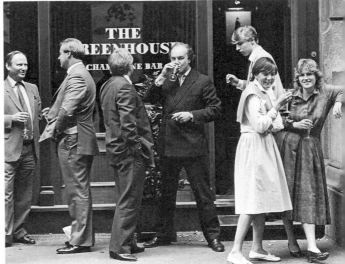

The down-and-out junkie (above left) and wealthy patrons of a champagne bar are all indulging in addictive drugs. On what logical grounds should alcohol be condoned while heroin is condemned?

Liza Harrison and her daughters (below left), around the time when she started taking benzodiazepines, and (below right) after she weaned herself off them.

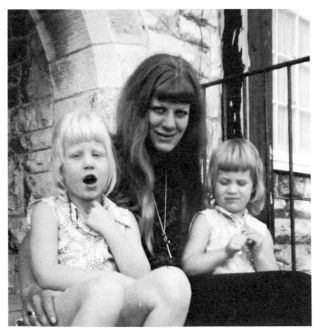

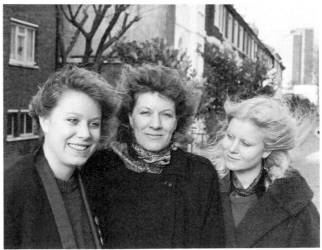

one in five of all women in Britain had taken tranquillisers for at least several weeks.

The warning signs were slow to appear. First, there were the unusual cases in which benzodiazepines taken in combination with other drugs did contribute to successful suicides. Judy Garland's death in 1969 resulted from an overdose of alcohol and Valium. Many people began to be worried about the reliance that such a large proportion of the population of the western world were placing on 'Mother's Little Helper'. And finally came the gradual realisation that benzodiazepines, like so many of the wonder drugs of former times, *can* be addictive. The American consumer champion, Ralph Nader, investigated the use of benzodiazepines in the mid-1970s and claimed that 1.5 million Americans were addicted to Valium. Senate hearings under the chairmanship of Edward Kennedy exposed the problem and by 1980 the rate of prescription of Valium fell to half that of the peak in 1975. There is little doubt, however, that millions of people around the world are still addicted to these drugs.

Liza Harrison, a teenager in the 1960s, when the fashion for Valium was exploding, was first prescribed tranquillisers because she was very depressed and under stress. After twenty years in the reassuring embrace of benzodiazepines, she tried to give up. Liza's experience was unusually extreme. While there is no denying the need that many Valium users have for their drug, withdrawal symptoms as serious as Liza's are rare:

> I would experience electric shocks going all over my body, and my skin felt as though I had been scalded with hot water. I felt as though my body was actually falling apart, that my arms and legs would come off, that my chest would just fall open.... It was as though my thought processes were rivers, and there were thousands and thousands of these.... There were so many thought processes ... and it was crazy. I couldn't cope with it. It was insanity.

Liza Harrison continued to take the capsules for a long time, unable to resist their reassuring shape and size. But each time, before taking a capsule, she pulled it apart, poured the white powder on to a piece of gold card and scraped a fraction into an ornate glass ashtray. Then she poured the remaining powder back into the capsule, resealed and swallowed it. On each successive occasion, Liza threw away just a little more of the drug, gradually cutting down on the amount that she was consuming. Now Liza has been off benzodiazepines for much more than a year.

Here is a group of drugs, the first-born of the new generation of designer drugs, with effects on the brain just as specific as those of the opiates. The lesson of Hans Kosterlitz and the opiate receptor immediately raised a similar question about the benzodiazepines. If these synthetic substances can so specifically reduce anxiety by their action on the brain, is it possible that they too act on receptor molecules? And, if so, could this mean that the brain produces its own anxiety-reducing substances, in the way that it produces its own morphine-like enkephalin? The answer to both questions may well be yes. There are certainly receptor sites on nerve cells in particular parts of the brain that bind benzodiazepine molecules selectively. These benzodiazepine receptors can be mapped out, and they are seen in very high concentrations in the very area, the hippocampus, that Jeffrey Gray believes is part of the punishment system of the brain. Indeed, the benzodiazepine receptor molecule seems to be closely associated with the receptor for an inhibitory transmitter substance called GABA, whose actions are also influenced by barbiturate sedatives. The jigsaw puzzle begins to fall into place. GABA receptors, especially in the punishment system of the brain, may well be the site of action of all the major anxiety-reducing drugs. Barbiturates certainly act there; and so do the benzodiazepines. Recent results suggest that alcohol, too, may have some actions on the same receptor site.

In the last few years, evidence has grown that the brain produces its own chemicals with actions similar to Valium, which act directly on the benzodiazepine receptors. Several candidate substances have been identified, some of them small peptides, like the enkephalins. Some researchers even speculate that there may also be natural substances that *increase* anxiety, and that the mood of a human being or an animal is determined by a balance between two rival chemical families, one reducing, the other increasing the state of anxiety.

• WHO GETS HOOKED? •

Around 1970, shortly after US Congressmen who had visited Vietnam raised the alarm about heroin addiction among the troops, Jerome Jaffe of the Addiction Research Center, at the behest of a worried President Nixon, set up a review committee to evaluate proposals for research on drug abuse. Lee Robins, a sociologist who had studied addiction among young blacks in St Louis, Missouri, was one of the people whom Jaffe invited to join the committee. Jaffe rapidly established a testing programme in which the urine of troops in Vietnam was analysed for opiates; if the tests were positive, the men were held in hospital in Vietnam to withdraw from the drug for a few days before they were sent home. He asked Lee Robins to follow up a group of these men who had returned in September 1971, to see how well they dealt with their addiction.

To Robins's delight, her interviews showed that although three-quarters of the men whose urine tests had been positive admitted to feeling that they were addicted while they were in Vietnam, only 7 per cent showed signs of dependence on drugs a year after they returned (and many of these men had been addicted before they even went to Vietnam). Out of the normal population of enlisted men who had not had their urine tested, half freely admitted that they had tried opium or heroin in Vietnam and about one fifth said that they had physical or psychological dependence. But a year after their return, fewer than one in a hundred showed signs of opiate dependence. Thousands upon thousands simply kicked the habit, all by themselves, when they came home. As Lee Robins said:

> People were very curious about how this could happen. It so violated all their expectations. One of the commonest beliefs was ... that these men ... couldn't get drugs easily in the States and that had explained the change.

However, Robins discovered that fully one-third of those who had had positive urine samples and 10 per cent of the general population of returning troops had used opiates *after* their return to the United States. It seemed that they had no difficulty in obtaining drugs but most of them simply gave them up.

The message that emerges is that addiction chooses its victims with care. Many people, perhaps even the majority, can try powerful drugs such as nicotine, cocaine or heroin on a few occasions and can walk away from them without serious ill effect. For some people, however, a single experience with a drug such as 'crack' can destroy their lives. Jim Sloan was well able to handle alcohol and heroin and gave up cigarettes without great difficulty after years of smoking. But he spent $100 000 on cocaine in his first year of addiction.

Could we predict who is at risk of drug addiction? Stanley Schachter, a sociologist in New York, coined the term 'addictive personality' in the 1960s, but diagnosing this characteristic in advance of a trial by drugs is not easy. Only a few clear facts emerge: the earlier the age at which drug-taking starts, the more likely it is to become a serious addiction; and a tendency to addiction seems to be highly correlated with delinquency, violence and many other kinds of anti-social behaviour.

There is only one addictive drug that has been freely available and socially acceptable for so long that its pattern of use can be followed from generation to generation, providing the essential information to determine whether the tendency to become addicted is inherited. That drug is alcohol. The statistical evidence is clear; severe alcoholism runs in families. The fact that the children of alcoholic parents tend to take to the bottle themselves does not, of course, prove that the tendency to drink is genetic. Children might simply learn the habit from their parents. However, a large-scale study in Sweden shows that even children who were adopted in the first months of life are much more likely to become alcoholics if their own biological parents had a drinking problem. This strongly suggests an inherited link.

Alcoholism falls into two types. Type 1 alcoholics start their heavy drinking when they are adults and they do not generally engage in criminal or seriously anti-social behaviour. Type 2s start when they are young and usually have a history of delinquency; this latter type of alcoholism is sometimes called 'male limited' and is apparently inherited only in the male line.

According to Robert Cloninger of Washington University in St Louis, both genetic and environmental factors influence the appearance of type 1 alcoholism. Adopted children of a type 1 father are no more likely than any other children to become alcoholic *unless* they are brought up by their adoptive parents in an environment of heavy drinking. By comparison, the sons of type 2 fathers are nine times more likely to become alcoholics themselves, even if their adoptive parents do not drink.

What biological factors could be inherited which might predispose people to becoming alcoholics? Henri Begleiter of the State University of New York in Brooklyn believes that the brains of the young sons of type 2 alcoholics are genetically different, even before they begin to drink. He got the clue for his current, controversial research by studying the effects of alcohol on the brains of rats and monkeys. He became interested in the specific effects of alcohol on the processing of incoming sensory information, deciding what events are important and what are not. He now measures brainwaves, with electrodes stuck to the scalps of human beings, as an indicator of the electrical activity of the cerebral cortex.

Whenever a pattern is flashed on a screen or a sound is played over a loudspeaker, a cascade of electrical responses sweeps across the brain, starting out in the region of the cortex that first receives the signals from the eyes or ears and then spreading over other neighbouring regions that process the signal, interpret it and assess its significance. About a third of a second after any unexpected, new sound or visual pattern, the brain responds with a large positive wave. This 'P3 wave' is generally taken as an indication that the brain has recognised the significance or novelty of some event in the outside world. After a few stiff drinks, most of us become less aware of our surroundings, less able to pick up important signals in the outside world – one reason why someone drunk is such a danger behind the wheel of a car. Not surprisingly, then, the P3 wave shrinks in size after a few drinks. Begleiter's first unexpected result was that the P3 response is almost absent in the brain of an alcoholic even after a long period of abstinence. In the last few years, Begleiter has been testing the young sons of type 2 alcoholic fathers, before the children start to drink at all. Nearly 90 per cent of these young boys have P3 reactions to novel stimuli that are detectably abnormal. The genetic predisposition that they carry has, apparently, already stamped itself on the organisation of the brain, before they even take a drink.

The source of the nerve activity that causes the P3 wave may well be the hippocampus and amygdala. These structures, buried under the lower lip of the temporal lobe, are thought to be involved in assessing the emotional significance of events in the outside world, constructing from them a kind of internal representation of the meaning of things and the storage of that information as memory. This region of the brain, which may be innately deficient in the sons of type 2 alcoholics, is itself particularly susceptible to damage from alcohol. In rats and mice, after a period of alcohol consumption, the cells of the hippocampus lose many of the tiny spines on their dendrites, which probably indicates a loss of synaptic input to those cells. Thus, Begleiter suggests that there may be a genetic abnormality in the brain of the son of a type 2 alcoholic which subtly and cruelly predisposes the boy to consume alcohol, which in turn causes further injury to the same brain area, perhaps making it even more difficult for him to resist this drug of destruction. It is surely significant that the limbic system, to which the hippocampus and amygdala belong, is intimately concerned with the control of mood and aggression. Perhaps the genetic defect that leads to early drinking also triggers the aggressive behaviour that is so characteristic of type 2 alcoholics.

• TRIGGERS IN THE WORLD •

So far, we have a simple view of addiction as the chemical subversion of the machinery of pleasure and punishment in the brain. It is easy to paint an attractively simple picture of craving for drugs, of the high they produce, and of tolerance and withdrawal symptoms, in terms of simple little circuits of nerve cells and the chemicals they contain. But the reality of a life of addiction is so much more complicated than that.

In 1857 the Victorian novelist Wilkie Collins, on holiday with his friend Charles Dickens, sprained his ankle. A doctor's assistant offered him that favourite cure-all of the time, the tincture of opium, laudanum; and Collins, who suffered from gout, continued to take it for the pain. In his novel *Armadale* he put his own thoughts into the mouth of a character:

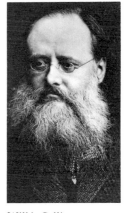

Wilkie Collins (1824–1889).

> Who was the man who invented laudanum? I thank him from the bottom of my heart, whoever he was. If all the miserable wretches in pain of body and mind, whose comforter he has been, could meet together to sing his praises, what a chorus it would be.

As Collins began work on his next and most famous novel, *The Moonstone*, the pain of his gout and his mother's serious illness, close to madness, drove him to consume laudanum by the glassful.

Collins admitted to an American friend, Mary Anderson, that he had written the book in a state dissociated from normal experience, because of the influence of opium. 'When it was finished,' Collins told her, 'I was not only pleased and astonished at the finale, but I did not recognise it as my own.' Collins had discovered 'drug dissociation' – the fact that the memories for actions and events that occur in a drugged state are poorly recalled when the drug has worn off. The discovery of this phenomenon is usually attributed, in the scientific literature, to a study performed on dogs in 1937. But Collins knew of it not only from his own experience but also from the famous textbook *Human Physiology* by John Elliotson, a physiologist and physician who was a friend of many Victorian writers, including Collins.

The Moonstone is a story of the effects of opium on the mind; a tale of drug tolerance and drug dissociation. A magnificent diamond, the Moonstone, given to Rachel Verinder for her eighteenth birthday, disappears during the night following her party. Suspicion falls on her fiancé Franklin Blake, though he protests his innocence. During the birthday dinner, a physician, Mr Candy, recommends that Blake, who is having trouble sleeping because he has recently given up smoking tobacco, should try laudanum. Blake refuses but Candy slips a dose of laudanum into his brandy, to prove its efficacy.

Acting under the influence of the drug, Blake, worried about Rachel's safety because of the interest of thieves in the Moonstone, takes the diamond from her bedroom and hides it. Not until a year later does Candy's assistant, Ezra Jennings, suggest that the truth might be revealed by exactly reconstructing the episode in all its details, including the administration of laudanum. He refers to Elliotson's *Human Physiology*, in which George Combe, past president of the British Phrenological Society, quotes an incident of drug dissociation:

> Dr Able informed me ... of an Irish porter to a warehouse.... On one occasion, being drunk, he had lost a parcel of some value, and in his sober moments could give no account of it. Next time he was intoxicated, he recollected that he had left the parcel at a certain house.

The scene is set; the birthday party is exactly re-enacted; but Collins was clever enough, through the character of Jennings, to know that the dose of laudanum should be increased a little to overcome the effects of tolerance, even though a year had passed since the last use of the drug:

> I shall run the risk of enlarging the dose to 14 minims. On this occasion, Mr Blake knows beforehand that he is going to take the laudanum – which is equivalent, physiologically speaking, to his having (unconsciously to himself) a certain capacity in him to resist the effects.

Collins's understanding of the complex relationship between expectation and tolerance is quite remarkable. It was not until the 1970s that Shepard Siegal of McMaster University in Ontario, Canada, demonstrated experimentally that rats which have become tolerant to large injections of opiates in one particular situation could even be killed by the same dose in a different setting.

The alcoholic's drinking and the effect it has on him depend as much on the environment of the bar, where he drinks, as on his deep physiological needs. The heroin addict and the heroin pusher know that all the extraneous cues and signals are as much a part of the mystique of fixing as the sensation produced by the drug itself. Abraham Wickler, working at the Lexington Addiction Research Center, was the first person to point out that 'cured' heroin addicts often succumb to the temptations of pushers, literally on their way home from the hospital; they report a fresh surge of withdrawal symptoms – nausea, shivering, watery eyes – as soon as they see a familiar pusher or pass an alley in which they have shot heroin in the past.

Charles O'Brien of the Veterans' Administration Hospital in Philadelphia once did an experiment in which addicts smelled peppermint while they were being injected with heroin, during treatment. One of his patients fell into the full 'cold turkey' of withdrawal while he was hanging peppermint chocolates on the Christmas tree, months after his release from hospital! O'Brien and Anna Rose Childress are trying out new ways of teaching addicts to deal with the enticements of the real world. They expose the addict to the whole ritual of taking a drug, short of the act of getting high. Attached to equipment that measures his breathing, his heart rate and his skin temperature, the addict sits in a small room. There, on a table, is all the apparatus needed for the drug of his choice. He has to go through the ritual of preparing the drug, but without consuming it, three times in a row, and then he watches a video tape of addicts getting high. O'Brien and Childress hope to desensitise their addicts by this ordeal of temptation. On the first occasion in the sealed room, the physiological reactions are usually frightening. Withdrawal symptoms rapidly develop; the skin temperature falls to less than 80°F. But after many sessions, these physiological reactions decline and the addict can contemplate facing the temptations of addiction in the real world. Jeffrey Gray, in London, is going a step further – taking heroin addicts out into the streets, to expose them to *all* the environmental cues associated with their habit, in the hope of producing a deeper cure.

The next group of experimental patients for the Philadelphia project will be compulsive gamblers, who share many of the problems of people addicted to chemical drugs. For gamblers, the triggers in the environment are just as strong as they are for a heroin addict. Estimates of the number of pathological gamblers in the United States exceed one million people.

Leonide Goldstein at the New Jersey-Rutgers Medical School has some evidence from the brainwaves of habitual gamblers that they have defects in the organisation of the brain very similar to those of children with attentional disorders, and adults who are alcoholic. Gambling, the repeating over and again of some behaviour that just occasionally results in a reward, is usually explained by psychologists in terms of that unpredictable pattern of 'reinforcement'. The behavioural psychologist Burrhus F. Skinner discovered that animals can easily be persuaded to perform extraordinary rituals of behaviour repetitively and with great enthusiasm as long as the rituals sometimes, but unpredictably, lead to a reward of food. The human habit of gambling has tapped into a fundamental mechanism that ties behaviour to reward. But Goldstein's results also suggest that the tendency to fall victim to the extremes of compulsive gambling is due to defects in the organisation of the brain.

Around the world, the consumption of cigarettes, alcohol and illegal drugs continues to rise. The black and white world of the law sorts addictive substances into categories largely on the basis of how long they have been used and how acceptable they are to respectable society, rather than on the grounds of their danger to health. It is difficult to defend, on logical grounds, a classification of drugs that accepts cigarettes (which are intensely addictive and which kill perhaps a quarter of a million people a week throughout the world) but outlaws marijuana. How can heroin-taking (which simply mimics the actions of a natural chemical in the brain) be wrong, when the consumption of alcohol (which is far more toxic) is right? Addiction cannot be solved by legislation or by more vigilant customs inspection. It is an illness like no other; an illness that blends imperceptibly with normal existence; an illness in which pleasure has become a disease.

Perhaps the cold, objective neutrality of science can eliminate some of the bigotry and prejudice that surround the phenomenon of addiction. The addict is not ill and is surely not committing a crime simply by seeking pleasure. Drugs of addiction break the normal, self-regulating cycle of need, action and satisfaction. They are chemical intruders in the power-house of pleasure, tinkering with the powerful but natural mechanisms for the regulation of hunger, anxiety and the urge for sex. Addiction is the other side of the coin of survival: a symptom of a society that has failed to come to terms with its needs.

MADNESS

GERRY cuts an imposing figure: over 6 feet tall and well built, with a shock of dark hair and deeply sunken, black, haunting eyes. He was living in the William H. White Building at St Elizabeth Hospital in Washington, DC, where, according to Gerry, he was working on a theory of psychological pain, a theory so all-encompassing that it could explain the nature of the universe. According to his doctors, Gerry was schizophrenic. He had been admitted to this particular hospital – an experimental branch of the United States Institute of Mental Health – because he was unresponsive to all the known antipsychotic drugs.

Gerry was a police officer patrolling the streets of a major American city when the illness overtook him. He began to isolate himself from his friends, to lose weight, to behave erratically. It slowly became clear to those around him – his family, his colleagues – that Gerry was undergoing a massive psychological change. Within a year, the metamorphosis was complete. The physician in charge of Gerry's case at St Elizabeth's, Darryl Kirch, describes his symptoms and paints a portrait of the disease:

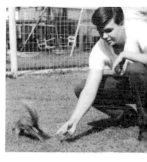

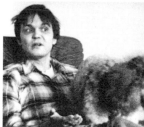

Gerry, before the onset of schizophrenia (top) and more recently, in his parents' home (bottom).

Gerry, in one patient, shows every one of the major features of schizophrenia. His thinking is disorganised; his thoughts are loosely connected. He has formed delusional ideas. Some of those delusions are grandiose, some are paranoid. He has disturbances in his moods – they are, in some cases, almost absent, in others, totally inappropriate. His behaviour is disorganised – he has mannerisms that are inexplicable. He has purposeless, aimless behaviour around the ward. He's a textbook case.

As far as we know, the human species is the only one that has to face the illness of schizophrenia – classical madness. The mind of the schizophrenic is a battleground of thought and emotion, of personality and perception. The disease disrupts logical and rational thought, triggers hallucinations and delusions, destroys its victim's ability to socialise, to understand the feelings of others, to love. As Daniel Weinberger, of the US National Institute of Mental Health, puts it:

> Schizophrenia seems to involve impairment of what we think of as the highest psychological functions, the most intricate, sophisticated, complex psychological functions people have – those aspects that separate the human species from the rest of the animal kingdom.

• POSSESSION •

Madness has been with us since the start of recorded history and, presumably, long before. The eighteenth-century English poet and hymn-writer William Cowper, who was committed to Dr Cotton's private madhouse in St Albans in 1763, gave an account of his symptoms which could have been written by a schizophrenic yesterday:

> Satan piled me with horrible visions, and more horrible voices. My ears rang with the sound of torments, that seemed to await me.... At every stroke, my thoughts and expressions became more wild and incoherent; all that remained clear was the sense of sin, and the expectation of punishment.

Compare Cowper's recollections with the pronouncements of Gerry in St Elizabeth's Hospital:

> I think and feel as though people have called me here to electrocute me, judge me, put me in jail ... because of some of the sins I've been in.... When a sperm and an egg go together to make a baby, only one sperm goes up into the egg.... And when they fuse, it's like nuclear fusion except it's human fusion. There's a mass loss of the proton; one heat abstraction goes up, and the electron spins around, comes back down into the proton to form the mind, and the mind could be reduced to one atom.

Even in the materialistic world of the twentieth century it is difficult to accept that such bizarre thoughts are the product of an organic disease of the brain rather than of a spiritually twisted mind. Yet as early as the fourth century BC, the Greek physician Hippocrates, the father of medicine, taught that *all* illnesses, including the sacred disease of epilepsy and madness itself, were due to imbalance in the four bodily fluids or 'humours' – black bile from the liver, yellow bile from the spleen, blood and phlegm. But the extraordinary symptoms of insanity, lying in the realm of reason and emotion, seemed, to ordinary people, to put that disease into a category quite different from bodily afflictions. At the time of Hippocrates himself, Greek drama gave a more spiritual account of madness; it was the result of the self-inflicted emotional conflicts of life – the traumas of love, desire, revenge and duty.

In pre-Christian Rome the mad were called *larvatum plenum* – filled with phantoms. The early Christian church saw the ravings of the insane as living evidence of the work of Satan, or, more rarely, as prophetic pronouncements. Until a few generations ago, this disease was interpreted by sane and insane alike in terms of possession by supernatural forces or agents. The hearing of voices, the mixed-up thoughts, the shocking lack of compassion – all of these were taken to indicate the occupation of the body by evil spirits. 'Witches' were burned; village 'idiots' were ostracised and ridiculed; the mad poor were incarcerated in notorious hell holes, such as Bedlam in London and the asylum of Charenton in Paris, chained like animals, their screams echoing around the bare stone walls.

• DIAGNOSIS •

Often in the history of medicine the understanding of disease has followed the classification of symptoms. Even today, schizophrenia is diagnosed on the basis of the symptoms rather than obvious pathological changes in the brain. From this standpoint the scientific story of schizophrenia began in England in 1809, when the British physician John Haslam gave the first accurate description of 'a state which cannot be termed maniacal: a state of complete insanity, yet unaccompanied by furious or depressing passions'. Benedict Morel, in Paris, coined the phrase *démence précoce* (early dementia) in 1852 to describe the kind of madness that so often appears in adolescence. But it was the German psychiatrist Emil Kraepelin who, in the 1890s, established the term *dementia praecox* and who distinguished it most clearly from that other family of psychotic disorders, the depressive illnesses. Kraepelin drew together, under this single title, the three major forms of madness that had formerly been thought of as separate – paranoia (delusions and fear of persecution), hebephrenia (emotional disorder) and catatonia (periodic stupor). He saw it as an incurable disease.

In 1911, Eugen Bleuler, the Medical Director of the Burgholzli Hospital in Zurich, Switzerland, called the illness 'schizophrenia', meaning *disintegration* of the mind (not the popular Jekyll-and-Hyde view of two personalities). Bleuler considered the central feature of the disease to be the disruption of personality, rather than the dementia and its incurability. In fact, he recognised that while most patients do deteriorate steadily, others improve, and some return to a state of near normality. Bleuler drew on the ideas of Sigmund Freud to account for the specific *content* of the delusions and hallucinations, but he, like Kraepelin before him, believed that some *organic* change underlies the disease, causing the associative 'threads' that link words and thoughts to be broken.

Bleuler's analysis led to a broader concept of schizophrenia, even extending to the idea of 'latent schizophrenia', characterised by a *tendency* to the disease without strong symptoms. This view has its echo in the work of some present-day psychiatrists and psychologists who see the bizarre symptoms of madness as merely an exaggeration of normal mental states. Gordon Claridge at the University of Oxford has reported that a surprisingly high proportion of normal young adults (albeit Oxford undergraduates) had, at some time, experienced one or more of the defining symptoms of schizophrenia, including hearing voices.

By the 1930s, the notion of schizophrenia as a single illness, a monolith, had faded even further. The discovery of antibiotics meant that certain infectious diseases that had often been classified as schizophrenia – including tertiary syphilis – could be cured and redefined. Better diagnostic methods meant that epilepsy originating in the temporal lobe, which sometimes produces symptoms remarkably like those of schizophrenia, could be distinguished from it.

Today, even true schizophrenia is seen as an umbrella definition that applies to a number of different clusters of symptoms. The course of each case of schizophrenia, and the precise behaviour of each schizophrenic, is like a fingerprint – following a certain general pattern, but unique in its detail. The individual twists to this disease and the variety of its symptoms have hindered classification, analysis and the search for causes.

Schizophrenia is surprisingly common and is universal in its occurrence. It attacks almost one per cent of the population, although the incidence does vary around the world. Until recently, differences in diagnostic criteria have led the recorded rate of madness to be much higher in Russia and the United States than elsewhere. But there are genuine variations too; the incidence of schizophrenia is unusually high in parts of Yugoslavia, Sweden and Ireland, which some see as a clue to an environmental contribution to the cause of the disease.

Among those who succumb to schizophrenia, the prognosis is initially hard to predict. Psychiatrists talk about a 'rule of thirds': a third of those afflicted will recover and not fall ill again; a third will suffer intermittently, spending some time under treatment in hospital, but more time outside; and the final third, the chronic schizophrenics, remain ill despite all attempts at treatment. Gerry belongs to the final third.

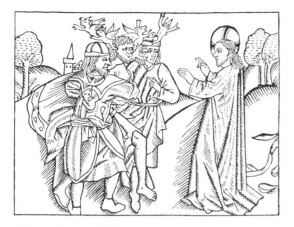

Jesus casting out devils.

Although asylums for the mentally ill were first established more than 700 years ago, until very recently they could offer little in the way of effective treatment for schizophrenia. Many patients were simply incarcerated behind barred windows (right) or subjected to extraordinary procedures, such as the electrical therapy practised at the French asylum at La Salpetrière towards the end of the nineteenth century (below).

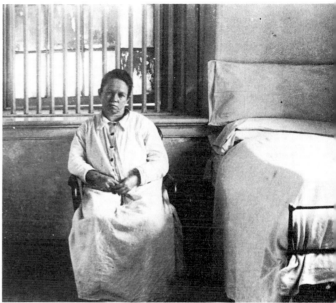

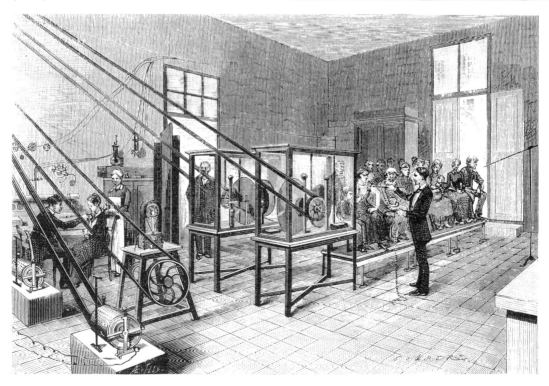

Those two, apparently contradictory views, which were already established in ancient Greece – that madness is the product of physical pathology, and that it is the result of spiritual crisis – can be traced to the present day.

With the emergence of psychiatry as a branch of medicine, and the proliferation of asylums, there began a search for methods of *treatment*. Maniacs were sedated with herbal drugs, were purged with enemas and emetics, were subjected to electric shocks, exhausting manual labour, scalding or freezing baths. Opium, blood-letting, confinement, restraint; all were applied as desperate remedies, with an underlying, implicit assumption that the disease itself had some cause in the organisation of the brain, which might be set right by these physical insults.

Sigmund Freud's attitude to schizophrenia was ambivalent. He tried to treat very few schizophrenic patients and concluded that psychoanalysis was not a valuable therapy. Nevertheless, he saw psychotic madness as a deep disturbance of the subconscious mind and some of his followers have pursued further a psychoanalytical interpretation of the origins of schizophrenia.

This particular school of thought reached its zenith in the 1950s, when Theodore Lidz, a psychiatrist at Yale University, contended that the key to the disorder was the 'schizophrenogenic mother', whose personality and techniques of parenting trigger the illness. Lidz believed that certain mothers place their children in situations in which they inevitably experience conflict no matter what course of action they take. His hypothesis was disputed and, ultimately, discarded when researchers examining the personalities of the mothers of schizophrenics could find no common characteristics among them. Nevertheless, the notion reverberated through psychiatry for years and left a terrible burden of guilt on many mothers.

In fact, schizophrenia devastates not only those afflicted, but their families as well. To lose a child to schizophrenia is a tremendous load to bear. To be told by a psychiatrist that this awful disorder is due to the way the child was nurtured is far worse. This attitude led to a breakdown in communication between families and certain psychiatrists, especially in the United States. Many professionals felt that the best treatment was to keep the patient away from the family, which, they believed, triggered the illness in the first place. The families, on the other hand, felt abandoned by the medical profession at the precise moment when they most needed help. The result was anger, fear, frustration, distrust – a mood which, in some areas, persists to this day.

Although it is now generally agreed that schizophrenia is not simply a product of traumatic emotional events in early childhood, there is, paradoxically, good evidence that the detailed course of the illness (the time and speed of onset and the probability of subsequent worsening or amelioration) influenced by the environment and experiences of a schizophrenic. However, over the past two decades, a growing mass of evidence, from both the clinic and the research laboratory, has pointed the finger of blame for this disease at a fault in the structure and the chemistry of the brain, and even at a defect in the genes.

Seymour Kety, a research psychiatrist, now at the US National Institutes of Health, had heard of the fastidious record-keeping practised by the government of Denmark. The Danes maintain a population register that includes the name, date of birth, and address of everybody in Denmark; a psychiatric register, with names and diagnoses of over 90 per cent of those who have sought professional help or stayed in an institution; and, most important, a record of every legal adoption, with the names of the adoptive parents, the biological mother and even the presumed father (who, in Denmark, must participate in the adoption proceedings). Kety realised that the Danish records contained all the elements for investigating the psychiatric history of people who had two separate pairs of parents – a biological pair, who had contributed very little to the environment in which the children had grown up; and an adoptive pair, who had contributed nothing to the children's genetic heritages.

In 1963, Kety's team began to compile an enormous sample of cases (over 5500 in Copenhagen alone) of people over the age of thirty who had been legally adopted by people who were not their biological relatives. By comparing the records from the three registers, they found 33 schizophrenics among the Copenhagen adoptees. To complete the experimental design, they selected a control group of 33 normal adoptees who resembled the schizophrenics in age, sex and social class.

The scientists now had four sets of relatives to investigate: the biological relatives and the adoptive relatives of each of the two groups. By finding out which groups of relatives suffered a higher incidence of schizophrenia, they hoped to determine which factor – genes or environment – played a more important role in the disease.

Out of 463 relatives surveyed, 21 were found to have a history of schizophrenia. When Kety's team broke the code that concealed from them the relatives' exact identities, they discovered that schizophrenia was concentrated among the true, *biological* relatives of the adopted schizophrenics; there were, in fact, about eight times as many as would be expected by chance among the general population. The team concluded that at least some types of schizophrenia must involve a significant inherited contribution.

Several other studies have supported Kety's findings. If both parents are schizophrenic, the chance of their offspring being schizophrenic is about 40 per cent. And the incidence of schizophrenia in *both* members of a pair of twins is much higher if they are identical than if they are not, whether or not they were raised in the same household. Clearly, this does not mean that every parent who has schizophrenia will have a schizophrenic child; the majority of people whose families have histories of schizophrenia do *not* suffer from the disease. Only half of those who have identical twins with schizophrenia are themselves schizophrenic. It is clear that factors other than genetics must be involved.

Indeed all the studies of the inheritance of schizophrenia, even the careful Danish survey, have been criticised on many grounds. For instance, since adoption often takes place between matched socio-economic groups, the home environment of an adopted child tends to be similar in some respects to that of the true parent. Even more significant is the fact that events *very* early in life, before adoption takes place – perhaps even before birth – may play a part in triggering schizophrenia later in life.

There is, for instance, a definite tendency for schizophrenia to be more common in people born in the winter months, which raises the possibility that infection or some effect dependent on temperature is involved. An old claim that many schizophrenics (more, at least, than among the general population) experienced difficult births has recently been confirmed. There is a high incidence of asthma and immunological deficiency in schizophrenics, which again suggests that infection or immune defects might be involved. The situation is obviously complicated, but the majority of researchers in this field do believe that there is a genetic contribution to madness. Indeed, Hugh Gurling and a team at the Middlesex Hospital in London have very recently used the techniques of genetic engineering to identify an abnormal gene in people with schizophrenia.

Tim Crow, director of the Division of Psychiatry at the Clinical Research Centre in Middlesex, has made the controversial suggestion that some kind of viral infection may play a part. There have been many reports of schizophrenia (or conditions like it) occurring shortly after attacks of viral encephalitis, measles, influenza and other virus infections, but what Crow now has in mind is something more sinister – an infection by a retrovirus, which (like the viruses that cause AIDS and certain kinds of leukemia) becomes incorporated into the DNA of the chromosomes of its human host, acting as a kind of genetic parasite. Crow points out that the incidence of schizophrenia among *both* members of a pair of *non*-identical twins is higher than among pairs of ordinary brothers and sisters, even though they share the same fraction of their genes. The twins are more likely to have grown up very close to each other (especially in the uterus, of course) and therefore to have shared contagious infections. The proposed virus might even be passed from relatives to children at a very early age producing the impression that madness is inherited.

But what might this virus, or the defective gene, if there is one, actually *do*? Tim Crow now suggests that it may interfere with the normal development of asymmetry of the cerebral hemispheres! The dissimilarities between the two sides of the cerebral hemispheres, which are so exaggerated in human beings, seem mainly to be associated with language. Speech (as well as thought) is usually very abnormal in schizophrenics, involving bizarre, almost poetic associations. Linguist Elaine Chaika quotes an example from a patient asked to identify a particular colour:

> Looks like clay. Sounds like grey. Take you for a roll in the hay. Hay day. Mayday. Help. I need help!

In most normal humans the upper part of the temporal lobe, near the auditory region of the cortex, is enlarged on the left side and much evidence suggests that the left temporal lobe is abnormal in many schizophrenics. As long ago as 1915, E.E. Southard, Professor of Neuropathology at Harvard, described 'atrophy' or degeneration, particularly in the left hemisphere, of schizophrenics. Modern brain scanning techniques confirm Southard's other finding that the fluid-filled ventricles inside the cerebral hemispheres are enlarged, and Crow's group have recently reported that the major change often occurs in the part of the ventricle within the left temporal lobe, suggesting shrinkage of the surrounding cortical tissue. Indeed, specific degenerative changes have been described in the parts of the temporal lobe that feed information into the hippocampus (concerned with memory formation) and other parts of the limbic system (which is concerned with emotional responses), as well as in the left hippocampus itself. It may all add up to a failure of the normal proliferation and migration of nerve cells early in life, in regions on the left side of the brain that are concerned with language, visual perception, emotion and memory for words.

The corpus callosum, the great cable of fibres that joins together the two cerebral hemispheres, is often abnormally thickened in schizophrenics. Remember Giorgio Innocenti's discovery that there is normally a huge *loss* of fibres from the corpus callosum during early development. Perhaps this loss is partly concerned with the establishment of cerebral asymmetry. This, then, might be another indication of a failure of normal dominance in the brains of some schizophrenics.

• ANOTHER POINT OF VIEW •

The search for drugs to help schizophrenics has thrown up a quite different but equally compelling picture of the pathology in a schizophrenic brain – a hidden defect in its chemistry. In the early 1950s, Henri Laborit, a naval surgeon at the Hôpital Boucicaut in Paris, was searching for ways to treat the syndrome of post-operative shock, which sometimes follows major surgery. He tried a newly discovered drug chlorpromazine, which was known to have calming effects. 'The substance put my patients into a state of psychic and physical relaxation,' Laborit now recalls. 'They displayed a real indifference to the environment and to the surgery. It struck me that these drugs must have an application in psychiatry.' A young surgeon who attended one of Laborit's conferences told his brother-in-law, a psychiatrist named Pierre Deniker, about Laborit's speculations.

Deniker injected chlorpromazine into ten agitated, uncontrollable psychotic patients, most of whom had been diagnosed as schizophrenic. Deniker's memory of what followed is still clear:

> We tried Laborit's famous cocktail, and very quickly we saw the restlessness of the patients begin to level off. They became calmer and calmer; and some were able to sleep normally. And the nurses, who had all the scepticism of old-timers about our experiments, came to us and said, 'This time you've really got something.'

The 'drug revolution' had begun with chlorpromazine. Other antipsychotic agents quickly followed. Immediately, scientists began to search for the chemistry underlying the effects of these drugs. It became clear that most of them influenced a specific system in the brain, a network of nerves that uses one particular neurotransmitter, dopamine. The cell bodies of dopamine neurons are found in clusters in the midbrain and they send their fibres up into the basal ganglia (part of the system for movement control), into regions of the emotion-controlling limbic system and into the frontal lobe, which seems to be involved in the highest of human faculties – responsibility, planning for the future, social behaviour, rational thought.

When dopamine is released by the terminal of a nerve fibre, it crosses the synapse and attaches to receptors on the next neuron, thus influencing its firing. The antipsychotic drugs seem to block the receptors, hence reducing the action of dopamine. It was, therefore, logical to assume that schizophrenia is caused by an excess of dopamine, especially in the limbic system and frontal lobes. This notion was strengthened when amphetamine – a drug that increases the amount of dopamine released from terminals – was found to exacerbate schizophrenic symptoms.

Interestingly, Parkinson's disease, in which patients have difficulty in making voluntary movements, is associated with degeneration of the dopamine cells that send their fibres to the basal ganglia. The drug L-DOPA, which *increases* the release of dopamine from nerves and alleviates the symptoms of Parkinson's disease, also tends to precipitate certain schizophrenic symptoms.

The 'Dopamine Hypothesis' has been a dominant theoretical basis for research into schizophrenia for the past two decades, but evidence for it (other than the effectiveness of anti-dopamine drugs) has been elusive. Indeed, the drugs alleviate symptoms dramatically in only about a third of the schizophrenic population – indicating either that the dopamine system is not the only pathway involved in the disease, or that schizophrenia is in fact a varied group of diseases – or both.

Measurements of nerve cell activity in the living schizophrenic brain with positron emission tomographic (PET) scans do indicate a slight decrease in the activity of the frontal lobes. But direct measurements of the dopamine pathways have produced mixed results. One thing seems certain. There is *not* a large excess of dopamine itself in the fluid of the ventricles in schizophrenics, nor in the brain tissue of schizophrenic patients, measured by chemical analysis after death. However, a number of studies, including one by Tim Crow's group, have revealed an increase in the density of dopamine receptors on cells in various parts of the brain, even in patients who had not been treated with drugs for long periods before their death. More recently, the PET scan technique has also shown a small increase in the density of dopamine receptors in the brains of living schizophrenics. It is generally accepted then, that some of the symptoms of schizophrenia may be due to overactivity of dopamine pathways, but through an excess of receptors on the receiving nerve cells rather than an overproduction of dopamine itself.

• PARADOXES AND RESOLUTIONS •

In just thirty years a state of utter ignorance has been replaced by an embarrassment of riches in the search for a physical basis of madness. We are now faced with two apparently unrelated physical defects in the schizophrenic brain – a problem in the dopamine pathway, ending mainly in the limbic system and the frontal lobe; and defects in parts of the temporal lobe, especially on the left side. Tim Crow has suggested that these two pathological changes may be associated with different aspects of the symptoms of schizophrenia. The negative symptoms (poverty of speech, emotional flattening), which are characteristic of chronic schizophrenia and are relatively unaffected by antipsychotic drugs, may be caused by the structural changes in the temporal lobe. The error in the dopamine system may account for the positive symptoms (delusions and hallucinations), which are particularly severe during acute attacks of madness and which do respond well to drugs. Crow's idea seems at first to reverse the attempts of Kraepelin and Bleuler to unify this disease but he does not believe that these two facets of schizophrenia are separate illnesses with fundamentally different underlying causes. They may both be linked by a defect in the genes.

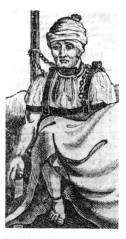

William Norris, an American who died in Bethlem Royal Hospital in 1815 after being confined there for twelve years, bound by short chains to an iron rod. His only crime had been to attempt escape.

But so many questions remain. What is the sequence of cause and effect? Do the degenerative changes in the brain appear early in life, before the disease is apparent? Or are they a secondary result of the disease itself? Do the defects in the temporal lobe *cause* the changes in the dopamine pathway, or vice versa? If the real start of the pathological change is very early in life, why are its effects delayed until adolescence or later? These questions are exciting challenges for brain research; they are sources of frustration and despondency for schizophrenics and their families, who wait in hope for the key to this terrible disease to be found.

In our cities, the drug revolution has had its own side-effects. The programme of 'deinstitutionalisation' (a proud product of the 'success' of scientific research, aided by governments grateful for an excuse to save public money) has put tens of thousands of victims of this disease out on the streets, discarded and ignored, in conditions that are different from the cacophony of Bedlam and Charenton but scarcely any better. It is a crisis not so much of science, but of societies that are delighted to find an excuse to shirk their responsibility for the most profoundly ill, the most helpless, of their members. But at least we are witnessing a fundamental change in opinion, which is slowly diffusing out from the research laboratories and hospitals, through the media to the general public. Schizophrenia is a disease of the brain, not a curse from the gods or an aberration of personality caused by an inadequate mother. It should not be a source of ridicule or shame, any more than Parkinson's disease, that tragic *neurological* condition which may be closely related to the *psychiatric* disorder of schizophrenia in its chemical origin. This slow change of public perception of the nature of madness challenges the dualistic view of the mind that our everyday language and our social prejudices give to us. That change of view will be good – not just for the mad, but for the rest of us too.

SIGHT
UNSEEN

A SINGLE ATOM of gas, baking in the unimaginable heat at the surface of the sun, suddenly shifts from one energy state to another, and spits out the surplus energy as a photon – the smallest, indivisible unit of light. This tiny pellet of energy is thrown into space at the highest speed that Einstein could conceive of. Eight minutes or so after its birth, our chosen photon slows down a little as it hits the atmosphere of the Earth and a fraction of a second later it reaches the surface. It strikes the wrinkled skin of an old woman but, as chance has it, the wavelength of our charmed photon of light is such that it is not captured by the pigments of her skin. It is reflected, and 10 microseconds later it shoots into a tiny black hole, just 3 millimetres across. This hole is the pupil of a man's eye.

The photon slips past the transparent window that covers the front of his eye, through the lens within it and on, between the particles of the gelatinous mass behind the lens, even across the membranes and cytoplasm of the nerve cells of the retina in the back of the eye. But time is running out. It penetrates a strange, thin cell at the back of the retina and its existence ends as it strikes a single molecule of pigment inside that cell, which captures the photon, destroying it by stealing its energy.

'Hello, Grandma.' The man, whose retina has caught our hero, the photon, has recognised his grandmother. He sees her wrinkled face and her blue gingham dress.

She smiles and opens her mouth. As she exhales, the folds of her larynx vibrate as the air rushes past them. Her breath rushes around her moving tongue as it darts skilfully back and forth within her mouth, occasionally touching her lips or her teeth. She is speaking. The rich mixture of tones and noises pulses through the air towards her grandson's head. Some of the vibrating particles in the air are caught by the crevices of his outer ear and funnelled into the narrow tube that leads to his eardrum. They beat on it, setting up a rhythm in a chain of minute bones, which rattle at another membrane, setting up waves in the liquid inside a tiny coiled tube. And these vibrations, in turn, tickle hairs on tiny specialised nerve cells that stand like a regiment of sharp-eared soldiers along the length of the tube. 'Hello dear.' The man hears his grandmother speaking.

This everyday scene sets the stage for a detective story. The detective is the human brain; the story is our perception of the world around us.

• KNOWLEDGE FROM MOLECULES • AND WAVES

To the inner eye and ear of the conscious mind, our senses give us windows through which we see, hear, touch, taste and smell the physical world. The job of the sense organs is to convert light, sound, heat, pressure and molecules into the tiny electrical impulses that scurry along nerve fibres – their currency of communication. We are blissfully unaware of the machinery of nerves within our sense organs and our brains; all that we know directly is the impression of reality. Perception is an invention of nerve cells inside our heads.

For more than 2000 years, philosophers and scientists have been deceived by the apparent simplicity of perception. The great Greek geometer, Euclid, who lived about 300 BC, thought that we see the world because light flows *out* of the eyes, like an invisible hand, feeling the reality of the physical world. But Plato, who lived 100 years earlier, realised that knowledge – even knowledge of the outside world – comes from *within*. He described a fable, told by Socrates, about people living in a strange underground world:

> Behold! Human beings living in an underground den, which has a mouth open towards the light ... Here they have been from their childhood ... Above and behind them a fire is blazing at a distance, and between the fire and the prisoners there is a raised path; and you will see, if you look, a low wall built along the path, like the screen which marionette players have in front of them, over which they show the puppets.

Socrates described the way in which the human beings trapped in the cave could see the people and objects that were out of sight behind the wall only by virtue of the flickering shadows of them thrown on the opposite wall of the cave by the light of the fire. In such a frightful world,

Socrates said that 'the truth would be literally nothing but the shadows of the images.' He went on to explain his allegory: 'The prison-house is the world of sight, the light of the fire is the sun.' And so it is; our understanding of the world around us comes from the merest echoes of reality – the photons of light that bombard the eye, the vibrations in the air that strike the ear, the floating molecules that rush into the nostrils.

Aristotle, the first great biologist, wrote that each sense organ 'receives the form of the object without its matter'. The immaterial qualities (such as colour, shape and smell) of physical things in the world strike the sense organs and evoke the perception of the world. Galileo's eyes, peering through his telescope at the heavens, changed our entire understanding of the universe, yet he wrote, in 1623, fourteen years before he lost his sight, that sensations 'are nothing more than names when separated from living beings, just as tickling and titillation are nothing but names in the absence of such things as noses and armpits'.

• PICTURES IN THE HEAD •

How, then, can nerve cells create our knowledge of the world? To start to answer that question, we can peer backwards in time and downwards through the animal world to simple creatures with no more than a few thousand neurons to help them find their food, avoid their enemies and manage their lives. Any animal that moves must understand something of the world around it. Many simple animals *detect* light but learn little from it: they merely move towards or away from the light, depending on their particular style of life. The light-sensitive nerve cells in the human retina, on which those photons that enter the pupil fall, can also do nothing more than signal the intensity of light. All the richness of our visual perceptions, all the information needed to recognise a grandmother's face, comes from those tiny cells in the retina that know nothing but the number of photons hitting them.

In 1637, in his book *La Dioptrique*, the French philosopher and scientist René Descartes described how he had taken the eyeball of an ox, cut a hole in the back and covered it with a translucent piece of paper. There, on this tiny screen, where the retina would normally lie, Descartes saw a little, upside-down image of his room, focused by the cornea and the lens of the eye. Descartes was not the first to observe the retinal image, but his interpretation of it went far beyond a mere comparison with optical instruments. For Descartes, this extraordinary little picture, painted with light on the retina of the eye, was the clue to our perception of the world.

As in a camera, the image in our eye falls on a sensitive film. The 'grain' of the retina is those tiny light-sensitive cells, the rods and cones: the detail in the message that passes to the brain depends on the tightness

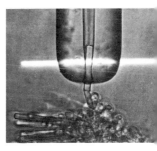

Dennis Baylor and his colleagues recorded the electrical responses of rods from a piece of toad retina, viewed under the microscope (top). One rod is sucked into a glass tube and illuminated with light. The trace (bottom) shows the signals recorded from the rod as a very weak light is shone on it every thirty seconds, indicated by the pulses underneath. The signal varies in size, depending on the number of individual photons captured by the rod.

of packing of those receptive cells. When we look directly at something to examine it in detail, we move our eyes so that the image of that object falls on a specialised patch in the centre of the retina, where the receptive cells are crowded together in unbelievable density – 200 000 or more in a square millimetre. Over the whole retina, there may be as many as 150 million rods and 10 million cones.

The rods are exquisitely sensitive, capable of converting a single photon of light into a detectable electrical signal. They are the receptors of low-light vision. They catch light only at the blue end of the visible spectrum and provide information only about the *brightness* of that light; hence the discrimination of wavelength – the basis of colour vision – is impossible in very dim conditions. On the other hand, the cones, which are concentrated in and around that specialised central region, function when the conditions are quite bright; and, as the physicist Thomas Young speculated early in the nineteenth century, there are three types of cone, each sensitive to light in a different part of the visible spectrum – blue, yellow-green and red. The white light that reaches the earth from the sun contains photons of all wavelengths. Indeed, the sensation that we call 'white' results from the stimulation of all three types of cone. A coloured object appears coloured because it absorbs light of some wavelengths, reflecting the rest.

Despite its superficial similarity to a camera, the eye is not a passive image-maker. The retina is actually part of the brain, derived from a bulge of tissue that pushes out on each side of the growing forebrain in the fetus. The retina consists of a complex array of four other classes of nerve cells, as well as the rods and cones, connected together in a layered arrangement. We do not see *in* our eyes, but our eyes begin that process of analysis that constitutes our understanding of the visual world. The signals that start in those myriad light-sensitive cells are channelled into the one million nerve fibres that leave the eye, bundled together as the optic nerve.

Descartes had seen the optic nerve; indeed, he knew that it contained many individual fibres. He suggested that they keep themselves in perfect order, like a well-disciplined bundle of spaghetti, as they pass between eye and brain and distribute themselves over the walls of the fluid-filled ventricles in the centre of the brain. Thus, the picture formed by light on the retina becomes converted into an internal picture created by the 'vibration' of those nerve fibres on the surface inside the brain. But, however attractive this idea, Descartes realised that a picture in the head is no explanation for a picture in the mind:

> Although this little picture still retains some resemblance to the objects from which it originates, as it passes to the back of our head, we should not fall into the error of thinking that it is by means of this resemblance

that we *see* the objects; for there is not another set of eyes inside the head with which we could see the images.

Descartes never resolved this disturbing paradox, but neatly side-stepped it by proposing that a third, and final, spiritual image is formed in the depths of the brain. He imagined that the array of twitching nerves, forming their picture on the walls of the ventricles, set up currents in the magical fluid. These, in turn, transmits the message to that mysterious organ, the pineal gland, at the back of the ventricles, which Descartes thought of as the seat of the soul. The pattern of vibration drumming on the surface of this little soul might be the medium of conscious perception.

• THE MANTLE OF UNDERSTANDING •

All the sense organs, from the eyes to the skin of the toes, send their telegraphic descriptions of reality through cables of nerve fibres, up to the huge puckered sheet of grey matter – the cerebral cortex – that swaddles the cerebral hemispheres. In humans, its total surface is a quarter of a square metre. It grows relentlessly during the development of the fetus, and it becomes wrinkled and twisted as it squeezes itself, concertina-like, into the confines of the skull. Though only 2 millimetres or so thick, this vast sheet probably contains almost 10 000 million nerve cells with 100 million million synaptic connections amongst them. If any part of the brain is the anatomical hallmark of mankind, it is the cerebral cortex.

Nowadays it is common knowledge that the cortex is probably responsible for perception and consciousness. Yet in the seventeenth century, Descartes, like every other philosopher and scientist from the time of Aristotle, thought that the clear liquid within the brain, the animal spirit (from the Latin *anima*, meaning soul), was responsible for those functions. But, around the same time, a physician, Thomas Willis, working in Oxford, was conceiving the revolutionary hypothesis that the inauspicious jelly of the brain itself might be the substance of mind. After the restoration of Charles II in 1660, most of the great Oxford scientists moved to London to help establish the Royal Society. But Willis stayed in Oxford and was rewarded by the University with the professorship of natural philosophy. Dissatisfied with the traditional injunction to teach from the writings of Aristotle, in 1661 he began a series of dissections of the brains of animals and people. He saw the huge size of the human cerebral hemispheres and it struck him that they must reflect our greater intelligence.

In 1664, Willis published his great work, the *Cerebri Anatome*, which was still used as a textbook until the middle of the last century. Drawing his evidence from dissection and from the symptoms of injury to the brain,

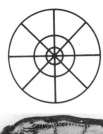

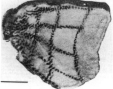

Russell DeValois provided this direct demonstration of the 'map' of the visual field in the cortex. Using one eye alone, a monkey stared at the very centre of a pattern of radial lines and circles (top), made up of flashing dots of light, after it had been given an injection of a radioactive glucose derivative. The radioactivity accumulated in the activated nerve cells, which are shown as black areas, forming a pattern corresponding to the image viewed by the eyes, spread across the cortex (below). The horizontal bar is 1 cm long.

Willis argued that perception, memory, intelligence and all voluntary functions take place in the cerebral hemispheres.

In the middle of the last century evidence began to grow that not only was Willis's general notion correct but different regions of the cerebral cortex could be assigned specific functions. By the beginning of this century, touch, vision and hearing, as well as the control of movement, had each been allocated to small patches of land in the vast territory of the cerebral cortex. At first, the evidence came from the effects of injury in man and animals. Damage at the very back of the hemispheres, in the occipital lobe, caused blindness. At the top of the temporal lobe or the front of the parietal lobe, injury interfered with hearing and bodily sensation, respectively. And at the very back of the frontal lobe was a strip of 'motor cortex', where injury caused partial paralysis of the body muscles. Between these kingdoms of sensation and movement lay a vast uncharted wasteland of cerebral cortex, to which (in the absence of any real evidence) the functions of 'association' and intellect were assigned.

When neurologists, anatomists and physiologists peered closer into these sensory and motor areas, they saw something that seemed to confirm the wildest speculation of René Descartes. In each region, there is a kind of 'map' of the job to be performed. Take, for instance, the primary visual cortex, at the back of the head. Henry Head, the eminent British neurologist, studying wounded troops in the First World War, noticed that tiny injuries in this region, caused by fragments of shrapnel, produced corresponding little patches of blindness in the field of vision. Electrical recording methods also suggested that there is a kind of picture of the visual field, albeit distorted, laid out across the surface of this part of the brain.

The two strips of cortex devoted to the surface of the body and to the muscles, lying side by side in the middle of the cerebral hemispheres, also contain maps of the body. Wilder Penfield, the Canadian neurosurgeon who developed methods for stimulating the surface of the brain in conscious human beings, found, when searching for the focus of epileptic seizures, that, if he stimulated a particular point in the motor strip, some part of the opposite side of the patient's body would twitch involuntarily: a finger, a toe, the corner of the mouth – depending on the position of the electrode. In each case, stimulating at the corresponding position in the neighbouring somatic sensory strip would produce a strange tingling feeling in the skin of the same general area of the body.

The auditory cortex too forms a map of a kind; however, what is represented there is not the position of sounds in space but their *pitch*. Like the keyboard of a piano, one end of the auditory cortex is devoted to the lowest tones, the other to the highest, with a steady progression of pitch in between.

The general rule that emerges is that the fibres entering and leaving the cortex maintain a regularity of order that is related to the arrangement of sensory cells in the sense organs or of the muscles in the body. Even the curious pattern in the auditory cortex falls into this mould, because those tiny, hair-covered cells that detect sound vibrations in the inner ear and convert them into impulses are arranged in a similar musical scale along the coiled tube that forms the inner ear: one end vibrates in sympathy with high tones, the other end with low.

But to find these maps in the brain does nothing more than resurrect the paradox of Descartes. Somehow the nerve cells themselves, within the sensory areas of the cortex, must capture the meaning of the messages from the senses.

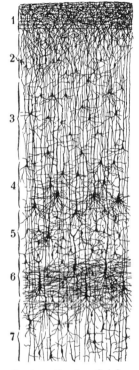

• THE NEURONS OF KNOWLEDGE •

In the late 1920s, Edgar Adrian at the University of Cambridge, later Lord Adrian, started to develop methods for recording the electrical activity of sensory nerve fibres in anaesthetised animals. He already knew that nerve cells generate tiny electrical pulses, about one-tenth of a volt in amplitude, which sweep along the fibre at a speed of between 0.5 and about 150 metres per second (depending on the size and type of the fibre). Everywhere that Adrian put his electrodes – in the nerves from the tongue, from the skin, from the eye – he found the same thing. The *stronger* the sensory stimulation, the more frequently those impulses would chatter along the nerve. We now see this as one of the most fundamental laws of the brain – that information is transmitted in the form of coded messages with impulses and their frequency as the elements of the code. But that was by no means the whole story.

When Adrian recorded from the optic nerve of a conger eel, he detected strong but *brief* bursts of impulses each time he increased or *decreased* the light. Although the rods and cones themselves are like photo-cells, simply signalling directly the level of light, the message has already been transformed by the time that it leaves the eye. What is signalled to the brain is mainly the *change* in illumination at each point on the retina. Though we are often unaware of it, our eyes are constantly in motion; and so they *must* be, for without the constant shifting of the image across the retina that each eye movement produces, vision would be impossible. The retinal image can be frozen by viewing through a special optical instrument, and under those conditions everything fades to a kind of formless grey within a matter of seconds.

In 1953, Horace Barlow, a young physiologist working in Adrian's department at Cambridge, recorded from individual nerve cells in the frog's retina, whose fibres make up the optic nerve. Each cell was connected to an array of rods or cones – called the receptive field of the cell. The

Santiago Ramón y Cajal drew this picture of nerve cells in different layers of the cortex, starting from the outer layer, labelled '1'. The dendrites and axons of the cells run up and down – an anatomical substrate for the systems of functional 'columns' found throughout the cerebral cortex.

cells fell into a number of distinct classes, according to the kind of visual pattern that would cause them to respond. One class responded best to any *movement* in the visual field and another to small black objects, about the size of a fly at tongue's length from the frog. Barlow suggested that the frog's retina may be processing the simple information from the rods and cones in order to detect particular distributions of light and dark and particular patterns of stimulation in time, so as to recognise *features* in the world of special importance to a frog.

Here, suddenly, was a transition in thinking. The senses are not slavish projectors of images; they are active searchers after meaning. The optic nerve describes the retinal image to the brain in succinct, symbolic terms.

Curiously, in higher mammals – cats, monkeys and presumably human beings – the process of extraction of meaning seems to be delayed until the cerebral cortex. The nerve fibres that run up into a cat's or monkey's visual cortex, carrying messages from the eyes, simply signal when a particular point on the retina brightens or darkens. When David Hubel, a Canadian, and Torsten Wiesel, a Swede, working at Harvard in the late 1950s, started to record with microelectrodes from the neurons of the visual cortex of anaesthetised cats, they tried flashing light on a screen in front of the animal's eyes or projecting the usual bright or dark spots. But nothing seemed to work. David Hubel takes up the story:

> One day, we were shining small spots . . . on to the screen and we found that the black dot seemed to be working in a way that, at first, we couldn't understand. We found that it was the process of slipping the piece of glass into the projector, which swept a *line*, a very faint, precise, narrow line, across the retina. Every time we did that, we'd get a response.

What Hubel and Wiesel had discovered was that most neurons in the visual cortex respond to edges or lines moving across the appropriate part of the retina. If the angle of the line is changed by more than a few degrees, the neuron becomes blind to it, and another cell takes over. These neurons may play a part in the analysis of the *shapes* of objects in the visual field. Moreover, these orientation-selective neurons are organised into their own microscopic map within each tiny patch of the visual cortex. They are arranged such that all the cells lying one above the other in a column, running through the entire depth of the cortex, respond best to the same angle of line or edge. On either side are neighbouring columns of cells, each preferring a slightly different orientation. Then on and on, across the cortex, an ever-changing preference for angle; until, half a millimetre or so away, the whole cycle of angles is completed.

So, a microscopic map of orientation is superimposed on the map of the visual field. And there are other regular patterns too. The monkey, with its acute colour vision, has clusters of nerve cells in the upper layers of the cortex that are sensitive to the colour of light: they form a kind of polka-dot pattern at half-millimetre intervals across the visual cortex. Also, the two sets of fibres entering the cortex, from the left eye and the right, form their own pattern. They terminate in narrow, alternating bands about a third of a millimetre across in the middle layers of the cortex.

In every other sensory area, the story seems to be the same. Within the overall picture-map, the individual nerve cells are organised into regular columns, blobs and patches, each representing a different feature of the incoming sensory information.

The fundamental anatomical organisation of the cerebral cortex is formed before birth and some of the neurons of the visual cortex already have their ability to recognise the angles of edges before the monkey or cat has seen anything at all. But visual stimulation early in life also plays a part. Hubel and Wiesel themselves showed that, if one eye is covered, even for a short time, during the first few weeks of life, the nerve fibres carrying messages from that eye fail to make normal connections in the cortex. Equally, if a kitten grows up in a visual world consisting entirely of vertical black-and-white lines, the microscopic map in its visual cortex becomes distorted and the majority of the nerve cells respond to vertical lines with only a few detecting angles that the animal has never seen. Though sketched in its important aspects by the genes, the precise representation of reality within each sensory area may well depend on the signals received from the sense organs.

Mike Merzenich, of the University of California at San Francisco, has recently shown that the map of the skin in the somatic cortex can even change in an adult monkey, as it learns to make fine judgements with its fingers. Merzenich carefully mapped out the territory devoted to each finger, in the somatic cortex of a monkey. Then, he trained that same monkey to touch a spinning disc with one particular spot on one finger. After an hour a day of training for three months, the region of cortex devoted to that finger had expanded by about a third of a millimetre in all directions, at the expense of the representations of the neighbouring fingers. Cortical nerve cells seemed to have switched their allegiance, changing their connections so as to increase the number of cells devoted to the much-used fingertip.

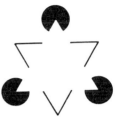

The perception of a line or edge does not always depend on the presence of a genuine light and dark boundary. This well-known illusion, discovered by the psychologist, Gaetano Kanizsa, produces a vivid impression of a central white triangle. Richard Gregory has called the edges of such shapes 'cognitive contours', since their presence is inferred from the interpretation of the meaning of the surrounding shapes.

Even at the turn of this century, anatomists had divided the vast regions outside the primary sensory areas of the cortex into a number of different zones, according to minor variations in their appearance under the microscope. Neurologists too, from time to time, described people with injuries outside those major sensory areas, who suffered from bizarre disturbances of perception, far more subtle than mere blindness or deafness. But it was not until about 1970 that physiologists and anatomists began to see that each major sensory area is surrounded by a patchwork of neighbouring regions.

There are more than twenty separate *visual* regions in the monkey's brain, stretching forward into the parietal lobe, and downward into the temporal lobe, occupying more than half of the entire surface area of the cerebral hemispheres. Each contains its own map of all or part of the visual field and each receives incoming nerve fibres from one or many of the other visual regions. Information from the eyes enters the cortex mainly through the primary visual area, but the signals then race through this array of maps, taking perhaps a twentieth of a second to sweep across the surface of the brain.

It now seems that hearing and somatic sensation also have their own arrays of secondary maps surrounding the primary region. Even the motor strip is flanked by a number of accessory motor regions that feed into it. One of the most remarkable revelations of brain research in the past twenty years is that the cerebral cortex seems very largely devoted to the analysis of sensory information and the preparation of movements.

Why should there be so many different regions of the cortex for each of the senses? What may be happening is that different aspects of the perceptual process are being handled in different maps. A grandmother, with her glowing cheeks and her blue dress, may appear to the mind's eye of her grandson as a single, fully integrated physical object. But, in fact, the outline and form of her body and face may be analysed in one set of areas, the colour of her dress and her skin in another, the three-dimensional, solid form of her in a different region, and the movements of her face and hands in yet another.

Mortimer Mishkin of the US National Institutes of Health discerns two major routes through the patchwork of visual areas: one, running forward and upward into the parietal lobe, may signal *where* things are in space and their position relative to the viewer; the other, running south into the temporal lobe, seems more concerned with *what* those objects are – their shapes, colours, movements and identities. These two functions cannot be completely separated; to know *where* something is, that object must be defined and identified. But, in terms of broad function, Mishkin's distinction has been very useful.

Semir Zeki of University College, London, who played a major part in the discovery of the multitude of visual areas, has concentrated on two of the attributes of vision-colour and movement. Each of these qualities, he argues, has its own special area or areas. Colour, for instance, seems to be analysed in a region labelled v4 (the fourth visual area), in front of the primary cortex. Many nerve cells in this region, which itself receives signals from the primary area, respond to patterns of a particular colour, regardless of their shape. Why, then, should an area of cortex be devoted to the analysis of colour when neurons in the primary area can themselves already respond selectively to the wavelength of light? Zeki has an answer that gives a clue to the value of multiple sensory representations. If a white piece of paper is illuminated with orange light (the light of the setting sun, for instance) it reflects those longer wavelengths. But it still *appears* white. Somehow, the brain is able to take account of the *overall* pattern of illumination of the scene in order to decide the real colours of objects. The colour-sensitive neurons in the primary visual area cannot perform this process of 'colour constancy'; they simply respond according to the range of wavelengths reflected from any surface. But, as Zeki has shown, the cells of v4 respond selectively to the *true* colours of surfaces, regardless of the light illuminating the scene. They seem to be capable (like a whole human being) of *comparing* the wavelength reflected from one point with the overall range of wavelengths reflected from the surrounding region.

A neighbouring cortical area, which Zeki calls v5, seems more concerned with the detection of motion, each cell responding preferentially to a different *direction* of movement of an object. Neurons in the primary area also respond to individual moving edges, but those in v5 are able to take into account all the different components in a complex textured pattern and to derive from them the true direction of the object of which those components form a part.

Vision starts with pinpricks of light and dark in the retinal image. Yet that simple information is analysed and re-analysed, again and again, to squeeze from it the last drops of knowledge about the outside world.

The very evolution of intelligence may have involved the piece-meal addition of extra sensory regions of cortex. The cerebral hemispheres of a mouse are very small – not only because each individual area is tiny, but because it has *fewer* sensory areas. The humble hedgehog has an eye and a retinal image not too different from that of a monkey, but presumably it *knows* much less about the visual world, because it has only two visual areas rather than twenty or more. Each new visual area added to the growing array during evolution may have provided an extra quantum of understanding.

With the discovery of this patchwork of visual areas covering the entire back half of the cerebral hemispheres came new insight into those strange syndromes of brain damage that had been reported in the past. Josef Zihl, a neuropsychologist in Munich, has recently been studying a woman who suffered a small stroke in the general area of the movement region v5 on both sides of her brain. She can see objects perfectly well, recognise them, see their colours and judge their distances. However, she seems almost totally incapable of perceiving *movement*: as she pours tea from a teapot into a cup, the stream of liquid appears to her 'to be frozen, like a glacier'. The level of tea in her cup does not visibly *rise*; it merely changes from empty to full. Damage lower in the occipital lobe, again on both sides of the brain, can produce a condition called achromatopsia, in which the perception of shape and movement are quite normal but the world appears virtually without colour. These extraordinary examples of disintegration of perception teach us that our apparently unified and instantaneous perception of the world is in fact an incredibly complex *parallel* analysis of the separate components of the scene.

The man on the doorstep sees his grandmother in a single glance, but his brain creates that understanding by first breaking down her image into its component shapes, distances, colours and movements. The same is probably true of our perception of sound. Separate regions of the brain may tell the man the *direction* from which the sound of her voice is coming and the pitches and changes of tone that make up the sounds she utters.

• PUTTING THE • PICTURE TOGETHER

How then is our perception unified? What part of the brain, if any, plays the role of Descartes's pineal gland in our modern view of the mechanism of perception? There is no clear answer to that and it is not even certain what would be needed to put the picture back together. To follow the line of argument originally proposed by Horace Barlow, one might expect to find a region of the brain in which individual neurons respond only when a particular, familiar *object* appears in the visual scene. Thus, the man might recognise his grandmother by having in his brain one or more nerve cells that respond to the sight of her and her alone. Indeed, this kind of theory has become known as the 'grandmother cell' hypothesis.

Attractive though this idea seems, it raises enormous logical problems. For one thing, with so much of the cerebral cortex now known to be dedicated to the *disintegration* of the image, are there sufficient numbers of neurons remaining for every distinguishable object that a person could recognise to have its own neuron or neurons? Also, what exactly constitutes an object? If the man's grandmother has a cell to herself in his brain, what about her gingham dress, her grey hair, her shoes and her nose? These are all individual *things*, to which the man could give a name. Would each individual *part* of an object have its own nerve cell, as well as the object itself? Then, the biggest difficulty of all: an object remains a recognisable object when it is viewed from different directions, at different distances and under different illumination. The man would recognise his grandmother whether she was sitting or standing, whatever clothes she was wearing and even if he saw her in a distant crowd. The retinal *image* of her would be quite different under each of these circumstances. How could a single nerve cell be able to adjust its connections so flexibly and so rapidly that it could respond to any view of the grandmother, yet not to anything else?

Though we do not yet know exactly *how* objects are recognised, we do at least have a good idea *where* the process of recognition takes place; it is probably in the lower part of the temporal lobe, below the auditory areas. When Wilder Penfield stimulated this region in conscious human beings, it often provoked strange hallucinations of complex objects or even entire scenes. Damage in the back part of this region in monkeys interferes with their ability to recognise objects; and injury further forward impedes their ability to *remember* visual tasks.

Some years ago, Charlie Gross, at Princeton University, began to describe the properties of nerve cells recorded in this region. Many do respond to visual stimulation and some also to sound or touch. Although most of the neurons can be stimulated with relatively simple patterns of moving lines presented almost anywhere in the visual field, Gross described a few that seemed to prefer complex shapes, such as the outline of a monkey's hand, or even solid objects. More recently Edmund Rolls and his colleagues at Oxford have shown that a substantial fraction of neurons, clustered in one region of the lower temporal cortex, respond fairly selectively to views of *faces*. Such neurons respond little, if at all, to simple patterns of lines or dots, but burst into activity when the monkey is presented with a photograph or even a line drawing of a human or monkey face. Some prefer full-face views, others profiles. Some respond strongly to one *particular* familiar face, others have little preference.

It is tempting to think that such neurons are well on the way to being 'grandmother cells', but nothing described so far has the selectivity, combined with an ability to tolerate variations in viewing distance and angle, that would be required of a true object-detecting cell. Indeed, recently, Rolls has shown that these neurons can change their properties as a monkey learns to recognise a new face and he suggests that, even for this highly specialised group of neurons, the information that allows the animal to distinguish one face from another is distributed over vast populations of neurons.

For social animals, such as monkeys and people, it is hard to imagine a more essential skill than distinguishing one face from another. Perhaps,

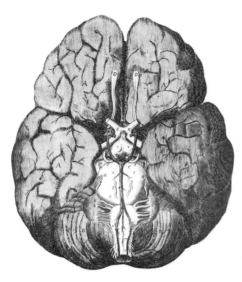

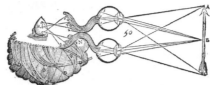

In the Traité de l'Homme *of 1664 René Descartes shows the image formed on the retina inside the eye and the corresponding 'maps' of activity on the surface of the ventricles and on the mysterious pineal gland (above). In the same year, Thomas Willis published the* Cerebri Anatome, *in which he proposed that the tissue of the cerebral hemispheres was responsible for perception, memory and intelligence. This illustration from the book (left), showing the undersurface of the human brain, was drawn by Willis's assistant. This young man was another eminent anatomist who was also Professor of Astronomy at Oxford, founded the science of meteorology, did pioneering research on insects and was called the foremost geometer of his time by Isaac Newton. He was also rather a good architect – his name was Christopher Wren!*

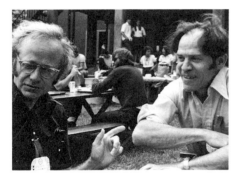

David Hubel and Torsten Wiesel (left centre), with records (below left), photographed from an oscilloscope, showing the impulses recorded from a single nerve cell in a monkey's primary visual cortex. A black line of different orientations, as shown by the bars on the left side, was moved back and forth across the screen in front of the animal. The nerve cell responded strongly to an oblique line but not to a vertical or horizontal one. Beyond the primary visual area, different visual regions in the cortex may be concerned with analysing different aspects of the visual stimulus. One region, in the temporal lobe, contains cells that respond specifically to faces. Aled Jeffreys, from Keele University in England, recorded brainwaves (below right) from this region in the human brain, in response to various pictures, shown on the left. The pictures were flashed on a screen for the

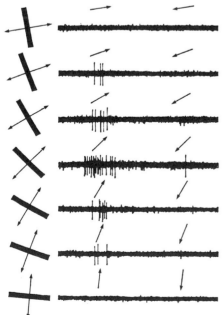

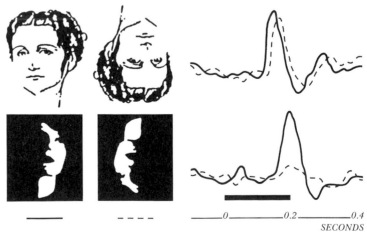

SECONDS

period of time corresponding to the thick horizontal bar below the brainwave traces. For a recognisable drawing of a face (upper row) there was a clear response, whether the face was upright or upside down (dotted line), but for the silhouette (lower row) only the upright version produced a response (continuous line); the inverted one, unrecognisable as a face, produced no specific brainwave.

then, it is no surprise that the important task of recognising faces has its own group of neurons and its own specialised region of the brain. David Perrett, who was formerly a student of Edmund Rolls and is now at the University of St Andrews, believes that the region of the temporal cortex within which the face-sensitive cells are found has as its general function the detection and classification of other animals moving in the field of view. He finds there cells that respond preferentially to the sight of a human being walking naturally in a particular direction across the visual field.

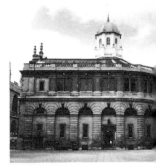

The Sheldonian Theatre in Oxford, Wren's second major building, was designed in 1663, the same year that he drew the illustrations for Willis's book.

• THE RIGHT SIDE •
OF THE BRAIN

A French lady, Paulette, sits watching slides on a screen in the office of Michel Poncet, a neuropsychologist working in Marseilles. On the screen flashes a full-face photograph of that best known of all Frenchmen, General de Gaulle, complete with the familiar peaked cap and military uniform. 'I'm searching for his name,' says Paulette. 'How old is he?' asks Dr Poncet. 'Over seventy. He has a little moustache and inquisitive eyes, with a mocking look.' She describes him perfectly but she has no idea who he is. She cannot recognise a slide showing the face of Dr Poncet himself, even though he is sitting next to the screen. Paulette had a stroke several years ago and she now has an extraordinary condition called prosopagnosia – an inability to recognise faces. This strange condition is associated with damage around the region occupied by face-sensitive neurons in the monkey brain.

Although the most obvious symptom of prosopagnosia (and the most devastating in everyday life) is the inability to recognise faces, the failure of understanding is often broader and applies to many tasks in which members of a large category must be separately recognised. For instance, people with prosopagnosia may have difficulty distinguishing different makes of car, even though they can recognise that they are all cars. It is as if the process of visual perception works rather like a dictionary in which the world is first divided into general groups, such as 'cars', and those are then subdivided into their component members, such as 'Ford', 'Rolls Royce', 'Honda'. Then, there may be even further sub-classifications – 'Sierra', 'Escort', 'Fiesta', etc. Damage to the brain may affect some step in this process of classification.

The similarity between perception and the *naming* of things is, perhaps, no coincidence. It could be that our understanding of the world, which we express through language, is derived from the description of the world created by the process of perception. Human language may have evolved as a final expressive step in the perceptual process of classifying and describing the world.

From the experiments on monkeys, there is no hint that the visual areas covering the back of the brain differ significantly between the right and left hemispheres. The whole structure seems to be quite symmetrical. Each hemisphere is simply concerned with the opposite half of the body and the opposite half of the visual field. Though we are entirely unaware of it, an invisible seam runs through the middle of our perceptual world dividing it into two halves, each the responsibility of a different side of the brain.

But in human beings there are, beyond the primary visual cortex, huge differences between the two hemispheres. Prosopagnosia, for instance, usually occurs only if there is extensive damage in the *right* hemisphere. In the normal brain, the two hemispheres are connected together by the corpus callosum, a huge cable of millions of fibres. These rich interconnections ensure that both temporal lobes have access to information from *both* sides of the visual field. It seems as if regions on the right side of the brain may be responsible for recognising the overall outline and pattern of a face, whereas those on the left side may be more concerned with detecting small details on that face.

Damage on the right side can also interfere quite selectively with the ability to recognise that two photographs of the same object, from different points of view, represent the same thing. Elizabeth Warrington, a neuro-psychologist working at the Institute of Neurology in London, has suggested that the right hemisphere contains a file of 'structural descriptions' of objects, allowing things to be recognised when seen from different directions, at different distances or under different lighting conditions.

Another difference in emphasis between the two hemispheres emerges when we look at that northerly route through the visual areas – the 'where pathway' that heads towards the parietal lobe. Vernon Mountcastle and his colleagues at Johns Hopkins University in Baltimore have spent many years studying the responses of nerve cells in the parietal lobe, recorded in awake monkeys trained to make hand and eye movements. The rear part of the parietal lobe is known to have strong connections with various structures in the brain concerned with movement, including the motor areas of cortex in the frontal lobe. This region, in the view of Mountcastle, is concerned with planning reactions to objects and events in the animal's own 'extra-personal space' – the area within reach of its hands. In monkeys, there seems to be no difference between the functions of the parietal lobe on the two sides of the brain, but in humans, damage to the *right* parietal lobe usually has much more dramatic consequences than injury to the left.

In 1967, Anton Raederscheidt, a well-known artist, had a stroke that involved his right parietal lobe. The paintings that he executed over the following few months give an insight into the disturbance of his perceptual world. He suffered a condition called hemifield neglect, a common consequence of injury to the right parietal lobe. The left side of space simply ceased to exist for him. He was not *blind* on the left, as he would have been if his right primary visual cortex had been injured; he simply *ignored* the left-hand side of everything that he saw. His first self-portrait after the stroke was little more than a few brush strokes drawn on the far right-hand side of a piece of paper, showing only the right-hand side of a face – one eye, half a mouth. Gradually, as Raederscheidt recovered a little from the effects of the stroke, he was able to force himself to add more of the left side of everything that he drew, though the right and left sides of the face that he painted still differed enormously. This strange condition of neglect seems, in the view of many neurologists, to be a defect of *attention*, as if the victim has lost interest in half of the world. Some of these patients even ignore the left-hand side of their own body and deny that it belongs to them. As they lie in bed they may constantly turn towards the right side – the focus of their remaining attention - until they roll off the edge of the bed.

• THE TWO BRAINS •

As methods have advanced for the analysis of function in the living human brain – brain scans, brainwave techniques, analysis of the result of damage – it has become increasingly clear that the anatomical similarity of the two sides of the brain belies their functional differences. The right side is more concerned with analysing the spatial arrangement of things in the world, recognising objects, appreciating music and, perhaps, in determining emotional reactions. But the left hemisphere, in the vast majority of people, is dominant for speech and, indeed, for most aspects of language.

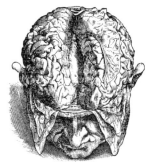

In this illustration from De Fabrica *(1543) by Andreas Vesalius, the corpus callosum ('L') is visible, joining together the two cerebral hemispheres.*

A relatively simple clinical test, often undertaken before a decision is made about brain surgery, amply demonstrates these differences in function. The test, the Wada test, involves the injection of a short-acting anaesthetic, sodium amytal, into the carotid artery on one side of the neck. This artery supplies blood to much of the cerebral hemisphere on that same side of the brain. The patient lies, fully conscious, on a bed and is asked, before the injection, to raise both arms and to start counting backwards. The anaesthetic is injected into the left carotid artery and, within seconds, the right arm flops on to the bed. In 95 per cent of right-handers and in more than half of left-handers too, the patient also stops counting and indeed remains speechless for several minutes.

Without doubt, the most dramatic demonstration of the division of labour in the cerebral hemispheres has come from a small group of patients in the United States, who have had the corpus callosum joining the two hemispheres completely cut through, in order to prevent the spread of severe epilepsy from one side of the brain to the other. These 'split-brain' patients, studied originally by Roger Sperry and Michael Gazzaniga, then at the California Institute of Technology in Pasadena, have two half-brains, each seeing and feeling the opposite half of the world and each working more or less independently, though sharing the same body.

The right hemisphere, though usually mute, has control over the left hand. The left hemisphere not only regulates the right hand but can also *speak*. Michael Gazzaniga, now at Dartmouth Medical College in New Hampshire, believes that the left side of the brain, with its mastery over language, has also been given (at least in a normal, whole person) the ultimate task of interpreting perception and deciding on action:

> There's some final system, which I happen to think is in the left hemisphere, that pulls all this information together into a *theory*. It has to generate a theory to explain all of these independent elements; and that theory becomes our particular theory of ourself and of the world.

The allocation of different functions to the two hemispheres of the brain can be seen as an evolutionary advance similar to the addition of extra areas for different aspects of each of the senses. Rather than wasting space by duplicating functions on the two sides of the brain, hemispheric specialisation makes it possible to squeeze more functions into the same space. It can, then, be seen as a further step along the road of intelligence.

• THE MOST DIFFICULT TASK •

When we look now at present-day maps of the cerebral cortex and compare them with the pictures of a century ago, it is as if an unknown continent has been largely explored and surveyed. Those 'association' areas, which were supposed to be responsible for the highest achievements of human intellect and thought, have now shrunk to a few strips of no-man's land between the vast territories occupied by the senses. Here is a lesson from the very anatomy of the brain; to use our senses to understand the world is much the most difficult thing that we do with our brains.

The complexity of perception is something that has been discovered the hard way by computer scientists attempting to make machines that can see or hear. Despite more than thirty years of effort, the most sophisticated robot vision systems, complete with their television cameras and mighty computers, are little better than a newborn child – and nowhere near as fast – in their ability to understand the things that they see.

David Marr, a brilliant mathematician from Cambridge, who

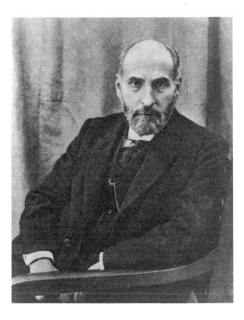

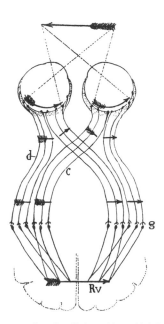

LEFT *The great Spanish neuro-anatomist Santiago Ramón y Cajal (1852–1934) was one of the giants of brain research. His diagram (right) of 1899 shows the way in which roughly half the nerve fibres from each eye cross over to the other side of the brain, so that each cerebral hemisphere receives visual information from the opposite half of the visual field.*

Visual perception is extraordinarily efficient. No artificial vision system, however enormous its computer, could recognise the dalmatian dog in this photograph (left).

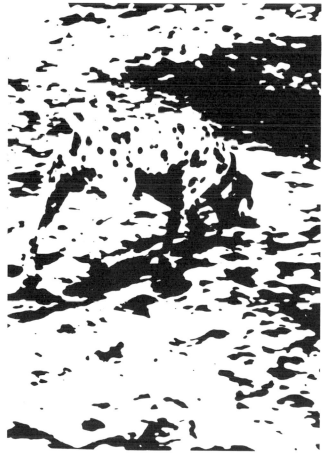

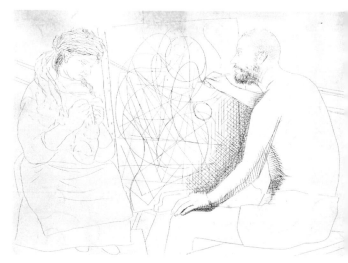

Painter with a Model Knitting (*1927*)
by Pablo Picasso. Perception, like art, is a matter of interpretation, not just making a direct picture of the outside world.

became interested in the brain in the late 1960s, had great insight into the sheer difficulty of vision. He taught us that vision is an immensely challenging *task* (or more accurately many different tasks) that can be defined in terms of essential operations, which could, in principle, be carried out by any machine. Marr saw that the problem of vision is basically one of reversing the optical process that forms the retinal image in the first place. The characteristics of the flat image must somehow be used to *compute* the shapes, distances, colours and movements of the solid objects in space that gave rise to those images.

But in order to synthesise that theory about the world, which we call perception, the brain must also apply its pre-existing knowledge of the nature of the world to the interpretation of the particular images and sounds that bombard it. Indeed, we use our general knowledge – our expectations and our prejudices based on previous experience – to *modify* our very sensations. When a person walks towards you, the image constantly expands on your retina, but you see the person as remaining the same size – person-size – because you apply your knowledge of the physical properties of people (particularly the fact that they do not change size rapidly) to your interpretation of the image.

As the great German nineteenth-century physicist Hermann von Helmholtz recognised, perception is even more than the difficult job of decomposing images and sounds. It is a process of 'unconscious inference' in which the true properties and names of things in the world are derived by analysis of signals from the senses combined with the application of the knowledge of past experience.

It would be fascinating to know, today, what Thomas Willis and René Descartes would think of our state of understanding of the cerebral cortex. Modern neurophysiology has not solved the paradox of Descartes, but perhaps the current attempt to produce artificial seeing systems will teach us how the brain can use information from the senses to guide the thoughts, the language and the actions of a person, without an internal set of eyes to look at the pictures within.

As John Ruskin wrote in his book *Modern Painters*, in 1856:

> The greatest thing a human soul ever does is to see something, and to tell what it saw in a plain way.... To see clearly is poetry, prophecy and religion – all in one.

PAIN AND HEALING

Nearly a century ago, Sir William Osler, Professor of Medicine at Johns Hopkins University in Baltimore and then at Oxford, arguably the finest clinician of his time, wrote: 'The care of tuberculosis depends more on what the patient has in his head than what he has in his chest.' He was simply expressing what folk medicine had long assumed: that people who are depressed, stressed, lonely or bereaved, become ill more easily than those who are content. And that the reactions of body and mind to injury or disease sometimes depend as much on attitude and character as they do on medical treatment.

At the core of this folk wisdom lies personal observation, intuition and a quintessentially human belief in the power of mind over body. Countless stories and legends relate our capacity to conquer pain, even to speed the mending of broken bones and to shrink deadly tumours. But anecdotes are not data; conventional science has had a hard time verifying these observations. Until recently, most of what has passed for research into the healing power of the mind has been left to quacks and charlatans. But in the past few decades research has begun to reveal what is true – and what is not – about our perception of the mind's ability to overcome injury and illness.

But before we approach the issue of whether the mind might conquer pain and heal the body we have to think again about the relationship between body and mind. Consider the following story. It is said that Bertrand Russell once went to his dentist with a toothache. The dentist looked in his mouth and asked, 'Where does it hurt?' 'In my mind, of course,' Russell answered. Russell's pain was real to him – real because

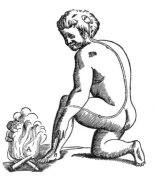

Descartes thought that the withdrawal of the body from a painful stimulus was an automatic response mediated by nerves connecting the skin to the brain and from the brain to the muscles. The sensation *of pain, however, involved the action of the signals on the soul.*

of his experience of it. The dentist might have called in a neurophysiologist to record impulses from the nerves in Russell's jaw; or a behavioural psychologist to catalogue Russell's reactions as the dentist poked around. But no one can measure pain itself objectively. Ultimately, we have to take Russell's word for it – a completely subjective account, buttressed, but not proved, by empirical evidence. In this respect, pain is rather different from the other senses; the things that you *see* or *hear* are also creations of the machinery of the brain, but the relationship between the physical properties of objects and the way that we perceive them is much more straightforward for vision and hearing than for pain. Ever since the time of Descartes, scientists have tried to press pain into the mould of the other senses, seeing it as a straightforward biological response to injury; but still it wriggles out of strict definition and defies a simple account in terms of cause and effect.

• THE PATHWAYS OF PAIN •

When the signals from it are fed through an amplifier and loudspeaker, you can actually hear the sound of a nerve in response to something that hurts. The impulses fire in a staccato burst, like a Geiger counter. Listening to it, you can almost feel someone else's pain.

In Uppsala, Sweden, Erik Torebjörk reduces the study of pain, as far as he can, to a laboratory exercise, trying to make this enigmatic sensation as reliable as the laws of physics and as predictable as a stopwatch. He comes as close as anyone can to tying pain down to nerves, chemicals and synapses. He studies the start of the pain process by implanting a tiny wire electrode into a nerve under the skin of a fully conscious volunteer. His technique allows him either to stimulate or to record from the smallest unit of a nerve bundle – a single nerve fibre whose fine endings terminate somewhere in the skin, and whose cell body lies close to the spinal cord.

Torebjörk is able to map the areas of responsibility of these tiny agents of sensation. When he *stimulates* an individual fibre in a nerve in the calf, for instance, his volunteer might feel pain over an area of skin 2 cm wide, on the top of the foot. Now, if he *records* the naturally occurring impulses in that same nerve fibre he finds that a pinprick, or the hot head of an extinguished match, sets off an angry burst of impulses if it is applied to just the same region of skin. Another fibre nearby might supply a patch of skin just next to the first area. A third fibre might be monitoring the next region of skin, and so on. The apparently seamless surface of the skin is, in reality, a patchwork of nerve endings, each waiting for the touch, the tickle, the warmth or the injury that will provoke its signals to the brain. Many of the fibres are remarkably specific in the kind of physical stimulation to which they will respond. Shake the hand of another person and different nerve fibres in your hand will inform your brain of the moment of contact, the movement of your hand, the temperature of the other hand, the force with which it grips and even the moment when that squeeze begins to hurt!

Torebjörk has found that, in the simplified conditions of the laboratory, the human brain is quite precise in its ability to convert nerve impulses into pain: 'It is the number of impulses per fibre and the number of fibres activated which will announce the amount of painful stimulus, which is then interpreted by the brain as intensity of pain.'

Two types of nerve fibre deal in the currency of pain. One set responds specifically and briefly to any damaging *mechanical* stimulation of the skin – a pinch or a pinprick for instance – but usually not to painful chemicals or heat. The other very numerous group consists of the tiniest fibres that ramify throughout the skin and almost all the internal organs of the body. They conduct their impulses very slowly; a message from the toes takes well over a second to reach the brain. These ubiquitous fibres disobey the general rule; each one responds to many different forms of stimulation – to light touch and warmth, for instance, as well as any painful stimulation. Nearly all of them respond to things that cause pain.

The existence of these two sets of fibres with very different speeds of transmission explains why the pain of an injury usually comes in two waves. As the hammer comes down on your thumb you first feel just the contact and almost simultaneously a sharp but brief stab of well-localised pain, as the larger fibres announce the injury. You have probably dropped the hammer and pulled away your hammered thumb before the next flood of pain arrives, courtesy of the smaller fibres: a nastier, longer-lasting, diffuse, deep, throbbing pain.

Impulses from the two types of fibre race up to and into the spinal cord, and on through their own pathways of interconnected nerves, through the brain to the cerebral cortex. Some of the messages reach the regions of the cortex, at the front of the parietal lobe, where the other sensations of the body are mapped out. But others end up in parts of the frontal lobe, which in turn connect with the limbic system – the network of structures at the heart of the forebrain that rules our emotions. That is the simple story; nerves, connections, reactions and sensations, all as automatic as the knee jerk or the contraction of the pupil of the eye in a bright light. But the algorithm of agony is more mysterious than that.

At first glance, Sarah Roberts from Sioux Falls, South Dakota, seems like any other seven-year-old girl. She plays happily in a room full of dolls. She is rambunctious, energetic, curious. Maybe a little too curious, for her leg is in plaster and her arm bandaged. And wherever she goes, her parents stay at her side, anxiously watching her every move. Her father explains why:

> She was something over a year old when her teeth began to loosen and eventually come out. Through a series of dentists, we finally came to the conclusion that she was biting them out. It was some time later that she had a significant burn on her foot and in treating that burn we realised that she had virtually no pain.

Sarah's parents brought her to Peter Dyck at the Mayo Medical School in Rochester, Minnesota. He diagnosed her as having a rare, congenital insensitivity to pain; Sarah had been born with 'a significant reduction' in the number of those peripheral nerves that transmit pain messages to the brain. Erik Torebjörk might say that without the full complement of nerves the information doesn't reach her brain with enough force to trigger the normal sensation of pain. As her mother says, 'As far as Sarah is concerned, there is nothing bad in her environment.'

In her short life, Sarah has burned off the tip of her right index finger; she has pushed a sharp pencil through her cheek; she has severely damaged many of the joints in her body. She must be closely watched wherever she goes. In a sense, her parents have to act as her surrogate system for pain, pulling her away from harm before she is too badly hurt. Life without pain is not the heaven that one might imagine; it is a hell with no warnings of danger. Pain is one of the most valuable aids we have in our struggle to understand what is beneficial and what is harmful in the world around us. Sarah is living (but injured) evidence that a major function of pain (or, more accurately, of our *reaction* to pain) is to help *prevent* serious injury.

• THE CONTROL OF PAIN •

But what exactly *is* pain? It is from the interpretation of the signals that we feel pain, not from the signals alone. There is an interesting paradox here. Pain is an essential sensation; without it, we would constantly risk death. But we also have the power to control and even invent it.

On 19 August 1987, Michael Ryan went to war. His was a personal campaign, the product of a twisted mind, against his fellow citizens in Hungerford, Berkshire. In his rampage through the streets of that little town he shot and killed fifteen people and injured many more. At the subsequent enquiry Jennifer Mildenhall described how she was preparing lunch for her daughter Lisa when Ryan passed by her house:

> We heard the shots, like loud cracks, and Lisa went round to the front of the house to see what was going on. Then Lisa came back into the doorway covered in blood, and the blood was running down her legs. She said: 'Have I been shot, Mummy?'

This harrowing tale reveals vividly the paradox of pain. Lisa had to *ask* if she had been shot. Why didn't her pain answer the question?

American Marine Sergeant Ken Kraus had a similar story to tell. He was stationed in the US Embassy in Tehran in February 1979 when Iranian guerrillas stormed the compound and captured 102 Americans, including Ambassador William Sullivan. Remarkably, Ken Kraus was the only American who was shot. He described his encounter with a guerrilla. 'He hit me in the chest with the gun butt and I fell to the floor. Next, I heard a blast and started to bleed.'

Again, a vivid report of the sounds and sights of the attack but not a word about the pain. It is a surprise to anyone who has not been in such a situation that in the frenzy of battle, the shock of an accident or even the excitement of a rugby match, injury goes almost unnoticed. Only afterwards, sometimes long afterwards, when the threat and stress have passed, does the victim 'allow' himself or herself to feel the pain.

H. K. Beecher described this phenomenon in his study of soldiers severely wounded during the Second World War: only one in three severely wounded men complained enough of pain to require morphine. After the war, he found that among civilians who suffered similar wounds, from voluntary surgery for instance, four out of five asked for morphine. He reached the conclusion that

> There is no simple direct relationship between the wound *per se* and the pain experienced. The pain is in very large part determined by other factors, and of great importance here is the significance of the wound.

The power to censor pain is not purely a human ability; indeed it can be even more dramatic among other animals. Of course, we cannot be *sure* that animals ever feel pain in the same way that we do, but they can certainly react *as if* in pain – with changes in heart rate, breathing and movement. However, when animals fight, they often seem to ignore terrible injuries as they get on with their strategy of attacking or fleeing to preserve their lives.

The 5th of June 1980. Derby Day. It was a thrilling race, closely contested until 300 metres from the finish, when a horse called Henbit stumbled and veered to one side, but then burst away from the rest of the field to win the race in the second fastest time in forty years. Henbit trotted proudly through to the winner's enclosure, £4 million of horse. But some minutes later he began to limp and became agitated. A vet examined him and declared that he had broken the cannon bone in his right foreleg during that stumble. He had won the Derby on a broken foot.

But there is something special about the ability of people to choose deliberately when to react to pain and when not. We can even ignore pain in pursuit of something as far from biological imperative as an artistic performance. For Lesley Collier, principal dancer with the Royal Ballet in London, strain and injury are a price she pays for her profession. She says that one key to a successful career in dance is to learn to distinguish among pains – to know when pain is caused by serious injury and when it is the outcome of asking the body to do something it wasn't really meant to do. For Collier, one of the pains she knows she must come to terms with is triggered by the *fouetté*, a dance step in which the ballerina spins on one leg. When the spin begins, the foot is flat on the floor; but as it continues, the dancer must go on point, then come down again, then push back up to her toes. Says Collier:

> Isolated, the *fouetté* is not very complicated; but in nearly every ballet, you never have to do *one fouetté*; you have to do a series. In *Swan Lake*, the series amounts to thirty-two. I've only really got to hear the *fouetté* music of *Swan Lake* (I can be anywhere; it can be on the radio while I'm driving my car) and I can really get a pain in my calf. But I think I've danced long enough to know that when one gets on stage, pain disappears, and Dr Theatre takes over.

Dr Theatre is, of course, a character in the human mind – a brave-faced disciplinarian who tells the body to bite its lip and press on despite the agony. It would be easy at this point to paint a simple picture. Somehow the heightened courage, need and expectation associated with fighting, performing or competing trigger a system to turn off the tap through which pain signals from the peripheral nerves flow to the brain.

Obligingly, science has recently discovered just such an adjustable pain tap. In 1969 neurophysiologist D. V. Reynolds reported that electrical stimulation, through a microelectrode, of the central part of the stem of a rat's brain induced analgesia as total as that produced by morphine; the animals showed no reaction of pain even during abdominal surgery. The similarity of this strange phenomenon to the pain-killing effect of morphine and other opiate drugs is no coincidence. It turns out that the analgesic effects of brainstem stimulation can be prevented by the drug naloxone, which also blocks the actions of opiates. Apparently the stimulation of the brain activates a system of nerves, some of which use as their transmitter substance the *natural* morphine-like substances, the enkephalins, which were discovered by Hans Kosterlitz in Aberdeen. Enkephalins *and* morphine act on the same specific receptor molecules in the membranes of nerve cells in the pathway for pain control. Indeed it is the imitating action of opiate drugs on this system in the brain that gives them their enormous pain-killing potency.

The pain-regulating pathway starts high in the brain, in the cerebral cortex and the hypothalamus, and it ends in a network of tiny enkephalin-containing nerve cells in the spinal cord, which can interrupt the flow of signals in from the smallest peripheral nerves. Eighteen different peptide substances with morphine-like action have now been identified in the brain, including β-endorphin, which is released from the pituitary gland directly into the bloodstream in situations of stress and which can be fifty times as potent in its pain-killing action as morphine itself.

It seems very likely that several systems producing natural opiate-like substances are employed by animals and human beings to turn off the tap of pain in moments of life-threatening danger. They may also be used by ballet dancers and rugby players, and by the performers in a thousand different religious rituals, around the world, in which people walk on hot coals, and cut, pierce or stab themselves in trance-like states, without apparent pain. The discovery of these systems of pain control has given anatomical reality to the concept of the influence of mind over body.

The Chinese have practised acupuncture for more than 2000 years. The value of this form of therapy for the treatment of organic disease is still hotly debated, but its pain-killing effects are now well established. Moreover, the analgesia produced by acupuncture is also prevented by administration of the anti-opiate drug naloxone. It seems that the stimulation produced by the twisting needles also turns on the morphine-like systems in the brain.

• THE PAIN-PERSON •

Even more amazing than the examples of pain suppression in exceptional circumstances is the report that 37 per cent of patients admitted to the emergency clinic of a large city hospital, with unanticipated injuries as a result of accidents in everyday circumstances, said that they felt no significant pain for minutes or hours after being injured. The first reaction of a machine-shop foreman whose foot had been torn off by a falling machine was to feel embarrassed rather than in pain; 'What a fool they are going to call me to have let this happen,' he said. 'There goes my holiday.' Patrick Wall of University College, London, who has spent much of his career studying pain, suspects that the conscious perception of pain has more to do with the need for recovery and convalescence than with the immediate reaction to injury. Pain, he argues, is the response to a situation in which treatment and cure are given top priority. This idea puts pain in an entirely unexpected light: pain is the result of a positive decision in the brain, not the inevitable consequence of an injury.

The view that pain is a choice to behave in a certain way illuminates the frighteningly common phenomenon of pain without apparent organic cause. The borderline between tragedy and malingering is difficult to define, but there is no doubt that many of the patients who fill the consulting rooms of pain clinics have chronic pains that dominate their lives, leaving them disabled, incapable of caring for themselves, yet without any injury or disease that could explain such suffering. They have become, in the words of Patrick Wall, 'pain-people'.

Fran Brooks was a 'pain-person'. A series of accidents in the early 1980s damaged her back, her shoulder and her legs. The damaged tissues healed, but Fran continued to feel the pain. In September 1987 she entered the Pain Clinic at the University of Washington in Seattle, which is run by John Loeser, a neurologist, and Wilbert Fordyce, a psychologist. Fordyce disagrees with the sceptics who doubt the validity of chronic pain without an obvious physical basis:

> Patients who come to a programme like this are clearly suffering. People will ask: 'Is the pain real?' That's a nonsense question. Of course the pain is real. The proper question is: 'Why is the person suffering?'

Not everybody responds to this clinic's particular regime of physical and psychological therapy, but Fran Brooks seemed a promising case. She was an anxious person, easily upset, who concentrated on her pain and was frightened by it. She tended to confuse anxiety, depression and fear with pain, and to exacerbate the pain by focusing on her state of suffering. Fordyce also believed that Fran might have acquired her chronic pain by overprotecting herself – by guarding the sites of injury too zealously, and under-using them, prolonging the expectation of healing. Fordyce and Loeser predicted that simply putting the painful areas to work again would ease her pain.

On Fran's first day at the clinic they tested her by having her walk as fast as she could down a hallway. She moved haltingly, limping badly. It took 56 seconds for her to move the short distance. For three weeks, Fran went through a demanding series of sessions of stretching, exercise and psychotherapy aimed at changing her awareness of pain. Gradually, she began to confront the true issue: that she might be in pain because she *expected* to suffer. And the physical therapy began to pay off. Her range of motion and strength increased and her pain began to dim. Finally, treatment was complete. Fran's family came to participate in the final day. And at the end, a repeat of the first day's test; the walk down the hallway. This time, there was no limp, no halting, no danger of falling. Fran's time was just 19 seconds. It is rare for a patient to leave the clinic completely cured of pain, but almost without exception, they finish the programme able to do more than they could when they began.

• THE PROMISE OF PLEASING •

The importance of expectation in our responses to pain and treatment for disease can be seen most clearly in a phenomenon known as the placebo effect (from the Latin meaning 'I will please'). A placebo is an inactive medication – a sugar pill, for instance – used to treat a disorder. But in a broader sense it describes anything without inherent healing properties that nevertheless combats illness. Many forms of primitive and unconventional medicine, faith-healing and, probably, some kinds of psychotherapy depend largely on the placebo effect. In each case the process seems the same; if the patient *believes* he or she is being helped, that belief triggers a healing response, which can be as powerful as more conventional therapies.

The placebo's effectiveness has been acknowledged in folklore for centuries. In the sixteenth century Michel de Montaigne wrote.

> Why do doctors begin by practising on the credulity of their patients with so many false promises of a cure, if not to call the powers of the imagination to the aid of their fraudulent concoctions? They know ... that there are men on whom the mere sight of medicine is operative.

Nevertheless, conventional medicine used to look on the placebo effect with scepticism. But nowadays it is seen as a potent contribution to therapy, with an explanation in the chemistry of the brain.

Jon Levine, at the University of California in San Francisco, is trying to discover how simple belief can alleviate pain. He works with healthy volunteers who have just had their wisdom teeth extracted. They are all told that they are going to be given intravenous injections to reduce their pain but in fact they receive only saline injections. Levine divided the suffering students into two groups. Half of them are given their placebo injections by an automatic pump controlled by a computer, without a doctor or a nurse in sight. The other half are injected by Levine himself, with all the ritual of attention that Sir William Osler knew is so important. Levine explains:

> I go in with my white coat on. I have a stethoscope in my pocket. I have the medicine drawn up in a big syringe. And I make sure that the patient sees me administering the medication. I think the white coat in this

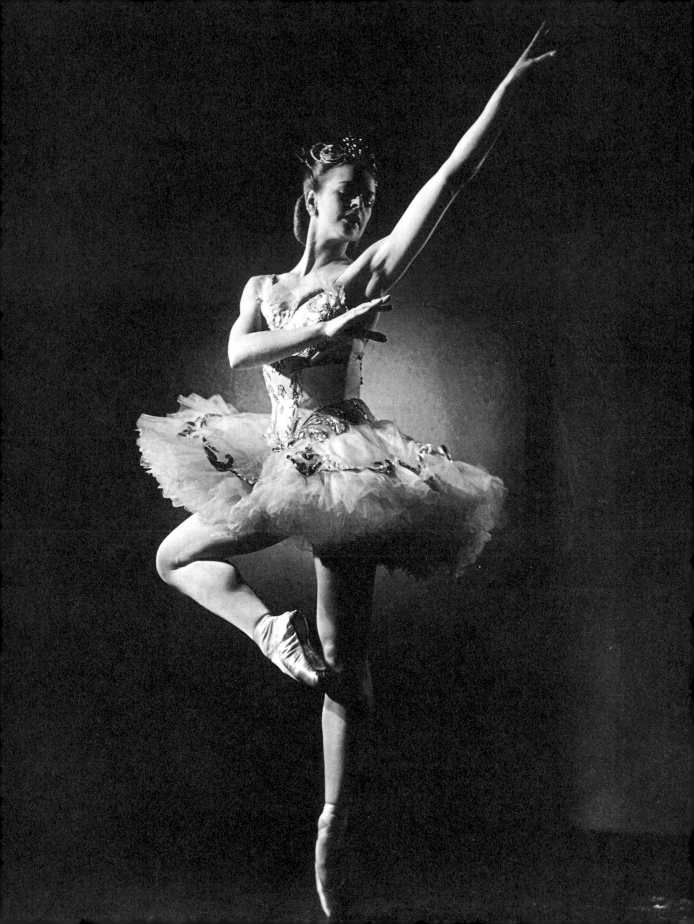

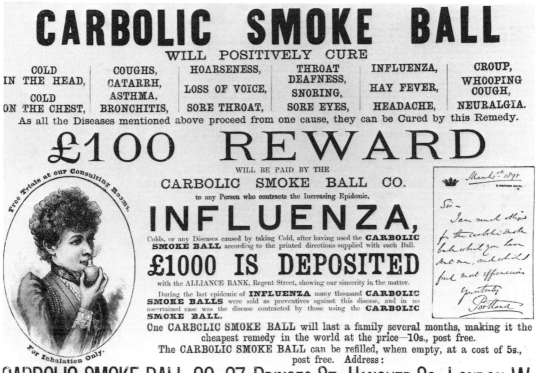

CARBOLIC SMOKE BALL

WILL POSITIVELY CURE

| COLD IN THE HEAD, COLD ON THE CHEST, | COUGHS, CATARRH, ASTHMA, BRONCHITIS, | HOARSENESS, LOSS OF VOICE, SORE THROAT, | THROAT DEAFNESS, SNORING, SORE EYES, | INFLUENZA, HAY FEVER, HEADACHE, | CROUP, WHOOPING COUGH, NEURALGIA. |

As all the Diseases mentioned above proceed from one cause, they can be Cured by this Remedy.

£100 REWARD

WILL BE PAID BY THE

CARBOLIC SMOKE BALL CO.

to any Person who contracts the Increasing Epidemic,

INFLUENZA,

Colds, or any Diseases caused by taking Cold, after having used the **CARBOLIC SMOKE BALL** according to the printed directions supplied with each Ball.

£1000 IS DEPOSITED

with the ALLIANCE BANK, Regent Street, showing our sincerity in the matter.

During the last epidemic of **INFLUENZA** many thousand **CARBOLIC SMOKE BALLS** were sold as preventives against this disease, and in no ascertained case was the disease contracted by those using the **CARBOLIC SMOKE BALL.**

One CARBOLIC SMOKE BALL will last a family several months, making it the cheapest remedy in the world at the price—10s., post free.

The CARBOLIC SMOKE BALL can be refilled, when empty, at a cost of 5s., post free. Address:

CARBOLIC SMOKE BALL CO., 27, PRINCES ST., HANOVER SQ., LONDON, W.

Free Trials at our Consulting Rooms.

For Inhalation Only.

OPPOSITE *Pamela May as Princess Aurora in* The Sleeping Beauty. *The pain of dancing on points may be suppressed by the action of the internal pain-controlling pathways in the brain.*

ABOVE *The 'placebo' effect of medication without truly effective ingredients also depends on the pain-suppressing system since it is abolished by administration of the drug naloxone, which blocks enkephalin receptors. Conceivably, even faith-healing (right) might depend on similar effects.*

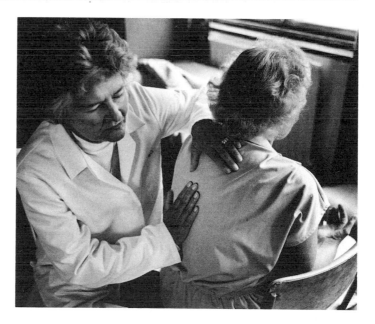

culture – as, say, a mask in an African culture – represents to the patient an image of an individual who has the power to provide a healing effect.

The volunteers were asked to judge their level of pain on a numerical scale, which revealed striking differences between the two groups. Those who were ministered to by the faceless computer had little alleviation of pain. But those who had the personal care of a doctor suffered much less.

Once again, those morphine-like substances produced by the brain itself are implicated in this vivid example of the power of the doctor-patient relationship. Naloxone, the drug that blocks morphine, also prevents the pain-killing effect of a placebo! A good doctor is able to use not only his own medical skills but also the chemistry of his patient's brain.

• STRESS AND ILLNESS •

The influences of expectation, emotion and arousal on the perception of pain are remarkable, but at least they can be understood in terms of influences within the nervous system itself. But what of the possibility that mental states can be communicated to the rest of the body and change its state of health? The idea that events in a person's life can affect their well-being began to achieve the status of scientific respectability in the 1930s. The psychiatrist Adolf Meyer introduced the concept of 'life events' – deaths, disappointments and problems – as factors contributing to psychiatric disease. Around the same time, Hans Selye began a series of experiments on the effects of long-term stress. The natural environment of an animal in the wild is full of problems that we would call stressful – the attacks of predators, shortages of food, extremes of climate. In such situations, the brain acts on the body to enable it to cope: endorphins, released from the pituitary gland, help the animal to avoid pain; adrenaline and noradrenaline, produced as a result of activity in the nerves reaching the central core of the adrenal gland, tone up the heart and direct blood towards the muscles; another hormone from the pituitary stimulates the outer rind of the adrenal glands to produce corticosteroid hormones, which help to mobilise reserves of fat and carbohydrate in the body.

All of these reactions are protective, indeed essential, for an animal in a demanding situation. They can, though, become dangerous under conditions of prolonged stress.

Doubtless, our hominid ancestors had to deal with horrific experiences from time to time, but modern life can place *chronic* demands on people, holding them in a constant state of stressful crisis: an air-traffic controller for whom each blip on the radar screen is hundreds of lives in his hands; a manager whose day-to-day decisions determine the fate of the company; workers who live under threat of redundancy; husbands and wives whose marriages are on the rocks. In such people, the bodily machinery of crisis creaks under the everyday load of stress.

As early as 1949, stress was implicated as a causal factor in diseases of growth and metabolism, in diseases of the eye, the lungs, the stomach, the intestines, the skin, muscles and joints, in headache and, most of all, in heart disease. It is now widely accepted that the stress of losing a loved one through death or divorce leads to an increased rate of pneumonia, tuberculosis and even cancer. Even more certain is the adverse effect that stress has on the *recovery* from disease.

William Mason, at the California Primate Research Center in Davis, California, discovered that the different personalities of two species of South American monkey seemed to cause them both to react badly, but dissimilarly, to the stress of isolation during quarantine. Squirrel monkeys are inquisitive and excitable; they have very fast heart rates and high levels of corticosteroid in their blood. Titi monkeys, by comparison, are shy and placid; their heart rates and corticosteroid levels are low. During stress, squirrel monkeys, like over-ambitious 'type A' people, are prone to high blood pressure and heart disease. By comparison, over half of the titi monkeys succumbed to pneumonia or intestinal infections during quarantine. For some reason, stress made them less able to fend off disease.

In the extreme, the brain even seems capable of terminating the life of its own body. Shock, depression and extreme fear can precipitate sudden death without obvious organic cause. In parts of Australia, the Caribbean, South America and Africa, the curse of a Shaman or witch-doctor can cause such 'voodoo death'. Such rare, rapid but dramatic effects of stress and fear are probably mediated through the brain's action on the heart. But research of the past few years has revealed a more subtle influence of the brain on the immune defence system of the body.

• LEARNING NOT TO COPE •

In the 1960s, Martin Seligman and Steven Maier, working at the University of Pennsylvania, coined the term 'learned helplessness' to describe the condition of animals that become submissive and even ill when put in situations in which they are not in control of their environments. Maier, now at the University of Colorado in Boulder, believes that this reaction is partly due to a suppressive influence of the brain on the animal's own immune defence system. He uses a very simple social challenge to examine the effects of loss of control. Two male rats, on excellent terms after living with each other for several weeks in their cage, are suddenly disturbed by a stranger, slipped into the cage by Maier. At first, the rats all explore each other. Then, invariably, one of the established males attacks the intruder, briefly but firmly. Most intruders give up very quickly and they are seldom injured. The invader simply flops on his back, legs in the air, offering no resistance. Within seconds, the fighting is over and he is allowed to get up and to move around the cage. But despite the apparent tranquillity of the scene, the intruder has suffered a terrible insult; he has lost his ability to control his environment. The effects on the health of such an animal can be dramatic, as Maier explains:

> The total outcome of the situation as far as physiology is concerned is determined by the way the intruder perceives the situation. It's specifically under the situation where there is no control that you see the deleterious consequences of stress. You see ulcer formation. You see a large steroid release. You see changes in metabolism. And, down the line, you see immune changes that are a result of these other changes.

The discovery that the brain can influence the immune system has led to the invention of a new discipline within brain research – psycho-neuroimmunology. The immune system is the security force of the body, patrolling it, defending it against attack. It does so through an extraordinary system of identification that allows it to distinguish between all the cells that are part of the body and any that are not. The organs of this widespread system are the thymus, lymph nodes, spleen and bone marrow; its vigilant agents are a host of white cells, including monocytes, lymphocytes, macrophages and killer cells, which wander through the blood and the tissues. They can recognise, attack and engulf invading bacteria and viruses. Certain white cells, the B lymphocytes, also produce antibodies – protein molecules that circulate in the blood, attach themselves to specific sites on invading cells and trigger various reactions that destroy them.

Until quite recently, the immune system had been viewed as a kind of privatised police force, acting to defend the body, independent of the brain and hormone systems. But evidence grows and grows that the brain can exert influence, both direct and subtle, on the agencies of the immune system. Direct control may come through the recently discovered peripheral nerves that run out to the thymus gland, the spleen, lymph nodes and bone marrow. The individual fibres spread out and ramify among the clumps of immature lymphocytes. But, in addition, various cells and components of the immune system are sensitive to the cocktail of hormones and transmitter chemicals that circulate in the blood. Corticosteroid hormones, from the adrenal gland, triggered during times of stress in response to a chemical signal from the hypothalamus of the brain, powerfully suppress the immune system. And it is now known that the surface membranes of lymphocytes, killer cells and other wandering patrollers of the immune system are studded with specific receptors that respond to the presence of various neurotransmitters in the blood, including nora-drenaline and β-endorphin, the pain-killing substance released by the pituitary gland during periods of crisis.

Steven Maier found that the activity of the crucial lymphocyte cells was reduced in rats that had learned to be helpless. At New York's Mt Sinai Hospital, Marvin Stein has detected the same kind of suppression of lymphocytes in widowers during the first year of bereavement after the deaths of their wives, and also in seriously depressed patients. Ronald Glaser and Janice Kiecolt-Glaser, at Ohio State University, have found that lymphocytes and killer cells are also sluggish and suppressed in people who are suffering the 'living bereavement' (as Kiecolt-Glaser calls it) of caring for a near relative with Alzheimer's disease. Even healthy medical students have the same kinds of reductions in immune activity during the stressful last month before their final examinations.

Animals and people can even *learn* to suppress their immune systems, through the classical conditioning procedure that Pavlov discovered. Some years ago, Robert Ader at the University of Rochester was shocked to find that some of his laboratory rats were dying for no obvious cause. On checking their records, he found that they had been involved in a conditioning experiment in which they had learned that the sweet taste of saccharin was followed by the administration of an immunosuppressive drug that made them feel nauseous. As expected, the rats had learned to avoid the saccharin, because of the learned association with the sick feeling. However, the rats that were dying were those that had started to drink the sweet water again. Ader and his colleague Nicholas Cohen found that the rats were suppressing their *own* immune responses as a result of the sweet taste, which they had learned to associate with the immuno-suppressive drug. That was the reason for the increased mortality. This bizarre phenomenon may possibly be of benefit to people who suffer from autoimmune diseases in which the patient's own immune system makes a mistake in its procedure for distinguishing between self and non-self and starts to attack the tissues of its own body. The Rochester group is now having success in teaching mice with autoimmune disease to reduce their immune attack on themselves.

Many of the experimental results in this burgeoning new field are controversial or are so small in magnitude that it is hard to believe that they are biologically important. And unfortunately the major effects of brain on immune system seem to be *suppressive*. While this may help us to understand the susceptibility to disease of people who have suffered emotional crises, it does nothing to explain the folklore that would have us believe that the mind can *heal* the body.

Last year about 4 million people visited a tiny town set in the misty foothills of the Pyrenees in south-west France. They came for their health; not because of the invigorating mountain air but because this town is Lourdes, a place of miracles and magical healing. In February, 1858, Bernadette Soubirous, the daughter of an out-of-work miller, claimed that she had seen the Virgin Mary standing in a niche, in a rocky grotto near the river Garve. Bernadette became a nun at the convent of St Gildard at Nevers, where she died in 1879. In 1933 she was proclaimed a saint.

What attracts pilgrims to Lourdes in their millions is not only the tale of Bernadette's apparitions, but the cures for which this place has become famous. Just two weeks after the first apparition a blinded stone mason who bathed his eye in the spring that Bernadette discovered found his sight miraculously restored. Bernadette herself suffered from the plague, asthma and tuberculosis, and died at the age of thirty-five. Nevertheless, thousands upon thousands of pilgrims believe that they have been cured as a result of their visits to Bernadette's town. All claims of miraculous cures are now rigorously examined by a local medical bureau and by an international committee. They apply strict criteria to distinguish between spontaneous remission or response to conventional treatment and true miracles. Sixty-four cures have been declared miraculous.

Science is not in the business of explaining miracles, but any visitor to Lourdes, whether a Roman Catholic or not, is struck by its extraordinary atmosphere and by the confidence that those millions of pilgrims have in its power. Everyone you speak to has a personal story of relief from pain or suffering. David Morrell, Professor of General Practice at St Thomas's Hospital in London, who has accompanied many groups of pilgrims from Britain, said, 'I have never known a sick person return from Lourdes who was not comforted, strengthened and happier.'

In my opinion, much of the power of Lourdes comes from the pilgrims themselves, and their families and helpers. They are bound in a fellowship of suffering, of common purpose, of belief and determination. No doubt the placebo effect is at work here too, aided by the squadrons of people in nurses' uniforms (most of them without any medical qualification, but adding enormously to the atmosphere of care and authority).

Science can start to make tentative statements about the everyday phenomenon of Lourdes, for there is growing evidence that a patient's attitude to disease can encourage the immune system and hence the powers of defence. Sandra Levy of the University of Pittsburgh describes a patient who was terminally ill with cancer in the 1950s and who was treated with a drug, Krebiozen. He underwent an amazing remission and began to lead a perfectly normal life. But soon reports appeared that Krebiozen had no therapeutic value whatever and the man immediately

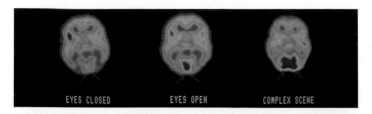

EYES CLOSED   EYES OPEN   COMPLEX SCENE

These three PET *scans show horizontal slices (forehead at the top) of the brain of a normal human volunteer. Colours indicate the degree of uptake of radioactive glucose, which is related to the level of activity of nerve cells, in different parts of the brain. Areas of high activity appear red, the least active regions blue. With closed eyes (left scan) there is very little activity in the visual areas, indicated by arrows, at the back of the brain. When the eyes are open, viewing an unstructured scene, activity is concentrated in the primary visual cortex (centre). When viewing a very complicated scene (right scan) strong activity spreads over a wider area.*

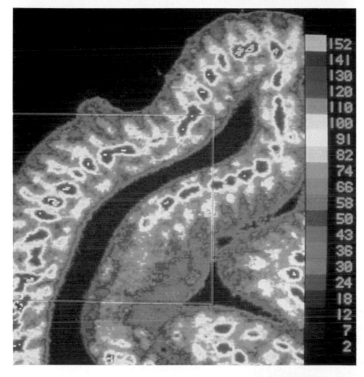

152	
141	
130	
120	
110	
100	
91	
82	
74	
66	
58	
50	
43	
36	
30	
24	
18	
12	
7	
2	

LEFT *Glucose uptake can be demonstrated in the brains of animals using a technique developed by Louis Sokoloff. After a tiny injection of a radioactive glucose derivative, a monkey viewed a normal visual scene, but with one eye covered. The glucose derivative was taken up by the most active nerve cells, revealed as red areas on this microscopic section through a fold of visual cortex. Small clusters of active cells spaced less than 1 mm apart are seen in the middle layers of the cortex, reflecting the pattern of incoming nerve fibres carrying information from the open eye. The gaps between these active regions are filled by relatively inactive fibres from the closed eye.*

RIGHT *Gary Blasdel made this computer reconstruction of a patch, about 5 mm across, of the surface of the primary visual cortex of a monkey, which had been stained with a dye that reacts when nerve cells fire impulses. Different patterns of lines, indicated by the coloured bars on the right, were moved in front of the animal's eyes, while a video camera viewed the surface of the cortex. Columns of nerve cells activated by the different orientations are shown as corresponding patches of colour.*

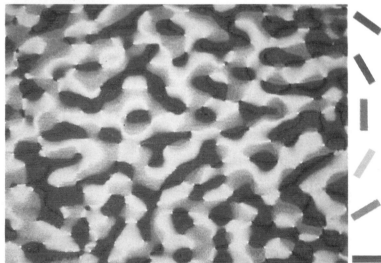

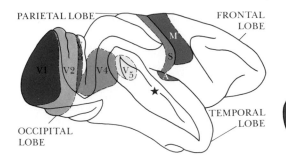

PARIETAL LOBE

FRONTAL LOBE

V1 V2 V4 V5 M S A

OCCIPITAL LOBE

TEMPORAL LOBE

Much of the primate cerebral hemispheres consist of a patchwork of sensory and motor areas, including more than twenty visual areas occupying about 60 per cent of the cortex. The picture above is of the right hemisphere of the primate brain (frontal lobe to the right), with some of the deep folds opened up, showing a few of the major visual areas, including the primary visual cortex (V1). The diagram on the right represents the entire hemisphere unfolded and flattened; all the areas concerned with vision are shown in shades of red and yellow, auditory areas (A) in green, somatic areas, dealing with touch, etc., (S) in blue, and areas controlling movement (M) in grey.

Some neurons in V1 respond selectively to reflected light, but those in V4 are often sensitive to the perceived colour of surfaces. Semir Zeki exposed different patches of colour within a 'Mondrian' pattern (below) to nerve cells whose impulses appear on the traces. The reflected light was made identical (containing more red light than green and blue) for every patch in turn. A red-sensitive cell in V1 (below left) responded to all the patches, detecting only the reflected mixture of light. But the cell in V4 (below right) responded strongly only to the true red surface.

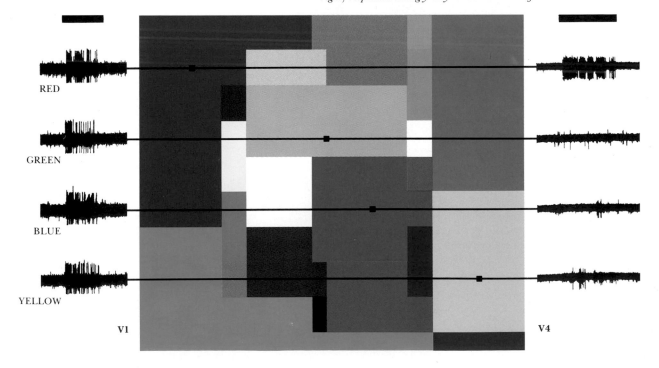

RED

GREEN

BLUE

YELLOW

V1

V4

The paintings of Anton Raederscheidt, made during the year following a stroke in 1967, reveal the
gradual but incomplete recovery of
his 'hemifield neglect'. The stroke
damaged Raederscheidt's right parietal lobe, producing a bizarre disturbance of space perception in which
the left half of any object seemed to
be missing. Raederscheidt was not
blind in the conventional sense, but
he ignored the left side of anything
that he viewed, even the image of his
own face in a mirror.

These self-portraits (from left to
right) show the initial virtual
absence of the left side of the image,
followed by progressive improvement
in the detail of that side of the face.

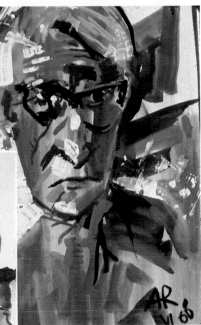

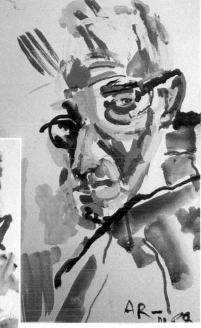

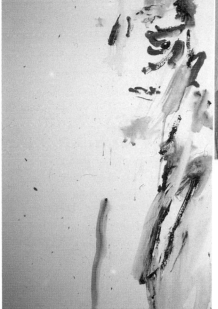

However, even in the final portrait,
executed a year after the stroke, the
two sides of the face are painted in
very different styles.

In January 1986, an American artist
'Jonathan I' was involved in a car accident
and suffered a head injury, which probably
damaged part of the visual regions at the back
of his brain. As a result, he is now virtually
colour blind. He painted these pieces of
fruit grey, except for a single orange, to
illustrate the appearance of his visual
world (right).

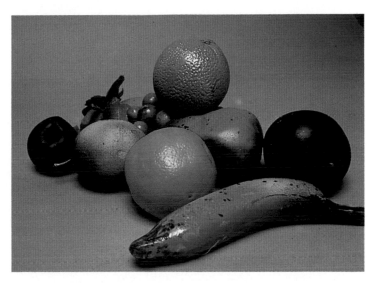

Firewalking at Madras, India, in 1908. Walking on hot embers is practised in many parts of the world as part of religious ceremonies and rites of initiation. Sometimes the participants achieve a trance-like state, by chanting or dancing beforehand. Conceivably, this may help to switch on the pain-suppressing systems in their brains. But also, if the pace of the walk is brisk enough, the contact with the coals may not be sufficient to burn the feet at all.

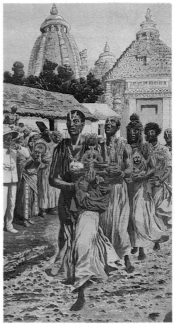

BELOW *The Barber Surgeon by Heinman Dullaert (1636–1684). Until the development of anaesthetics, surgery must have been a horrifying experience.*

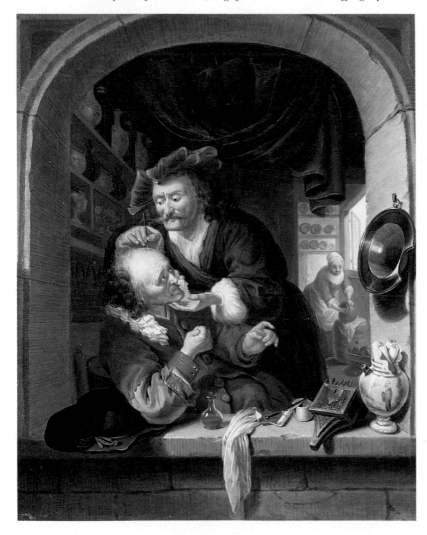

The power to control pain may depend on several systems in the brain. Acupuncture (opposite, top) can certainly produce analgesia and this effect is blocked by naloxone, a drug that also interferes with the action of morphine. Acupuncture probably influences the brain's own pain-suppressing system involving the enkephalins and other peptide substances produced by nerve cells. Lying on a bed of nails (opposite, centre) may also involve this morphine-like system in the brain. The placebo effect, which may play an important part in primitive treatment of disease (near right), is also prevented by naloxone. On the other hand, the reduction of pain by hypnosis (far right) probably works by a different mechanism, since that effect is not blocked by naloxone.

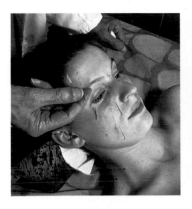

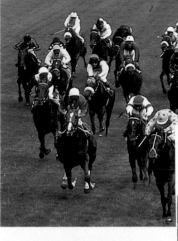

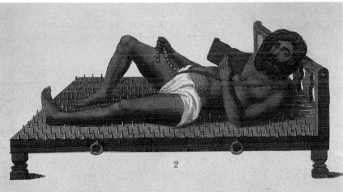

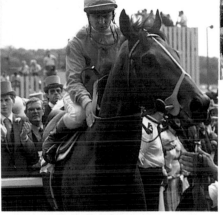

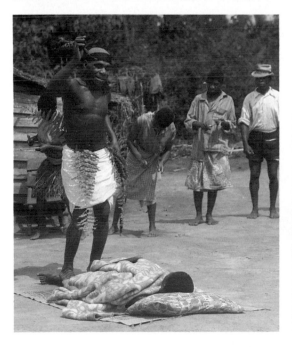

ABOVE *300 metres from the finish of the Derby in 1980, Henbit, ridden by Willie Carson, stumbled and broke a bone in his foreleg. Nevertheless, he won the race and showed no signs of pain until after he had been led into the winner's enclosure.*

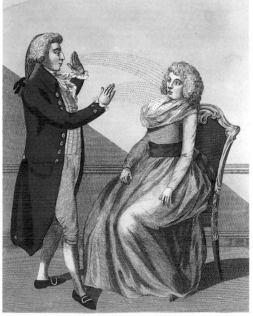

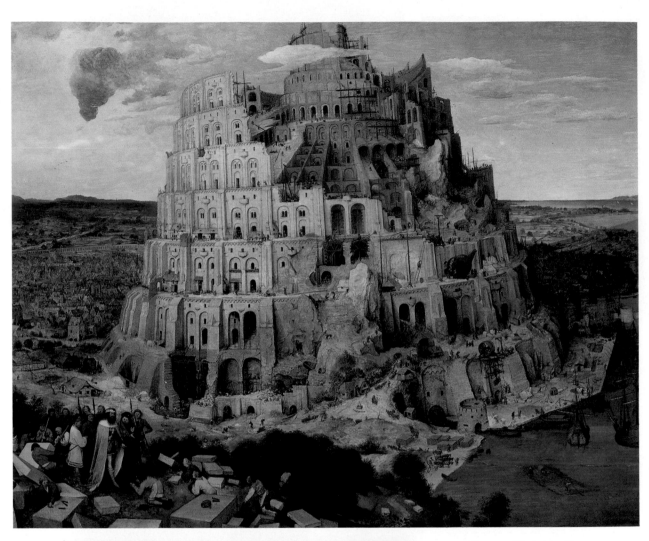

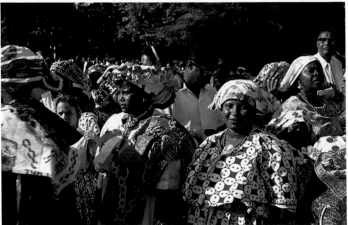

ABOVE Tower of Babel *by Pieter Brueghel the Elder (1525–1569). According to Genesis, Jehovah caused the builders of this tower, which was intended to reach heaven, to speak different languages, so that they could not communicate and therefore had to abandon the work.*

LEFT *In the former Dutch colony of Surinam in South America, the descendants of slaves and indentured labourers from many different West African tribes now speak a rich creole, invented by the children of slaves.*

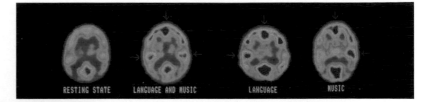

Vervet monkeys in Africa (below) use distinctive cries as 'words' to warn others of leopards, snakes or eagles.

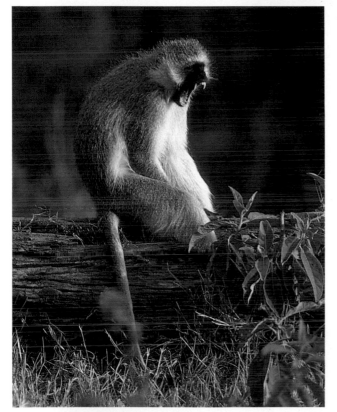

PET scans of the normal human brain (above) show the uptake of glucose reflecting the degree of activity of nerve cells in different parts of the brain. In these computer-constructed horizontal slices through the head (forehead at the top), highly active areas are shown as red, the least active regions as blue. In a quiet room (left-hand scan) there is very little activity in the auditory areas of the cortex in the temporal lobes, at the sides of the cerebral hemispheres. As the volunteer listens to both music and spoken words, the auditory regions on both sides of the brain become active; so too does the frontal cortex, which is probably involved in the interpretation of the sounds. Spoken language alone activates primarily the left side of the brain, while music alone stimulates mainly the right auditory areas.

Colwyn Trevarthen at the University of Edinburgh believes that mothers and very young babies conduct 'conversations', involving gestures, facial expressions and vocalisations, each responding to the other in turn. Language of a sort begins before a baby can speak.

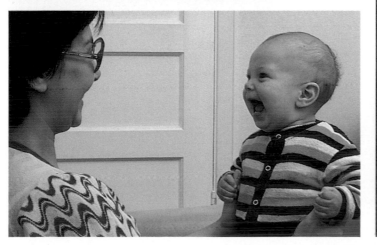

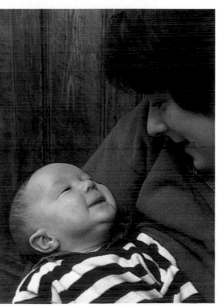

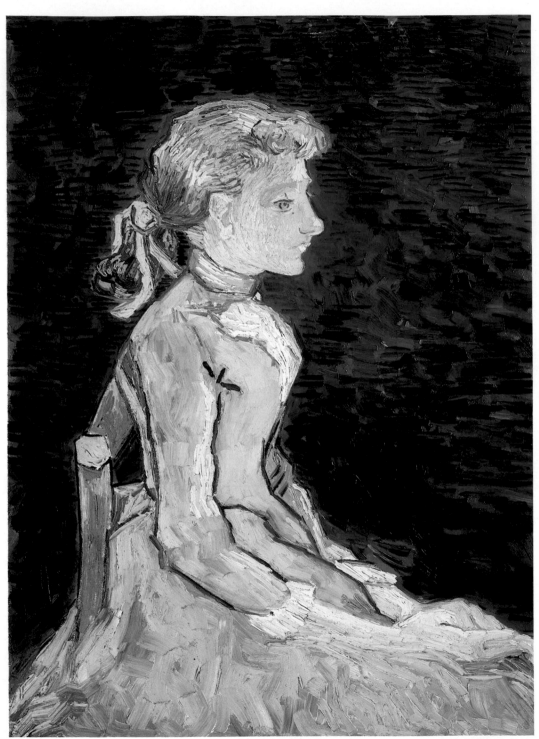

Portrait of Adeline Ravoux *by Vincent van Gogh (1853–1890)*.

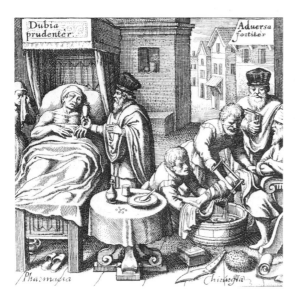

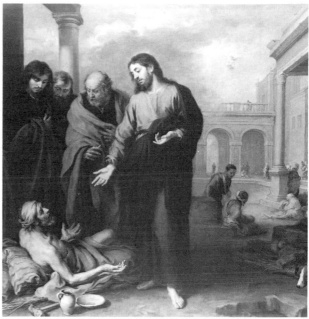

In medieval times (above left), treatment of illness through drugs and surgery was very primitive and must have depended largely on a mixture of good luck and the placebo effect.

Christ healing the paralytic at the pool of Bethesda *(above right) by Bartolomé Murillo (1618–1682).*

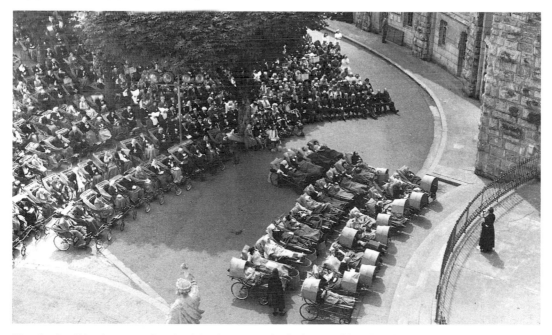

Very few invalids who come to Lourdes (above) expect a miracle, but something about the place makes most of them feel better. Does this healing power come from God or from the patients themselves?

relapsed into serious illness. His doctor, in desperation, gave the man distilled water, telling him (falsely) that it was a special, pure form of Krebiozen, which was known to be effective. The man again made a remarkable recovery but two months later a damning government report on Krebiozen was published and the man died a few days later. Levy is convinced that attitude is a vital factor in the personal fight against cancer. Her recent study of women with breast cancer showed that those who were angry about their disease, who had good social support and who were determined to fight had more active killer cells (cells of the immune system that specifically attack cancerous tissue).

Steven Greer, now at the Royal Marsden Hospital outside London, began a study of sixty-nine women with early operable breast cancer in 1971. He too has found that attitude correlates strongly with survival:

> The women who had an active attitude, mainly 'fighting spirit', had the best outcome. They were twice as likely to be alive and well ten years later than the women at the other extreme who showed helplessness or hopeless attitudes, who seemed to be overwhelmed by the disease.

Studies like these begin to provide a firm, scientific framework for folk wisdom. But caution is essential. The effects described are small compared with the well-established benefits of many conventional forms of therapy. One of Steven Greer's patients, Rachael Beales, who has been fighting against secondary cancer after breast surgery seven years ago, says, 'I think you're crazy if you don't use conventional drug treatment; it works, and it has worked in my case. But ... you have got a body and a soul and a spirit; and you've got to use all of them.'

There is another, more subtle danger in putting undue emphasis on the role of mind and brain in the cause of, and reaction to disease. It would be heedless and wrong to make people feel *responsible* for having become ill in the first place. As Greer points out:

> The attitudes towards cancer cannot be a cause of cancer. And we cannot cure patients with psychological factors. But what we can do is firstly improve the quality of their lives. And we hope to provide evidence that we may, in some cases, prolong their lives to a certain extent, to increase the duration of their survival.

Quacks and hypnotists, herbalists and faith healers – *and* the practitioners of conventional medicine; all of them appeal to a basic need in human nature. We need to believe that we are in charge of our own destinies. Science cannot yet give a convincing account of the power of a 'fighting spirit', but it may bring us an understanding of the way in which determination and belief can help the process of healing.

THE
LIVING
WORD

> Do not let us speak of darker days; let us speak rather of sterner days. These are not dark days. These are great days, the greatest days our country has ever lived; and we must all thank God that we have been allowed, each of us according to our stations, to play a part in making these days memorable in the history of our race.

WINSTON CHURCHILL spoke those words to a group of boys at Harrow School on 19 October 1941. Edward R. Murrow, the American journalist, commented that Churchill 'mobilised the English language and sent it into battle'.

About twenty years later, during a televised interview in the United States, David Susskind told the Soviet Premier Nikita Khrushchev that he was 'barking up the wrong tree'. The Russian interpreter, sweating profusely, translated the phrase with a Russian idiom and told Khrushchev that he was 'baying like a hound'. And when Pepsi-Cola expanded its market into Taiwan, the English slogan 'Come alive with Pepsi!' became 'Pepsi brings your ancestors back from the grave!' Language may be our supreme social skill, but it also defines and limits the social group to which we belong.

Language is the clearest evidence we have of the minds of other people. It cements the bonds between parents and child, allows us to convey explicit beliefs and intentions, to impart knowledge and emotion. Through language, we can leave the present behind and speak about the past or invent the future. Without language, history, art, science – the whole of culture – would be unthinkable.

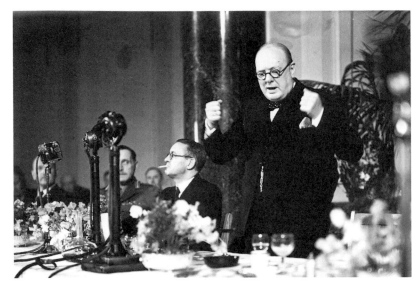

ABOVE *Winston Churchill speaking in 1941.*

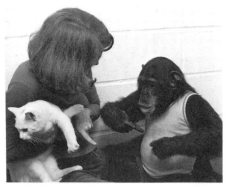

RIGHT *Chimpanzees can learn to make gestures in sign language and to string them together in simple sequences. Herbert Terrace's chimp 'Nim' signs (from top) 'Me hug cat' to his teacher, Susan Quinby.*

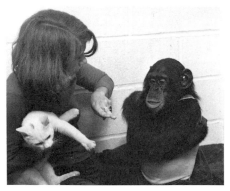

BELOW *The diagram of the left side of the human brain shows the two main areas involved in the interpretation of spoken and written language (Wernicke's area) and the production of speech (Broca's area).*

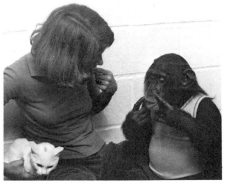

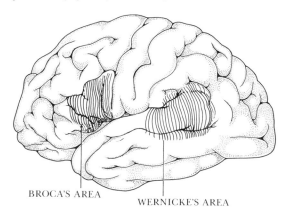

BROCA'S AREA   WERNICKE'S AREA

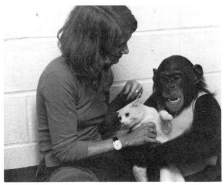

• THE STRUCTURE OF LANGUAGE •

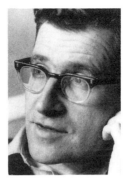

Noam Chomsky.

In 1950, Noam Chomsky, professor of linguistics at the Massachusetts Institute of Technology, set out to revolutionise our understanding of the nature of language. Since the end of the eighteenth century the focus of linguistic study had been the *differences* between languages. Chomsky preached that such an avenue of thought was a dead end, and that linguists should search for 'language universals' – the *similarities* among all languages. This deceptively simple proposal hid a fundamental change in philosophy; for Chomsky contended that the capacity for language is uniquely human and is *not* learned through experience (as was then commonly believed) but is innate.

If each child comes into the world 'preprogrammed' by its genes to learn a language, it must be supplied with plans for the acquisition of language. And if the genetic instructions for language are like those for other aspects of development, similar for everyone in our species, then *all* human languages ought to have a common structure. Obviously different languages vary enormously in their surface structure – the actual words and their arrangement in sentences. Even in a single language, different groupings of words can express a single idea ('The cat chased the mouse' and 'The mouse was chased by the cat'). Chomsky suggested that beneath the superficial outpouring of each utterance lies a deep structure – a simple arrangement of words that unambiguously specifies the meaning ('Cat chased mouse'). A single explicit statement can even have more than one underlying meaning ('Visiting relatives can be boring'). According to Chomsky the brain must, inherently, possess not only the apparatus for establishing the meaning or deep structure of sentences but also a universal grammar that determines much of the surface structure.

Chomsky's ideas were enormously influential and have stimulated a fresh interest in the biological basis of language. But the search for truly universal similarities in all languages has revealed very few, and rather unimpressive ones at that (all languages have nouns and use vowels). There do seem to be many common grammatical rules, but they are not absolutely universal and the exceptions raise doubts about just how much of the essence of language is specified in the genes.

Even the concept of a linguistic deep structure has run into problems. Many psycholinguists nowadays think of the representations in the brain that underlie sentences to be in a non-linguistic form, expressing the general meaning of the events in mind.

What then of the notion that the urge to use language is built into the human brain? Suppose we could take people who speak completely different languages and force them together in a cauldron of conflicting cultures. Suppose that we could demand that they work together and communicate with one another. We might find ourselves witnessing the birth of a new language, comprised of elements of the original languages, but with its own rules, its own grammar, its own syntax. In that event, we might be able to tease out of that raw, new language qualities inherent to *all* languages. The slave trade and the transportation of indentured labourers in past centuries unwittingly set up just such a bizarre experiment. Anthropological linguist Derek Bickerton has been studying the languages that evolved from this polyglot traffic.

One of Bickerton's interests is in the languages of Hawaii where a revision of the US tariff laws in 1876, allowing importation of sugar, stimulated a massive influx of indentured workers from as far afield as China, the Philippines, Portugal and Puerto Rico. After about 1900 the native Hawaiian language declined and the dominant true language on the island was English. The imported labourers had no common tongue and to communicate they improvised a makeshift language, called pidgin speech, which had a limited vocabulary and no true grammar.

The *children* of these pidgin speakers had no real language of their own. Bickerton believes that the children automatically brought innate grammar to their parents' rough methods of communication. In doing so, they created a completely new language – called a creole language – in one generation. In Hawaii this all happened so recently that both second-generation creole speakers and some of their pidgin-speaking parents are still alive.

Take, for instance, the following sentence in English:

In those days, unlike today, there were no washing machines and no piped water in homes.

In Hawaiian pidgin this would be rendered:

Now days, ah, house, ah, inside, washi clothes machine get, no? Before time, ah, no more, see? And then pipe no more, water pipe no more.

It is virtually a string of nouns, verbs and adjectives with almost no prepositions and no real grammar. The well-known information comes first and the new idea later. Compare the Hawaiian creole version:

Those days bin get no more washing machine, no more pipe water like get inside house nowadays, ah?

Bickerton has shown that creole has a much fuller structure with a rich syntax:

The adults who create pidgin speech are not able to provide it with any structure; they're past the critical age at which syntax develops. The children, however, are not. Syntax develops in them just as naturally as any other part of their bodies. It's natural, it's instinctive, and you can't stop them from doing it. I think the only explanation you can have for the way syntax works is that, somehow, it is built into the hard wiring of the brain.

Creole languages are essentially the inventions of children. It is significant that Bickerton and others have found grammatical similarities among creoles spoken everywhere from the Caribbean to the South Pacific, from Malaysia to West Africa. This evidence is the best yet that people have in their brains the inherent machinery to make language.

• WORDS WITHOUT SPEECH •

The capacity for language is a fundamental part of being human. The seventeenth-century philosopher René Descartes wrote that language 'belongs to man alone'. Certainly no other type of animal communication begins to approach its sophistication, its richness of meaning, its complexity. But this raises a paradox: true language seems uniquely human, yet it comes from the structure of our brains, which are built by genes that are largely shared with other animals. Spoken language depends on the special structure of the human larynx, tongue and mouth, but it also needs remarkable organisation in the brain – to house the rules of grammar as well as the vast lexicon of words; to conceive perceptions and thoughts in linguistic terms; to understand speech and writing. For Darwinian evolution to have invented this entire, elaborate machinery within the era of hominid species seems almost inconceivable. If language has emerged through natural selection, surely we should see its seeds in other animals.

Animals grunt, emit chemicals, sing, gesture, dance or even urinate to transmit information vital to their survival. Some have systems of vocalisation that can almost be labelled 'words'. Vervet monkeys in Africa, for instance, have specific, distinct calls that warn others of danger. When a vervet monkey gives the 'leopard call', its fellows climb high into the trees. When it gives the 'snake call', they scan the grass for signs of sinister movement. The 'eagle call' makes them all run for cover.

Chimpanzees are our closest animal relatives; they share as much as 99 per cent of our genetic material. Obviously they do not *speak* in the wild, but perhaps they have a capacity for language that is normally channelled into other forms of communication, or even just used internally as the basis of perceiving, thinking and planning. That is the speculation behind research that started more than sixty years ago – research that asks whether apes can learn to use a language to communicate with people.

Early attempts to train chimpanzees to *talk* were singularly unsuccessful; they simply do not have the throats and mouths for speech. But they do have free hands and nimble fingers. In 1966 Allen and Beatrice Gardner, two psychologists at the University of Nevada, adopted an eleven-month-old chimpanzee called Washoe and began to teach her the *gestural* sign language used by the deaf in the United States. In four years she learned to recognise and use 132 signs from American Sign Language, and the initial claims for her linguistic ability were a shock to those who valued the concept of the uniqueness of human language. She could do things that implied that she was not merely *associating* gestures with actions and things, but was thinking linguistically too. She *generalised* in her use of signs, employing the sign for 'dog', for instance, to indicate not only real dogs of various breeds, but also pictures of dogs and even the sound of a dog barking. She seemed to be using words as symbolic categories. She even invented new signs by combining simpler ones. A refrigerator became 'open-food-drink'.

But language is much more than the arbitrary stringing together of words. The essence of human language is *grammar* – the way in which words are assembled to make sentences, whose *meaning* depends as much on the sequence as on the words themselves. As Chomsky pointed out, grammar exists independent of content. Even nonsensical strings of words can instantly be judged as grammatically correct ('Colourless green ideas sleep furiously') or incorrect ('Green sleep furiously ideas colourless'). To create and interpret true sentences, the rules of grammar must be applied, although that process is normally entirely subconscious.

Washoe certainly put signs together in ways that were remarkably similar to the primitive grammatical sentences of young children, such as 'time drink', 'there shoe'. Jane Goodall, who has studied wild chimpanzees in Tanzania for nearly thirty years, tells the story of Lucy, another chimpanzee, who was brought up in a human household at the University of Oklahoma and taught sign language: 'She ... was treated just like one of the family ... watched television, had access to magazines, her own bedroom, everything.' After ten years, her adoptive parents sent her to a wild chimp reserve in the Gambia. She was terrified. 'It was rather like sending a somewhat pampered Western adolescent out to live with some Australian Aborigines.' When Lucy had been in the reserve for about two years, someone from her former life came to visit. Lucy ran up to the fence of her enclosure, looked her visitor in the eye, and signed, 'Please help. Out.' Such stories of the apparently spontaneous use of signs in a truly linguistic way to express needs and emotions abounded in the early years of the chimp language projects.

The Bible says that God took away from Adam and Eve their ability to talk with the beasts when He banished them from the Garden of Eden. By the early 1970s scientists began to think they might regain that ability. If only the right medium could be found, chimpanzees might express their innermost thoughts.

David Premack, now at the University of Pennsylvania, thought that plastic symbols arranged in order on a magnetic board might be the best way into the chimp mind. One of Premack's star pupils was Sarah, who became remarkably adept at using her plastic vocabulary. Not only could Sarah describe situations and make requests; she even grasped abstract notions, like 'same' and 'different'; she would choose the symbol for 'same' when presented with half a glass of water and half an apple. She could also make complex associations between causes and effects; at one point, she chose a knife from a pile of tools when presented with a whole apple and a sliced apple.

But as Sarah's ability to write her plastic messages increased, Premack's doubts grew. Even though Sarah realised that 'Sarah give apple Mary' had a different meaning from 'Mary give apple Sarah' there seemed to be little chance that she could learn that a single *thought* (that Mary should give Sarah an apple) could be expressed in many ways. There was no evidence that Sarah had mastered the formal structure of language – the grammar and its syntax. Herb Terrace at Columbia University came to the same conclusion on the basis of careful analysis of videotapes of his chimpanzee Nim Chimpsky, who had been taught American Sign Language. For one thing, most of his strings of signs were simply copies of sign statements made previously by his teachers. There was little use of signs to indicate anything beyond immediate needs. And again, there was no evidence of real grammar. Terrace thinks that everything chimps can do is explained by the rote learning of sequences. Signalling 'Mary give apple Sarah' to get an apple might, in principle, be no different from punching the correct 4-digit identification code into a bank cash dispenser to get some money; and no one would call that language.

But far from relegating animals even more certainly to a thoughtless universe, these experiments have stimulated psychologists to look in other ways at the wisdom of animals, at their ability to understand the world and represent it symbolically within their heads. Pigeons are the unlikely subjects of Richard Herrnstein's experiments at Harvard, aimed at discovering the limits of animal intelligence. Pigeons seem to be able, without specific training, to *classify* things as if they had internal 'words' to represent them. Herrnstein showed pigeons a series of eighty slides of ordinary scenes, half of them containing images of *trees*. They included oaks, maples, white pines; some were in the foreground, others far away; some were fully lit, others merely silhouettes. If the pigeon pecked a small panel when one of the tree pictures was on the screen it received a food reward. Most pigeons learned this game before the end of the first full presentation of the eighty slides; next day when the slide show began again, they pecked only for the tree pictures. Even more remarkable, if the pigeons were now shown completely new slides, they continued to peck only for those containing trees, even of different species. The pigeons seemed to have grasped the general *class* of things that was associated with the reward.

Herrnstein and others using similar techniques have shown that pigeons can recognise such classes as 'bodies of water' (slides of lakes, oceans, rivers), 'human beings' (faces, full torsos or even distant groups of people), 'fishes' (in underwater photographs), 'dogs' and even the letter 'A' (in any one of eighteen different typefaces)! Such skill reflects the need of every animal to divide objects and events into a limited number of *categories*, in order to decide how to respond to the world. What is remarkable is that even a pigeon has the capacity to form categories in the brain – internal 'words' – for things, such as fishes swimming, that it has never seen before.

Animals must have the power to represent the important features of their worlds in a symbolic form in their brains. Surely that is the first step on the road to language. But what they (even apes) seem to lack is the capacity to *express* themselves through the use of grammar. Being able to combine words according to rules to convey meaning may indeed be uniquely human. That ability requires the right machinery, not only in the brain but in the throat and the mouth.

• FREEDOM OF SPEECH •

Though language can certainly exist without speech (in writing, for instance), the emergence of the human larynx was surely an essential early step in the evolution of our language. At Brown University in Rhode Island, Philip Lieberman studies the fossils and skulls of primitive hominids to uncover clues to how they communicated. By examining bones and reconstructing missing vocal tracts, and by comparing them to the anatomy of modern man, Lieberman now estimates that modern human speech was physically impossible until only 100 000 years ago – a moment in evolutionary time.

In Neanderthal people (who shared Europe with *Homo sapiens* until they died out about 30 000 years ago) the physical structures for speech as we know it did not exist. Their necks were much shorter, their tongues longer; they had a high-placed larynx and an inflexible throat. These physical constraints would have made many of the subtleties of human speech impossible – sounds like 'ee', 'oo', and 'ah', or consonants like 'kuh' or 'guh'. Nevertheless Lieberman believes that Neanderthal was capable of language: 'The evidence of Neanderthal culture, which is apparent in their tools and tool-making techniques, their rituals and a social order which included care for the infirm, all point to the presence of language.' Neanderthal language was probably a combination of limited vocalisations and hand gestures.

Our direct ancestors, *Homo erectus*, living a million years ago and more, had the beginnings of the anatomy needed for modern speech, though they too could probably do little more than grunt. Over time, the human tongue became rounder, the neck elongated to accommodate it, and the larynx dropped to its present position. These changes allowed the precise co-ordination of tongue, lips and larynx needed for the elaborate, high-speed choreography that results in clear, rapid speech – about ten times faster than any series of sounds a chimpanzee can make. Lieberman doubts that these anatomical changes were merely a by-product of an evolving system designed for eating and breathing:

> We ended up with an airway that causes us to choke much more easily than any other animal; it crowds the mouth so that we can die from impacted wisdom teeth; it makes it hard to breathe. The only thing it really is good for is speech, which means that the selective advantage for speech must have outweighed everything else.

The transformation of the human larynx and mouth was driven by natural selection. The improving power of speech must itself have bestowed an advantage that drove the throat further towards its present state of extreme specialisation. But that change could not have happened without parallel evolution of the brain, building on its animal inheritance of classification and understanding – developing the machinery to control the throat and use it as the beacon of the mind.

• THE ANATOMY OF LANGUAGE •

Perhaps the strongest evidence that the capacity for language is genetically determined *and* that it has its precedents in animals comes from the study of the anatomical machinery of language in the brain and the effects of injury to it. In 1861 a French surgeon, Pierre-Paul Broca, encountered a patient who had suffered for years from weakness on the right side of his body and who, though he could still understand language, could say little more than the single syllable 'Tan', the name by which he is known in the annals of medicine.

When Tan died, Broca performed a post mortem and discovered that a portion of the frontal lobe of Tan's left hemisphere had degenerated. Over the following few years Broca gathered several similar cases; all of them shared injury in the region of the frontal lobe directly in front of the

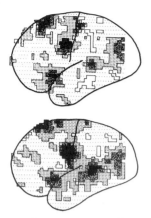

Computer reconstructions of blood-flow through the cortex of the left hemisphere of a human. The darker the region, the higher the blood flow, reflecting the degree of activity of nerve cells. In the top picture, the volunteer was reading silently, and there was activity in the visual regions (at the back of the brain, to the right), the 'supplementary motor area' (at the top of the frontal lobe), the 'frontal eye field' (in the middle) and Broca's speech area (lower left). In the other illustration, the person was reading aloud, which also activated the auditory regions in the temporal lobe.

part of the motor cortex responsible for movements of the mouth and tongue. And in every case the damage that caused near speechlessness was on the *left* side. He concluded that this region, now called Broca's area, was responsible for the production of speech; neurologists now believe that it is crucial for linking words together in grammatical fashion.

In the 1870s, a German neurologist, Carl Wernicke, located a second area, about the size of a hen's egg, in the left temporal lobe, which seems to be involved in the ability to understand the *meaning* of speech and writing. Wernicke's area sits between the visual and auditory regions of the cortex, perfectly positioned to do this job. In simple terms, a circuit seems to link the machinery of vision and hearing to that of understanding and speaking. Signals from Wernicke's area pass along a huge bundle of fibres that sweeps up and forwards into Broca's area, where intended meaning is somehow programmed for speech. Messages then travel to the adjacent area in the motor cortex, which controls the muscles of vocalisation.

Since the time of Tan, other brain-damaged patients with aphasia (speech problems) or alexia (inability to read) have enabled the pathways of language to be mapped. Aphasics with damaged Broca's areas can usually understand what is said to them, as long as the grammar is simple, and they know what they want to say; but often, their speech is a kind of verbal telegram. Those with injury to Wernicke's area, on the other hand, have greater difficulty in understanding language, but none in *producing* speech. On the contrary, words pour out of them, but their sentences (though grammatical) have little meaning. 'Carol', a patient of Antonio Damasio of the University of Iowa, has symptoms of Wernicke's aphasia:

> I woke up in the dark and my right foot was numb and just fell around. My ... under one leg so I changed and went back to sleep and worked a little bit with the laundry and things, and all of a sudden I just couldn't do anything. My husband put me on a chair and my hands just fell apart all the time. And he called the doctor, and this doctor knew and he said 'Take me to Grenelle Hospital'.

Carol's disability seemed mild at first. Her speech was jumbled, but not utterly incomprehensible, and its grammatical construction was quite good. She did not use many meaningless 'jargon' words, as some Wernicke's aphasics do. But when Damasio tested her for comprehension, the real depth of the problem became clear. In one examination, Damasio asked Carol to listen to this sentence: 'The bird that the cat watched was hungry.' He then showed her a picture of a cat watching a bird and asked: 'Who is hungry?' Carol pointed to the cat. 'The cat is hungry for the bird. The cat wants to eat the bird.' She could not interpret the subtleties of grammar and was left with commonsense and guesswork to help her interpret the meaning of sentences.

Twenty years ago the psychology and neurology of language seemed to fit hand-in-hand. Wernicke's and Broca's areas were seen as the central factories of understanding and speech respectively. But language enlists much more of the brain for its production. Perception, memory, thought and emotion all contribute to the full use of language. Positron emission tomography (PET scanning), a form of brain imaging that produces pictures of the living brain in action, shows that much of the cerebral cortex is galvanised into activity during reading or speaking.

Furthermore, the careful study of brain-damaged people has revealed a much more complicated picture of the processing of language. For instance, severe brain damage in the general region of Wernicke's area can produce a bizarre condition called deep dyslexia in which the internal representations of the sounds of words and of their written appearance seem torn apart, and they remain linked only via their common connection to some form of representation of *meaning*. A sufferer from this condition reads the word 'dinner' as 'food', and 'close' as 'shut'.

Other brain-damaged patients, exhibiting surface dyslexia, can read simple words but seem to be able to discover their meaning only by translating them purely *phonetically* into internally represented sounds, and then analysing these conceptually. For instance, asked to identify the word 'bury', someone with surface dyslexia said 'a little fruit on a tree' and another said 'a kind of hat'.

Broca's and Wernicke's original suggestion that the left side of the brain plays a special role in language has stood the test of time. In the vast majority of right-handed people, and in about half of left-handers too, the left hemisphere takes the lead in interpreting speech and writing, and in producing them. Brain-imaging techniques, the recording of the local electrical activity of the brain with electrodes on the scalp, as well as the effects of brain damage, all suggest that the left hemisphere is usually dominant for language.

However, the rhythm and melody of speech (which convey so much of its emotional meaning) depend more on the right hemisphere. Indeed, the right side of the brain seems to be the home of the interpretation and reading of *music* – skills that in some ways are very similar to language. An eminent Italian conductor had a massive left hemisphere stroke in 1977, which left him almost totally unable to read, write, speak, do calculations or copy gestures, and his right hand seemed weak and clumsy. Yet he could still read music well and could play the piano and many other instruments. He resumed conducting, though he could not speak to the orchestra, and his performance of Verdi's difficult opera *Nabucco* received great critical acclaim. When a similar disaster recently struck a well-known French organist and composer who had been blind since the age of two, he was robbed of his ability to read *words* in braille, but he could still read braille *music* and compose in braille too, even though the patterns of dots used in braille to represent musical notes are identical to those representing letters of the alphabet!

The dominance of the left hemisphere for language can even be *seen* with the naked eye. The part of Wernicke's area that lies in the deep fissure that separates the temporal lobe from the parietal lobe – the temporal plane – is usually much larger on the left side than the right. Broca's area is also often visible as a slightly oversized fold of cortex in the left frontal lobe. However, these anatomical lumps of language should not be taken too seriously: *Homo habilis*, our hominid ancestor of 2 million years ago, who could almost certainly not speak as we do, also had a visible Broca's area; and even chimpanzees usually have a larger temporal plane on the left side.

Despite the fact that an enlarged left temporal plane is usually detectable by about two months before birth in a human baby, the commitment of language to the left side is probably not complete until many years later, and is never total. Children under the age of about eight usually recover much better than adults after brain damage on the left side, even after complete removal of the left hemisphere. It is as if young children retain the ability to switch the control of language to the right side during those early years.

The most extraordinary living evidence of the division of labour in the human brain is that famous group of 'split-brain' patients, whose cerebral hemispheres have been deliberately disconnected from each other to prevent the spread of epileptic fits. Most of them are quite unable to say or write down, with the *right* hand, what they have seen after the name (or a picture) of an object is flashed briefly on a screen so that it falls to the left of the point they are staring at, and therefore ends up trapped in the right hemisphere. However, they can use the *left* hand (controlled by the right hemisphere) to pick up the same object from a number of things on a tray in front of them, which implies that the right side of the brain can *understand* at least simple non-abstract nouns.

Michael Gazzaniga of Dartmouth College found that the right hemisphere of one of his split-brain patients, whom he refers to as 'Paul', was unusually active. Paul had suffered from severe epilepsy all his life, and the earliest seizures had damaged parts of his left hemisphere. As a teenager, he underwent surgery to separate his left and right hemispheres, and his epilepsy improved dramatically. When Gazzaniga began to test Paul he found that the early damage to Paul's left hemisphere seemed to have forced his right hemisphere to assume some linguistic responsibility. Gazzaniga could actually communicate with each half of Paul's brain *independently*, and the two halves had distinctly different notions about the world. At one point, for instance, Gazzaniga flashed a question to Paul's left visual field (connected to his right hemisphere): 'What do you want to be?' Paul used his left hand to arrange letters from a *Scrabble* game to spell out 'automobile racer'. When the left hemisphere was asked the same question, the answer came back: 'draughtsman'.

Gazzaniga then presented the two hemispheres simultaneously with different visual information to see how Paul would explain it. He flashed a drawing of a chicken's foot to the right visual field (thus to the left hemisphere) and of a snow-covered cottage to the left visual field (and right hemisphere). Then he gave Paul a set of cards with pictures of a variety of objects – a rake, an apple, a hammer, a toaster, a shovel, a chicken's head – and asked him to point at the picture that corresponded to what he had seen. Paul chose the chicken's head with his right hand, but with his left he chose the shovel. When Gazzaniga asked him what he had seen, he combined his answers: 'I saw a claw and I picked the chicken; you have to clean out the chicken shed with a shovel.' The dominant left hemisphere had taken charge of the business of answering the question; and it solved the mystery of the right hemisphere's choice by creating a bit of fiction – by fabricating a story to link the two, unconnected choices.

• THE DRAWING BOARD •
OF LANGUAGE

At the University of Edinburgh, a mother sits in a curtained room, singing to her baby, who squirms and gurgles in time to the song. Observing the scene through a one-way mirror is Colwyn Trevarthen, who studies what he calls 'proto-language', the communication between mothers and infants. What looks at first like random activity is revealed, on closer examination, to be a choreographed interplay between mother and child. Mother speaks; baby responds by cooing and waving his arms. Mother takes the outstretched hands and claps them together rhythmically; baby picks up the rhythm and continues it without her urging.

The word 'infant' comes from the Latin *infans*, meaning 'without speech'. Speechless they may be, but Trevarthen believes that babies have an inbuilt urge to communicate:

> To an astonishing extent, a six or eight-week-old baby can perform what seems very much like conversational behaviour. The timing, the use of voice intonation, the combining of gestures with facial expressions, the attempt to make utterances with the mouth: all these are present in the infant.

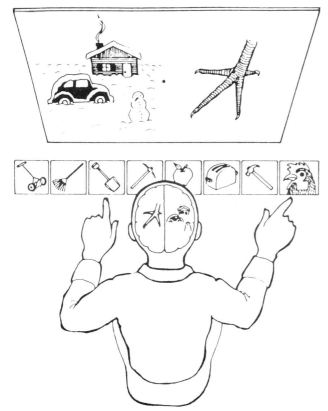

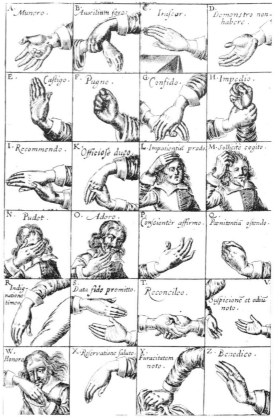

BELOW *Illustration from John Bulwer's* Chirologia, *or the Naturall Language of the Hand* (*1664*). *The sign languages used by the deaf, which have evolved over long periods, have rich grammatical structures.*

ABOVE *Mike Gazzaniga's split-brain patient 'Paul' stares at the dot in the centre of the screen and sees the picture of a chicken's foot with his right hemisphere and the snowy scene with his left. Each hand, controlled by the opposite hemisphere, points to an appropriate card.*

BELOW *In a school for the deaf in Newcastle, an animated discussion is conducted in complete silence.*

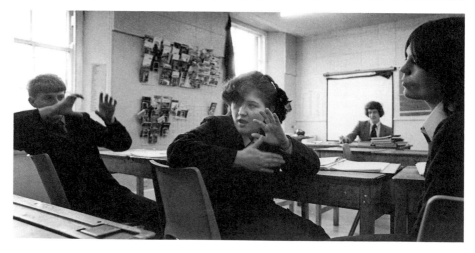

This precocious striving towards language implies that its foundations are indeed 'hard-wired' – built into our brains. But whatever is in the brain at birth is obviously not equivalent to a dictionary and a grammar textbook for one *particular* language. There are 4000 or so different spoken languages in the world (20 per cent of them in New Guinea!) and, as far as we know, any normal baby can learn any one of them if exposed to its sounds early enough. In order to understand words, whoever is speaking, the baby must recognise each particular speech sound – a certain vowel for instance – regardless of the pitch, stress and quality of the voice of the speaker.

Patricia Kuhl of the University of Washington is trying to pinpoint those stages of child development specifically involved in the perception of speech. Infants as young as six months old are capable of distinguishing among vowel sounds like 'ee' and 'ah'. Furthermore, they can make these distinctions no matter *who* is speaking. 'Once babies are trained on a particular speaker's voice, the training generalises to the voices of all different kinds of speakers,' says Kuhl. 'Babies are able to ignore all the variables in male, female, and children's voices and pay attention only to the *difference* in vowels.'

Categorising speech sounds in this way is essential to understanding spoken language, for if words were processed differently for each speaker, learning language would be impossible. But it is still a remarkable achievement. We can judge just how difficult it is by the fact that, despite enormous effort, computer scientists, motivated by the commercial importance of making machines that can understand human speech, have so far failed to crack the problem of making a machine that can recognise the *pattern* of each speech sound regardless of its pitch and timbre.

• LEARNING THE RULES •

All languages are based on particular rules. Paradoxically, the *mistakes* that children make as they start to speak often reveal that they have learned such general rules (before they learn the exceptions). For instance, in English, most nouns become plural with the addition of an 's'. A child who hears that 'more-than-one-toy' is called 'toys' and 'more-than-one-car' is called 'cars' learns that general rule, and is likely to talk of 'sheeps' and 'gooses'. Such errors demonstrate the generative power of the child's mind – the ability to learn rules and apply them to new situations.

Until the 1970s the simple language of two-year-olds was taken to reflect a poverty of understanding, of both the world and of the rules of grammar. But analysis of videotapes of children talking revealed that they can use single phrases to mean several things. Depending on the situation, 'Daddy out' may be a description of father's location, or a request that he leave the room. Cognition – the understanding of the world – runs ahead of expressive language in the growing child. And so it may have done in animal evolution. The difference between human language and animal communication may be our ability to acquire certain linguistic rules and use them to get knowledge efficiently from our brains into other people's.

• A CRITICAL PERIOD •

The spontaneous emergence of creole languages is powerful testimony to the presence of linguistic skill eager to burst out of the minds of children. But obviously the environment must contribute something to the emergence of language. At the very least it provides other people! Humpty Dumpty said to Alice, behind the Looking Glass, 'When I use a word . . . it means just what I choose it to mean – neither more nor less.' But what would be the use of words that no one else understood. Surely, language would have no value in a world of one.

Since the beginning of the fourteenth century, some forty-seven cases of 'wolf children' – children raised in isolation – have been described. The best documented include Victor, the 'wild child of Aveyron' (who was captured in France at about the age of eleven in 1799), Kaspar Hauser of Nuremberg, Germany (who was about seventeen when he was found in 1828), Amala and Kamala in Midnapore, India (discovered in 1920 at the ages of two and eight) and Genie, an American girl (who was found chained in an attic in 1970, after thirteen years of inhuman neglect and isolation).

The older children failed to develop linguistic abilities; and even the younger ones never gained full command of speech and grammar, despite great efforts to teach them. It seems that there is a *sensitive period*, lasting until seven or eight years of age, during which a child must be exposed to other people and to some kind of language if a true language is ever to be learned. During that period we can use our inherited capacity to acquire a language, or even more than one, without apparent effort. But after that sensitive period even the learning of a second language becomes an intellectual labour.

The Mogul Emperor of India, Akbar the Great, performed his own experiment to see whether children kept in isolation would learn to speak, which is described in the *Akbarnama* of Abu'l-Fazi:

> The newly born were put into that place of experience, and honest and active guards were put over them. For a time, dumb wet-nurses were admitted there. As they had closed the door of speech, the place was commonly called the Gan Mahal (the dumbhouse). On the 9th August

1582 he went out to hunt. ... The next day he went with a few special attendants to the house of that experiment. No cry came from that house of silence, nor was any speech heard there. In spite of their four years, they had no part of the talisman of speech, and nothing came out except the noise of the dumb.

Perhaps they did not speak but, according to the Jesuit Father Catrou, writing in 1705, 'they merely expressed their thoughts by *gestures* which answered the purpose of words.' If this is true, Akbar's poor imprisoned children may have acquired a true language.

• SIGNS OF LANGUAGE •

At the Salk Institute in California, Ursula Bellugi has spent many years studying American Sign Language, the gestural form of communication that is widely used by the deaf (and a few chimps!) in the United States. It was previously thought to be a primitive system of telegraphic symbols – little more than semaphore. But Bellugi's analysis has shown it to be a completely autonomous language, not simply derived from English, but with its own rich rules of grammar, expressed through the sequence of signs, the directions in which they are made and slight modifications of the individual signs.

Bellugi is now exploring how deaf children acquire sign language. Far from being 'wolf children' who, cut off from the hearing, speaking world, never fully learn language, they develop in a society filled with human interaction, human communication, human culture. At the Fremont School for the Deaf in California, students and teachers alike come from deaf families, and signing is the only language they have. The classrooms are quieter than most; but they are alive with the movements and gestures of sign language – a language that seems to be a remarkably satisfactory replacement for spoken language. 'We know by now from experiments that deaf people rehearse in signs, plan what they are going to do in signs, even dream in signs,' says Bellugi. 'We've seen little children signing to themselves. So to the extent that hearing people think in words, it's perfectly clear that deaf people equivalently think in signs.'

Helen Neville, also working at the Salk Institute, has been recording the electrical activity of deaf people's brains as they watch someone signing and has found that they process the information in their left hemispheres. In spite of the huge differences in the production of gestural and spoken speech, they both make use principally of the left side of the brain.

If language is so central to our mental life, might it also influence the very nature of thought? William Wang, a linguist at the University of California at Berkeley, considers it a possibility: 'Language must play a major role in shaping the mind. How we relate to others, how we see things, how we represent reality to ourselves – all are critically influenced by the choices that our language makes available to us.' Language teachers are fond of the proverb, 'Another language, another soul.' Certainly, having a second language usually means knowing something of another culture; and that gives the speaker another way of looking at things. Could this mean that the character of a society is moulded in part by its language – that so-called Germanic militarism and French romanticism, Italian flamboyance, Russian melancholy, and British phlegmatism are all products of the respective languages?

In the 1930s, ethnolinguist Benjamin Lee Whorf believed just that. He was studying the Hopi Indians, a peaceful tribe of farmers in the American south-west, and claimed that their language (and therefore their world view) differed radically from the European. Among other things, Whorf asserted that the Hopi language ignored one of the most fundamental elements of our world – the concept of *time*. He wrote that the Hopi language 'is seen to contain no words, grammatical forms, constructions or expressions that refer directly to what we call "time", or to past, present or future, or to enduring or lasting'. In Whorf's opinion, if the Hopis had no *expression* for time, they could have no *concept* of time.

Fifteen years ago, Ekkehart Malotki, a linguist at the University of Northern Arizona, began to test the 'Whorfian theory', that language determines thought. The topic he chose to study was Whorf's own – the question of time in the Hopi language. Within a few years, Malotki had accumulated dozens of Hopi references to time, some from within Whorf's own notebooks. But he also discovered why Whorf might have been mistaken:

> The Hopis are living with time in every moment of their lives – but not necessarily in the way *we* perceive time today. Before their encounters with the white man, there had never been a need for naming hours or minutes. In Hopi society, time is probably experienced as a more organic or natural phenomenon.

The Hopi concept of time thus springs from the Hopi environment, with its long seasons, imperceptible movement of the sun across the open sky, rhythms of planting and harvest. Whorf missed the implicit connotations of time in seemingly 'timeless' words.

Whorf may have been wrong about the Hopi language; but he was not necessarily wrong about the power of language in general. Most scientists today believe that uncovering the true relationship between thought and language depends at least partly on the way the question is framed. As George Miller, a psychologist at Princeton University, has written:

> Some scientists believe human language is what it is because it reflects the way the brain works; others believe our brain works the way it does because language has shaped it so. I believe they are both right. Human brains and human language have shaped each other. Children must be born with brains capable of learning language, and language must be the kind of thing that children's brains can learn. To ask which is the cause and which is the effect is like asking whether running is the result of the action of the right leg or the left.

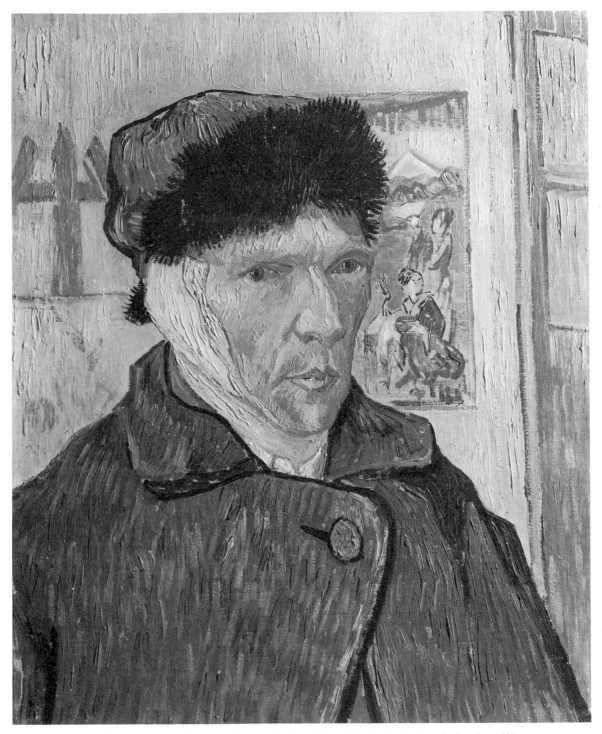

Self Portrait with Bandaged Ear, *painted in 1889 by Van Gogh. He slashed off a piece of his own ear after a foolish quarrel with Gauguin, shortly before his voluntary internment at the asylum of St Rémy.*

PORTRAIT
IN BLUE

IT WAS A MIRACULOUS year for van Gogh. First, a version of *Sunflowers* sold at auction for nearly £25 million, followed by *Irises* at a record price of more than £30 million. Then, on 11 May 1988, at Christie's in New York, a 'minor' work, a portrait of a thirteen-year-old girl dressed in blue, went for £7.3 million. In his lifetime, van Gogh sold just one painting.

The girl in the portrait was Adeline Ravoux, daughter of the owner of the Café Ravoux in Auvers-sur-Oise, north of Paris, where van Gogh lived for two months before his death on 29 July 1890. No doubt Adeline sat at his bedside as he lay dying in the tiny attic room that he rented for three francs a night.

Vincent Willem van Gogh, born in 1853, son of Theodorus, a pastor of the Dutch Reformed Church, and his strong-willed wife Anna Cornelia, was unusual from an early age; often taciturn and unsmiling, but with outbursts of temper or high spirits. His sister Elizabeth wrote, 'Not only were his little brothers and sisters like strangers to him, but he was a stranger to himself as well.' He took a job as a clerk at an art gallery in The Hague and at the age of twenty he was sent to the gallery's London branch. He fell passionately in love with his landlady's daughter Eugenie, but was crushed by her rejection of him. After further stints of work with the same company in Paris and London his obstinate, impatient attitude led to his dismissal, and he took a post as an unpaid teacher in Ramsgate. He was obsessed with religion and in 1876 became an assistant to a Methodist minister in Isleworth.

He returned to Holland and started to study theology at Amsterdam. Impatient to pursue his vocation, he transferred to a shorter course in

Brussels where his extraordinary swings of mood between warm generosity and foul temper soon gained him a reputation. His extreme self-denial became a passion and, when he failed the course and went as a lay preacher to the coal mining district near Mons, he gave away most of his possessions and ate almost nothing. It was here that he began to draw and paint; art became his new, and lifelong, obsession.

Much of the rest of the saga of one of the most innovative and sensitive artists of the nineteenth century is well known – the liaisons with prostitutes; the fights with Gauguin; the severed ear; the drunkenness; and finally the year-long incarceration at the asylum in St Rémy, which preceded his arrival in Auvers.

There is little doubt that Vincent was 'mentally' ill, though we cannot know exactly how he would be diagnosed today. At one stage he suffered paranoid delusions of being poisoned and heard voices – symptoms typical of schizophrenia. Several doctors who examined Vincent thought that he was epileptic. But what is certain is that he was the victim of his own extreme moods. 'Emotions are the great captains of our lives,' he wrote from St Rémy to his brother Theo, on whose love and financial support Vincent was totally dependent.

Vincent suffered a number of intense emotional crises, during which he was almost unable to work. 'Sometimes moods of indescribable mental anguish,' he wrote, 'sometimes moments when the veil of time and the fatality of circumstances seem to be torn apart for an instant.' Depression was one of the captains of Vincent's life.

• WHEN MOOD BECOMES ILLNESS •

We all experience fluctuations of emotion. Joy, frustration, sadness are intrinsic parts of being alive, of being human. Our moods are in tune with the events in our lives: a lovers' tiff elicits feelings of emptiness, guilt and depression; the company of good friends triggers a strong sense of happiness. Whether intense or mild, we can usually trace our feelings directly to our experiences.

Human beings are creatures of mood. True, the lives of other animals have their moments of fear, passion and anger – natural and adaptive reactions to the demands of their environments. But people's emotions come as much from *within* as from the world around them. They come from contradictions between expectation and achievement, from intellectualised ambition, from thoughts, memories and beliefs. The ancient emotional powerhouses of the brain – the hypothalamus and limbic system, which lie between brainstem and cerebral hemispheres – have been recruited in the service of human consciousness, adding colour to experience.

To a biologist, looking for adaptive value in the functions of the human brain, mood is something of a mystery. Perhaps our feelings – of sadness, pleasure and anger – help us to appreciate and predict the reactions of *others* to situations in their lives, and hence to deal with the complexity of social interaction. Whatever their function, in biological terms, for most of us our shifts in mood, like the changing seasons, are an essential part of the variety of life – a scale against which pleasure and sadness can be judged.

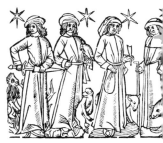

The four humours (from left to right: choleric, sanguine, phlegmatic and melancholy), from an early sixteenth-century edition of the Shepheard's Kalendar. *Hippocrates, about 400* BC, *thought that temperament depended on the balance of these four humours in the body.*

But the mechanisms of mood can go wrong and become dictators of the brain. By the latest estimates, one in five of the population (more women than men) will experience some kind of serious *affective* or mood disorder during their lives. Much the commonest form of mental illness is unipolar depressive psychosis, which usually strikes in early middle age (though the glimmerings of illness can appear much sooner). It imposes on its victims a cycle of intense episodes of sadness, lasting months or even years, interspersed with periods of normal experience. George Gray, an eminent British anatomist of the brain, who suffered a serious breakdown in 1979 and now lives with a hateful rhythm of sadness, said:

> I sometimes scream to myself; why can't I understand depression? It feels as if it's outside your brain, though I *know* it's inside.... In the core of my brain there seems to be a sort of muzziness, which stops me feeling pleasure, or thinking lucidly; and above all it stops me feeling I'm ever going to get better. It's terrifying. I'm on the edge of weeping all the time.... Life seems hopeless for me at the moment. Meals? Why eat? My wife – the only thing in my life worth having? Does she matter? But in my depressive breakdown I went much further down than this. I turned into a cabbage, an automaton. I felt dead.

In the less common bipolar or manic-depressive psychosis, which affects up to one per cent of the population, the pendulum of mood swings further, alternating between deep depression and the breathtaking euphoria, boundless energy and crazed thoughts of mania. Kay Jamison, psychologist at the Johns Hopkins University, School of Medicine, quotes a manic-depressive who describes his own suffering:

> There is a particular kind of pain, elation, loneliness and terror involved in this kind of madness. The fast ideas are far too fast and far too many; overwhelming confusion replaces clarity. Memory goes. You are irritable, angry, frightened, uncontrollable, and enmeshed totally in the blackest caves of the mind. You never knew those caves were there. It will never end. Madness carves its own reality. Which of the me's is *me*? The wild, impulsive, chaotic, energetic and crazy one? Or the shy, withdrawn, desperate, suicidal, doomed and tired one?

• THE KNIFE-EDGE •
OF CREATIVITY

Van Gogh arrived in Arles in February 1888. During the following 444 days, before his voluntary commitment in the asylum at St Rémy, he wrote 200 letters, and produced over 100 drawings and about 200 paintings, including many of his most famous works. All this, despite the unproductive interludes of mania and melancholy. It was as if the time *between* the extremes, when the pendulum of mood was resting on its knife-edge, gave him a power of creativity and a stamina sufficient to accomplish superhuman feats. The manic-depressive studied by Kay Jamison talks of this magical state of hypomania:

> When you're high, it's tremendous. The ideas and feelings are fast and frequent, like shooting stars, and you follow them until you find better and brighter ones. Shyness goes; the right words and gestures are suddenly there, the power to seduce and captivate others, a felt certainty.

The exhilaration of a lifting depression often seems to drive the sufferer into a period of enormous productivity. Indeed, it seems very likely that creativity and affective disorders, especially manic-depressive psychosis, are somehow linked. Saul, Nebuchadnezzar, Lincoln and Churchill; Coleridge, Hemingway, Sylvia Plath and Virginia Woolf; Handel, Schumann, Berlioz and Mahler: the known behaviour of each suggests that all experienced monstrous swings of mood typical of manic-depression.

Aristotle firmly believed that insanity fuelled creativity. He wrote: 'All who have been famous for their genius, whether in the study of philosophy, in affairs of state, in poetical composition, or in the exercise of the arts, have been inclined to insanity, as Hercules, Ajax, Bellerophon, Lysander, Empedocles, Socrates, and Plato.' More recently, Jamison sampled a large number of successful writers and artists in Great Britain. Her findings, that 38 per cent had been treated for mood disorders – almost double the incidence among the general population – have led her to wonder whether feelings of elation and invincibility, the fast flow of ideas, the contrasting extremes of highs and lows, help fuel the creative process. As the philosopher Nietzsche said, 'One must harbour chaos within oneself to give birth to a star.'

• THE CHEMISTRY OF •
ELATION AND DESPAIR

The neurons of the brain communicate with each other chemically. A neurotransmitter substance released by the terminals of a nerve fibre drifts across the tiny synaptic gap and comes to rest, fitting into receptor molecules in the surface membrane of the next neuron, that cause it to increase or decrease its firing of impulses. Neurotransmitters and receptors have complementary shapes – shapes that permit the receptor to accept only certain kinds of neurotransmitter. The neurotransmitter is then released back into the synaptic gap, where it is either broken down by an enzyme specifically designed for that purpose or reabsorbed into the terminal that produced it.

Affective diseases, like so many disorders of brain and mind, are now seen, at least in part, as errors in the balance of the chemistry of transmission in certain areas of the brain. The clue came from drug research. In the early 1950s, clinicians using a substance called reserpine, extracted from an Indian root plant, for the treatment of high blood pressure, noticed that some patients taking the drug became depressed. About the same time, other patients suffering from tuberculosis and prescribed a drug called iproniazid seemed to become inexplicably happier. Experiments on animals revealed that both these drugs act on synapses that use the amine transmitters noradrenaline and serotonin. Reserpine causes these transmitters to leak precipitously out of neurons into the synaptic gap, where they are destroyed by an ever present enzyme, monoamine oxidase. Iproniazid inhibits the production of monoamine oxidase and hence prolongs the action of amine transmitters. Thus a beautifully simple picture evolved: when amine synapses have their stocks of transmitter depleted, depression results; when the synapses are flooded with too much noradrenaline and serotonin, mania begins.

The new anatomical methods for staining neurons according to the transmitter substances within them revealed that serotonin and noradrenaline are used in two very particular but enormously widespread pathways in the brain. The cell bodies of both systems lie in small clusters deep in the brainstem, but they send their fibres to fan out across much of the cerebral cortex and indeed to many other parts of the brain. In normal animals, including humans, these diffuse networks may play a part in regulating attention, arousal, sleep and memory, as well as mood.

According to the amine hypothesis, depression is due to underproduction of serotonin and noradrenaline, and mania to overproduction, especially of noradrenaline. The hypothesis was fruitful in that it prompted the development of highly effective antidepressant drugs. The tricyclic antidepressants block the reabsorption of amine neurotransmitters into the releasing nerve terminal, so that more remains in the synapse; and the monoamine oxidase inhibitors destroy the enzyme that breaks down the neurotransmitter. The ultimate effect of both kinds of drugs is the same – to increase the amount of amine neurotransmitter in the synapse.

As so often happens in science, the beauty of this hypothesis has become a little blemished with age. The main contradiction is that anti-depressants do their chemical work in the synapse within a matter of hours; but the symptoms of depression often take weeks to lift. Currently, researchers are turning their attention away from the neurotransmitters and exploring the sensitivity of the receptors – looking, as it were, at the keyhole instead of the key. Antidepressant drugs do cause slow changes in the density of these receptors.

Whatever the risks of over-prescription and side-effects, anti-depressant drugs have transformed the prospects of the majority of sufferers, dissipating at least some of the cloud of despair that surrounds the diseases. Another drug, lithium, a naturally occurring salt, helps to calm wide swings of mood. Lithium treatment stretches back to the Greeks, who sent manic patients to partake of alkaline springs which contain high concentrations of lithium. Its precise mechanism is still unknown, although it certainly affects the sensitivity of neurons.

Before the era of drug treatment, unipolar depressives could expect to spend a quarter of their adult life in hospital, manic-depressives about half. Now almost 80 per cent of those afflicted are helped by drugs. But what of the remaining 20 per cent – those who are resistant to medication, or suffer severe side-effects? Some respond, surprisingly, to deprivation of sleep. And then there is electroconvulsive therapy, ECT, one of the most feared procedures in medicine, but the form of physical treatment that has been used longest in psychiatry – for fifty years.

Born out of the erroneous view that epileptics never suffer from schizophrenia, ECT was introduced as a way of providing artificial seizures. It did not help schizophrenics, but did seem to benefit depressive patients. Its use is still controversial, but its effectiveness is now undeniable: two-thirds or more of patients are helped and it is especially valuable where there is a serious threat of suicide, because its actions are faster than those of drugs. Moreover, the modern procedure is far from the medieval technique portrayed in *One Flew Over the Cuckoo's Nest*. It is performed painlessly and without gross convulsions, under the influence of anaes-thetic and muscle relaxant. Recent research begins to provide a rational basis for ECT; it produces a change in the density of amine receptors similar to that caused by antidepressant drugs.

The worst side-effect remains memory loss, the severity of which is hotly contested. Most of the psychiatric community contends that if permanent memory loss does occur, it is confined to a few days around the time of the treatment. But some former ECT patients assert that the loss can be devastating.

The choice becomes one of assessing a risk-benefit equation, for those considered the best candidates for ECT are among the most depressed patients – those most likely to commit suicide. For them, even the most profound memory loss may be considered a mercy.

• THE GENES OF MOOD •

Van Gogh's mother's family had a long history of depression, epilepsy and neurosis. The tendency for affective disease to run in families is clear to see. Samuel Johnson, another depressive, wrote, 'I inherited a vile melancholy from my father, which has made me mad all my life.' In the 1960s, methodical studies of family histories established beyond doubt the familial link. If one of a pair of identical twins is depressed there is a 50 per cent or more chance that the other will be too, even if they are adopted and reared apart.

Since then, researchers have been looking for a genetic contribution to affective disease. A clue has been discovered amongst the Old Order Amish of Lancaster, Pennsylvania, a Mennonite sect that seems to have forgotten time. Dressed in sombre, black garb, avoiding such modern conveniences as electricity, plumbing and automobiles, they live much as they did when their thirty ancestors first emigrated to the United States in the early eighteenth century. They lead isolated lives of subsistence farming and religious practice, with large families and marriages kept strictly within the boundaries of the community.

The Amish provide a unique human laboratory for studying the relationship between genetics and behaviour; a large, inbred population that keeps detailed family records and is almost completely free of such complicating factors as alcohol, promiscuity and drugs. In 1959, Janice Egeland, a young graduate student, began to study the relationship between cultural beliefs and health-care practices in the Amish community. When she shifted her focus to the incidence of manic-depression, in collaboration with a group of researchers from Yale University, the community was ready to help. Egeland had realised something that the Amish had known all along – that manic-depression was not spread evenly throughout the community, but was concentrated in certain families: 'I learned from the Amish that this disease is "*in bleut*" – in the blood.'

For ten years, Egeland and her colleagues took blood samples from 12 000 Old Order Amish and examined the chromosomes of the cells using the techniques of genetic engineering. When they cross-referenced the information with family records, they discovered a 'strong predisposition' to manic-depression in subjects who exhibited a certain genetic marker near the tip of the short arm of one of the twenty-three pairs of chromosomes, chromosome 11. The correlation was powerful. The incidence of manic-depression among the Amish is no higher than among the population at large, but if someone in the sect has the specific genetic marker, the chances of them developing the disease are as high as 80 per cent. Moreover the site on the chromosome seems to be related to the gene responsible for making an enzyme involved in the synthesis of the amine neurotransmitters.

The discovery of a probable guilty gene on chromosome 11 sent waves of excitement through the psychiatric community; Trevor Silverstone of St Bartholomew's Hospital in London called the finding 'a bull's eye hit'. But within weeks of the original announcement, Miron Baron, a professor of psychiatry at Columbia University in New York, reported that he had isolated a different genetic marker also correlated with manic-depression – this one on the X chromosome – in a group of Israelis. And shortly afterwards groups based in London and Bethesda, Maryland announced that another gene location might be responsible for affective disorder in families in Iceland and North America. Depressive illness may surface as a result of a host of genetic triggers: 'Different biological defects may lead to the same clinical picture,' Baron says.

Tim Crow, director of the Division of Psychiatry at the Clinical Research Centre in Middlesex, has even suggested that all the psychoses (depression, manic-depression and schizophrenia) may form a continuum with a single underlying genetic origin. Part of his evidence is the fact that schizophrenia is surprisingly common among the relatives of those with affective disorder. Van Gogh's youngest sister was in an asylum for thirty-eight years, almost certainly schizophrenic. George Gray also has a schizophrenic sister.

The depressive psychoses are extremely common yet deeply debilitating. If they do have a genetic origin, one must ask how the genes responsible have been preserved during human evolution. It is true that the symptoms often do not appear until after the beginning of child-rearing, so the disease does not directly hinder the propagation of genes. However it is surprising that genes that cause such problems for the family as a whole should have been conserved. Perhaps the relationship with creativity is no coincidence: the same gene or group of genes that place the curse of psychosis on a family may also bless it with exceptional creative ability, which helps it survive more than the illness puts it at a disadvantage.

We have entered a new era of psychiatric research; for the first time, we can examine the basic causes, not just the symptoms, of mental illness. As diagnostic techniques grow more sophisticated, the new genetic markers may make it possible to detect individuals who are *predisposed* to psychosis; and with detection comes the possibility of prevention. But such technology also comes with its own sizeable risks. If the psychoses develop

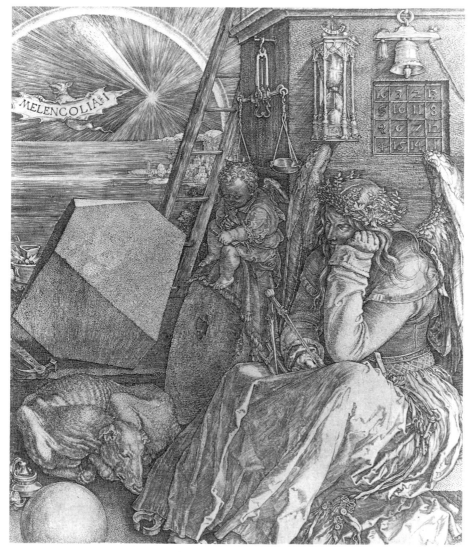

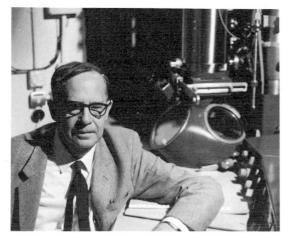

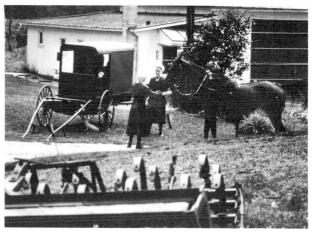

LEFT Melancholia I by
Albrecht Dürer (1471
1528) – an allegory on the
melancholy humour.

BELOW LEFT George Gray
at the electron microscope.

BELOW RIGHT The farm
of an Amish family in
Lancaster County in
Pennsylvania.

from an interaction between genetic and environmental events, might a person's knowledge that he or she is predisposed to the illness alter the 'environment' and trigger the disease? Is there a possibility that the knowledge alone can generate a self-fulfilling prophecy?

• WORDS AND THE BRAIN •

With the development of an effective armamentarium of treatments, it is tempting to assume that the Holy Grail of psychosis lies purely in the domain of physical intervention and that the *psychology* of depression need no longer be discussed. In fact, some of the so-called 'talking therapies' should not be taken lightly.

The efficiency of physical treatments, such as drugs, is not too difficult to test scientifically, but psychotherapy is notoriously difficult to assess. In 1981, however, the US National Institutes of Mental Health began a large comparative study of four types of treatments: interpersonal therapy, which focuses on personal relationships; cognitive therapy, which teaches people how to interpret their experiences more positively; imipramine, an antidepressant drug; and a placebo tablet, without any active ingredient. Nearly 300 outpatients with unipolar depression were randomly assigned to the four groups. After about sixteen weeks, the researchers found that imipramine was far more effective for the most severely depressed. However, over half of the first three groups – those receiving either of the talking therapies *or* the drug – recovered quite well, with no significant difference in the results. (Interestingly, nearly 30 per cent of those taking placebo alone also improved!) This result is surprising, but largely because we tend to put the psychological and the physical sides of mental illness into different categories. Talking to someone (and even giving them a placebo) influences the brain. Certain 'psychological' therapies may affect precisely the same parts of the brain as drugs or ECT.

Certainly many people who suffer from mood disorders claim that the support of their families is as important as their drugs. There were no antidepressant drugs or ECT for Vincent van Gogh. And in July 1890 the last line of defence seemed at risk; his beloved brother Theo was having financial difficulties and had decided to move back from Paris to Holland. Vincent feared the loss of the 50 francs that Theo sent him each week and the isolation that lay ahead. Some of his paintings reflected the depth of his feelings. He wrote to Theo: 'I have painted three more big canvasses since. They are vast fields of wheat under troubled skies, and I did not need to go out of my way to express sadness and extreme loneliness.' Vincent began to think about something that he had contemplated, and even attempted, in the past. Suicide.

On Sunday 27 July, after lunch with the local doctor, Vincent rushed out, as if anxious to continue painting in the wheat fields. A peasant heard him muttering 'It's impossible' as he wandered to the edge of the village. In his pocket was an old revolver that M. Ravoux had loaned him to shoot crows. Only four days earlier he had written to Theo asking for more paints; but his work was over. Vincent took the gun from his pocket, turned it to his chest, and fired.

The decision to live or die is a real one for many victims of depression. Until recently, it was assumed that opting for suicide constituted a purely psychological decision based on despair. But an extraordinary research project indicates that certain types of suicide can be traced to an imbalance of chemicals in the brain – of the same substances that seem to be involved in depression.

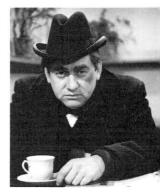

Tony Hancock, the British comedian, who suffered from severe depression and took his own life.

In the mid-1970s, Marie Åsberg, a psychiatrist at the Karolinska Hospital in Stockholm, was exploring the chemical composition of the fluid from the cavities of the brains of depressed patients. Among other things, this cerebrospinal fluid contains evidence of the activity of neuro transmitters in the brain, in the form of metabolites – products of the breakdown of neurotransmitters. Åsberg noticed that a third of the depressed patients in the hospital had low levels of 5-HIAA (5-hydroxy-indole acetic acid), a metabolite of serotonin. Åsberg wondered whether 5-HIAA might be a chemical marker for serotonin, the fall in the metabolite indicating the decline in brain serotonin that many believe to be associated with depression.

Åsberg continued her work, with little to show for it, until July 1975, when two depressed patients committed suicide. Analysis of their cerebrospinal fluid showed low levels of 5-HIAA. A remark from one of her colleagues, 'All these low 5-HIAA patients kill themselves,' prompted Åsberg to review the psychiatric case records. She soon discovered that more than twice as many depressed patients with low 5-HIAA levels had attempted or committed suicide than patients with normal levels. In addition, those with the lowest levels tended to kill themselves by violent methods – hanging, gunshot wounds, drowning. Those with only mod-erately low levels of 5-HIAA attempted 'milder' forms of suicide, such as taking sleeping tablets – often in amounts too small to be lethal.

In the thirteen years since her initial discovery, Åsberg has followed the cases of hundreds of depressed patients who have attempted suicide at least once, and her assertion has held true. 'Among people who have attempted suicide and survived, you can expect 2 per cent to be dead within one year,' she now says. 'But among people with low levels of 5-HIAA, in addition to a previous suicide attempt, the figure jumps to 20 per cent.'

The correlation of suicide rate with levels of chemicals from the brain raises a crucial issue in the search for the relationship between brain and mind. Surely all our behaviour, however extraordinary, must have physiological underpinnings in the machinery of the brain.

The bullet that van Gogh fired missed his heart and he managed to drag himself back to the Café Ravoux and up the stairs to his sad little room. The doctor decided not to operate, as if respecting his wish to die. Theo arrived the next day and sat talking with Vincent of paintings and the past. 'There is no end to sadness,' said Vincent. That night the two brothers lay side by side on the bed, bound by an inheritance of despair. At about one o'clock in the morning of 29 July 1890, Vincent cried out 'I want to go,' and he died in Theo's arms. In his pocket was a letter to Theo; not a suicide note but a confused account of the value of art. 'My own work', he wrote, 'I risk my life for it and my reason has half gone because of that.'

Theo contracted a kidney disease that made him uncontrollably violent. He survived Vincent by only five months and died in an asylum. They now lie side by side in the cemetery of Auvers.

THE
SEVENTH
AGE

HULDA CROOKS doesn't crochet or own a rocking chair; she climbs mountains.

> I have climbed ninety-seven peaks above 5000 feet since I entered the old-age category of sixty-five. I am now ninety-and-a-half. I never expected to last that long. I remember one elderly lady saying to me, 'Why do you waste your strength climbing mountains?' I said, 'I don't waste it; I gain strength.'

In 1987, at the age of ninety-one, Hulda Crooks became the oldest woman to climb Mount Fuji.

Is old age a time of weakness, of deteriorating ability? Or, as Mark Twain put it, is being old no different from being young, as long as you're sitting down? What determines whether or not we age well? And for those who escape the horror of dementia, what kind of mental life lies in store?

• THE AGEING WORLD •

In the coming century we face a global dilemma – a crisis that has grown out of the spectacular advances this century in hygiene, diet and health care. More of us are living longer than was ever thought possible. By the year 2051 Britain will be home to more than 6 million people over seventy-five, double the figure in 1985. The number of men over ninety will

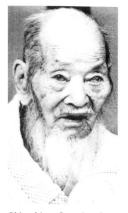

Shigechiyo Izumi celebrating his 119th birthday in Japan in 1984. He was the oldest man on record in the world.

increase by more than 600 per cent. The over eighty-fives are already the fastest growing age group in the United States.

This explosion of the elderly will bring a higher incidence of age-related illness and infirmity – an enormous drain on the national purse and a potential social catastrophe of imponderable proportion. Seen against this backdrop, the scientific investigation into the effects of ageing on body and brain is a race against time. This former backwater of research is growing in size and I am certain that it will soon assume a status as central as the fight against cancer and AIDS. The objective, at worst, is to minimise the misery of the elderly and, at best, to eradicate their own special diseases and keep the minds of the old young.

In ancient Rome, citizens were permitted to be appointed judges only after they had reached the age of sixty. In the Orient, the elderly have long been treasured as final arbiters in family decisions and as the guardians of tradition. Japan even names its most illustrious old artists and performers as 'Living National Treasures'. Societies throughout history, including our own, have recognised that wisdom can grow with age and experience. George Bernard Shaw wrote, 'Men do not live long enough. They are, for all purposes of higher civilisation, mere children when they die.' His message was clear: with the ebbing of material ambition, we may gain an ability to think more clearly and shed some of the emotions that distort our perceptions; we may accumulate experience, distil it, and donate it to future generations.

But with the disintegration of family life, with the emphasis on youth, physical fitness and financial productivity, our society has put the elderly, like out-of-date furniture, in the attic of life. They often feel themselves to be unwanted strangers in a world of the young, resented for the burden that they place on the community, and ridiculed because of their infirmity. We hide the old away like social lepers, pulling them out, blinking, like wrinkled moles, into the brief limelight of publicity when they turn one hundred or win the football pools. We have lost our respect for the old and must see the importance of regaining it. For we shall be them one day.

• FACING FACTS •

The proliferation of the aged will at least bring them power of a sort. The retired are already a major force in elections and they are an influential group of purchasers. In the United States, particularly, political groups have sprung up to influence and to represent old people. Madison Avenue is also in on the act, creating its own idealised image of the 'senior citizen' – a contented, active, utterly independent person, finding a moment now and then to pat the head of a grandchild between rounds of golf and trips to Florida. Above all, the image is eternally healthy and perfectly preserved.

The reality of ageing is not so pretty, but it is not all gloom. There is at least some solace in the growing evidence that ageing is not synonymous with total deterioration of the brain. That well-known story of tens of thousands of nerve cells throughout the brain dying every day of our lives – one-third lost in a lifetime – is probably science-fiction. Old age, like every other season of life, has its own special risks and diseases; but just as it is possible to escape infancy without autism, adolescence without schizophrenia and middle age without depressive psychosis, many old people do *not* succumb to dementia, stroke or degenerative diseases of the brain.

It would, however, be just as foolish to pretend that decline in the structure and function of the brain can be entirely avoided as it would to suggest that the rest of the body can remain perfectly preserved. But the very fact that there *are* and have been elderly people who have retained so much of their intellectual ability – the Rebecca Wests, Pablo Picassos, Lord Dennings, Bertrand Russells and Deng Xiao-pings of this world gives us hope that neither severe decline nor incapacitating disease is inevitable. The challenge is to define the best that we can expect in old age and to help everyone to approach that optimum.

Science has begun that process by exploring the nature of ageing. It is now clear that experience, the environment and mental effort all contribute to the health of the ageing brain and the mind that it makes. Successful ageing may not be a matter of chance, but a goal that science can help create.

In 1955, Warner Schaie of Pennsylvania State University began a long-term survey of more than 4000 people from the State of Washington, to find out what happens to cognitive abilities as we age. Scientific dogma at that time predicted that they would decline steadily. Schaie's study has already covered more than thirty years – a full generation – and it has painted a complex portrait of the ageing mind. He has found that, in the absence of specific disease, cognitive abilities change very little before the age of seventy-five; but then the decline usually becomes evident. For instance, 'fluid intelligence', which includes the capacity of short-term memory and the ability to process information quickly decreases significantly around that age, as do the sense of space and some elements of language. But 'crystallised intelligence' – the ability to use an accumulated body of knowledge to make judgements and solve problems (loosely what one would call wisdom) – was unimpaired in many of his subjects, and even seemed to improve in some.

Paul Baltes, working at the Max Planck Institute in West Berlin, has also found that, as long as they have enough time, old people can be as good as the young in using the ancient mnemonic trick of associating the

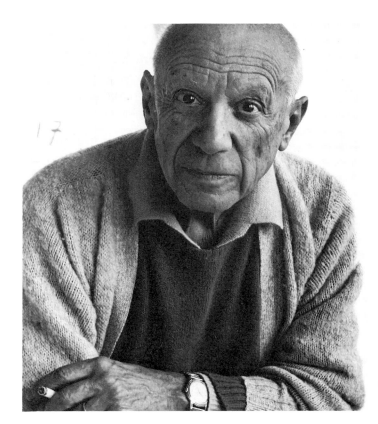

Some of us can look forward to the kind of long active old age enjoyed by Pablo Picasso (left) and Queen Victoria (below left). Others have less happy prospects: patients in the Day Room in the Victoria Cottage Hospital in Portsmouth in 1984 (below).

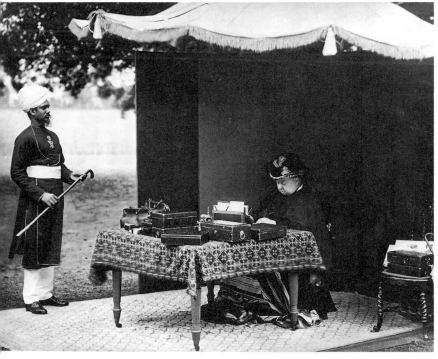

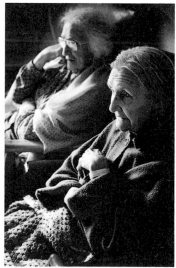

images of things to be remembered with the existing memories of familiar landmarks. Many older subjects could memorise as many as twenty words in the correct order, in less than a minute. But a good young performer could do the same in only ten seconds! The study of animals has revealed the probable cause of the inevitable decline in speed of memory and thought: nerve cells in old animals transmit impulses more slowly along their fibres.

Despite the biblical promise of 'three-score years and ten', widespread longevity is a very new phenomenon. Throughout the Middle Ages, ordinary people were lucky to survive to see the maturity of their children. Even at the beginning of this century, life expectancy in the western world was under fifty. The cruel rigours of the natural world do not give an opportunity for many animals to reach the equivalent of senescence. But in zoos and laboratories, protected from disease and supplied with a good diet, animals can live much longer than in the wild. The study of such geriatric animals is and will be crucial in the scientific investigation of the ageing brain.

At Johns Hopkins University in Baltimore, Maryland, Donald Price has assembled a colony of the oldest macaque monkeys in the world; some are more than thirty years old – the human equivalent of ninety or more, according to Price. He tests both old and young monkeys on simple tests of cognition and memory. Then he waits until his ancient subjects die natural deaths and examines their brains for changes which might correlate with any deficits in performance.

One of Price's monkeys, Gilbert, is a wizened, greying monkey of thirty-one. He watches as an inverted egg-cup is pushed towards him on a tray. He knows that it conceals food and lifts it to find the peanut underneath. The tray is removed and a few seconds later another one is pushed in, with both an inverted egg-cup and an upside-down beaker. This time the peanut is under the *beaker*; the task is called 'delayed non-matching to sample', and animals with damage to the frontal lobe or the region of the hippocampus do badly on it. So does Gilbert, even though he has been trying to learn it for days; he picks up the egg-cup.

Gilbert also has problems, much like those of very old people, in understanding the spatial relationships of things. He tries, with slightly trembling hands, to remove a boiled sweet shaped like a ring from a twisted piece of wire on which it has been threaded. He has great difficulty in retrieving the prize, compared with a young monkey. To Price this specific defect indicates a possible failure in the parietal lobe (the region of the cerebral cortex above the ears, where damage in humans can cause total spatial disorientation).

The difficulties of old monkeys and old people seem, then, to signify specific problems in the frontal and parietal lobes and in the memory system of the hippocampus and temporal lobe. But the defects may be more subtle than wholesale degeneration or attrition of neurons. The question of whether nerve cells *die* in significant numbers during normal ageing is still very controversial. But if there is substantial loss of cells it is certainly 'not ubiquitous. A recent study of the human brain showed only a tiny overall loss of cells in the frontal lobe, one of the areas that seem to be *most* affected in old age. There may be a somewhat greater loss in the hippocampus, that vital structure within the temporal lobe which is probably the printing press of personal memories. But any evidence for the death of nerve cells must be put into perspective; the loss is undoubtedly minute compared with the death of probably more than half of all neurons in the human brain before birth!

Neuronal death, by itself, may not be the cause of cognitive change. Like so many of the disasters that can beset the brain, some of the failures of old age may lie in the chemistry of individual nerve cells. Price himself suspects that the internal skeleton of the neuron – the system of tiny tubules and filaments that supports the structure of the branches of the cell – starts to break down in normal old age. These internal threads are essential not only for the growth and structural integrity of each nerve fibre, but also for the transport (all the way from the factory of the cell body along to the most distant terminals) of the chemicals needed to synthesise the transmitter substance, which is released at the terminals to carry messages across to the next neurons in the chain. Any disintegration of the skeleton might then interfere with vital chemical transmission.

There may also be failures in the chemical factory itself, in the mechanism of packaging and delivery of transmitter substance in the cell bodies of certain nerve cells, and hence a decline in the efficiency of communication at the synapses. Several systems of neurons, each with a distinctive chemical signature, may be affected: groups of cells in the midbrain that use dopamine or serotonin as their transmitter; a tiny structure, called the locus coeruleus, deep in the brainstem, that contains the brain's entire population of cells that use noradrenaline; and a mass of neurons that use the transmitter acetyl choline, which lie in the lower part of the forebrain, below the cerebral hemispheres. These systems are crucial because they all send their fibres (and therefore their transmitter substances) over vast areas of territory within the brain, and they all seem to act as modulators of activity and attention, turning the sensitivity of their target neurons up or down, making them responsive to other inputs or switching them into a mode in which they are ready to store information and lay down new memories.

Another avenue of research examines the *numbers* of dendrites that each cell has. Young, healthy neurons resemble vigorous trees, bristling with branches. But old ones look as if their branches have been pruned, probably because there are fewer connections between neurons. The implication is that essential circuits of nerve cells, on which all the actions of the brain depend, start to fail. The death of neurons; the loss of efficiency in those still alive; the pruning of the connections in the brain: these seem to be the prospects that face all of us who survive beyond those three-score years and ten. One crucial question is whether this general decline is inevitable, or whether it can be slowed or halted.

At one level, each new discovery of a mechanism that starts to run out of steam in the ageing brain is another blow to those optimists who would like to believe that the cognitive problems of the elderly are merely a matter of laziness, lack of motivation or inadequate stimulation. There *are* deteriorations in the brain, just as inevitable as those in the body. However, the fact that some of the most profound (and probably most significant) changes are essentially chemical offers at least the hope that these deficits may be treated by drugs that substitute for the missing transmitter.

The evidence for a literal loss of neurons and of the branches and connections of those that remain is, of course, more alarming. For the conventional wisdom is that, beyond the earliest stages of development, the brain loses its capacity to repair itself and form new connections. Recent research is, though, casting doubt on that view.

At Washington University in St Louis, Dale Purves and his colleagues have developed a method for staining individual neurons in a ganglion lying outside the central nervous system, which can easily be exposed under anaesthetic in the living adult mouse. One cell is injected with a fluorescent dye, so that it can be photographed under the microscope. That same cell can be found, re-stained and re-photographed at intervals over a period of several months, and there are definite changes in the exact shape and number of branches of the tree of dendrites that sprout from the cell body, on which incoming nerve fibres form their synapses. So, nerve cells can continue to grow and form new connections even in the adult animal.

William Greenough, at the University of Illinois in Champaign-Urbana, believes that growth and repair of neurons is also possible within the brain and can be switched on by the demands of the animal's own environment. In a remarkable experiment, Greenough took old rats who had lived drab, monotonous lives alone in uninteresting cages, and moved them to a large enclosure filled with fellow rats, and with a playground of slides, ramps, wheels and swings – what Greenough calls 'the rat equivalent of Disneyland'. At first, the old, overweight rats hid under the toys. Then, gradually, they recognised that they were in no danger and began to explore, to socialise and to play. They became fitter, lost weight and, as Greenough put it, they looked as if they were 'really enjoying life'.

The real revelation came not from looking at the *behaviour* of these old rats, when suddenly faced with a stimulating environment, but from seeing the effect on their *brains* after a few months. When Greenough

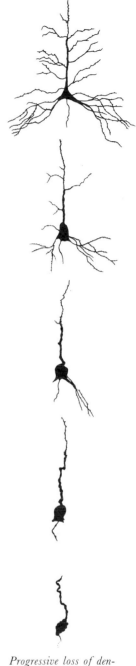

Progressive loss of dendrites of neurons in the cerebral cortex during ageing.

examined neurons from the cerebellum – thought to be involved in the co-ordination of movement and the learning of skills – he found a substantial restoration of the small side branches on the dendrites, where synapses are normally found. He concluded that each cell of this type may have as many as 2000 extra synapses compared with those from old rats kept in small cages. Cells from the cerebral cortex also seem to benefit in similar ways. Apparently activity and stimulation might save or restore billions of connections!

• THE SPECIAL HAZARDS •

Creaking joints, blurred vision and fuzzy memories face us all as we grow older. But to age is to be an unwilling contestant in a cruel lottery with some of the ugliest diseases as the unwanted prizes.

The human brain accounts for only 2 per cent of the body's weight but its frenetically active cells consume 20 per cent of the oxygen carried in the blood. Up to a litre of blood rushes through the blood vessels of the brain each minute, percolating into the tiniest capillaries to bring that vital oxygen within reach of every neuron. Deprived of blood, cells die within minutes. Unfortunately the huge network of vessels is vulnerable to clogging with blood clots or fatty deposits, and to rupture. These are the causes of stroke – the injury of part of the brain because of the loss of its blood supply.

In Britain there are 100 000 new cases of stroke each year, 95 per cent of them in people over sixty-five. The current cost of treating stroke victims (not including social security benefits and home care) is £565 million a year – about a quarter of the entire budget of the National Health Service. The effects of stroke range from a minor and transient disturbance of movement or speech to a devastating paralysis of body and mind.

The causes of stroke are complex and not well understood – diet, blood pressure, genetic disposition; all may play a part. But the variation in the incidence of stroke around the world at least offers hope that environmental factors (probably mainly nutritional) can be identified and preventive measures implemented.

Equally feared among the elderly are the dreadful degenerative diseases that prey on the old. Parkinson's disease affects one in 400 of the population, and in more than half of all cases the symptoms appear after the age of sixty. The hands and head shake uncontrollably and the muscles are stiff. But worst of all, there is an uncoupling of will and action that traps the sufferer in a strange kind of paralysis. Through research in the 1950s, mainly conducted in Sweden, we now know that one of the major defects in this disease is a massive loss of cells containing dopamine in one small cluster called the substantia nigra in the midbrain. These cells distribute their fibres into the basal ganglia – structures involved in the control of movement, lying below the cerebral hemispheres. The loss of dopamine is thought to prevent the normal selection of movements and their initiation. This discovery provided the rationale for the subsequent introduction of L-DOPA treatment for Parkinson's disease, for this substance is a chemical precursor of dopamine that can cross from the blood into the brain and help the remaining cells to produce more of the transmitter. L-DOPA treatment is not always effective and it can cause serious side effects, but it remains one of the most encouraging examples of the application of chemistry to therapy.

The statistics for stroke, Parkinson's disease and all the rare degenerative diseases of the brain, horrific though they are, are eclipsed by those for dementia of the old, including a condition that was first described in 1906 by a German neurologist Alois Alzheimer, and which now carries his name. The first patient Alzheimer described was in his early fifties – Alzheimer's disease can strike in middle age. It starts with poor memory for recent events and confusion about time and place, but it progresses inexorably, insidiously destroying language, thought, all kinds of memories, and finally the ability to eat, dress and control bladder and rectum. Alzheimer realised that this disease is not merely an exaggeration of the symptoms of normal ageing.

Dementia of all sorts now affects about 10 per cent of over sixty-fives, 20 per cent of eighty-year-olds. It is the main cause of hospitalisation and the fourth leading cause of death among the elderly. The full cost of this condition in the United States is estimated at $25 billion a year. It traps the wives, husbands and whole families of the patients in its web of suffering for years on end. It is, quite simply, one of the most disgusting diseases of the human species.

Hugh Bigelow is an eighty-one-year-old New Englander. He's having trouble with the lock to his room; his key simply won't fit the way it did yesterday. Soon an attendant takes him gently by the hands and leads him down the hall. He has forgotten where he lives. Hugh is in the early phase of Alzheimer's disease. He is embarrassed by any hint that he is not as quick as he used to be; and he has developed tricks to conceal his problems with memory and language. He fills sentences with 'they', 'the thing' and 'it' when he can't remember a word. He calls tasks 'dull' and 'boring' when he knows he won't be able to do them.

Hugh is just one of millions of people with Alzheimer's disease in the United States. What makes his case very special is that he has an identical twin, Bert, who is his mirror image, but who, so far, has given no indication that he will succumb to the disease that is killing his brother. These twins are genetically identical and only one has the disease. But they are an exception that proves a rule. Alzheimer's disease often has an inherited

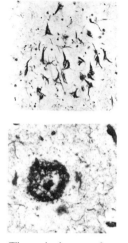

The cerebral cortex of people with Alzheimer's disease is characterised by 'tangles' (top) — twisted masses of fibres inside the nerve cells — and by dense 'plaques' (bottom) lying between the neurons.

pattern; indeed Hugh and Bert's father died with dementia and their older sister has been in a nursing home for six years.

Very recently, clues have emerged about the possible genetic basis of this disease. There is evidence that some families with a high incidence of dementia have an abnormal gene on chromosome 21, though this result is now rather controversial. (Interestingly, people with Down's syndrome, almost all of whom develop a condition very similar to Alzheimer's disease if they live to be more than thirty, have three of this same chromosome, rather than the normal two.) Nearby on the same chromosome is a gene that is responsible for making a protein that forms part of the membranes of nerve cells. This protein can break down to a smaller protein called amyloid, which may play a central role in the disease.

The brains of patients with Alzheimer's disease have a number of abnormal features, but the most obvious are tangles of filaments inside the larger nerve cells (evidence of a disturbed cell skeleton) and strange structures called plaques, lying in the space between nerve cells. Plaques are ugly lumps of amyloid protein wrapped around the swollen terminals of nerve fibres, which have been pushed away from their synapses. Plaques and tangles are seen occasionally in normal old brains but they pepper the demented brain, as distinctive in a cross-section as the spots on the face of someone with measles. No one can yet be sure of the sequence of events in Alzheimer's disease but a possible scenario is that something triggers a fault in chromosome 21, which makes neurons produce too much of the cell membrane protein, which becomes extruded to form the amyloid plaques. The original trigger may be a spontaneous reaction in the mutant gene, or could even be a virus infection or a toxic chemical in the environment.

James Edwardson and his colleagues at Newcastle General Hospital think that the level of aluminium in drinking water plays a part. They and others have shown that the incidence of severe Alzheimer's disease correlates well with local levels of aluminium, which is found concentrated in the cores of plaques in the brain. It is not yet clear whether aluminium might actually precipitate the disease or simply exacerbate it by being deposited in the growing plaques.

Though the plaques and tangles in the cerebral cortex and the hippocampus are the most visible features in Alzheimer's disease, they alone may not be the cause of the intellectual decay. That may be due to a more subtle change in a cluster of cells in the basal forebrain, below the cerebral hemispheres, which use acetyl choline as their transmitter and which send their fibres to the whole of the cortex and the hippocampus. As many as 90 per cent of these neurons of the basal forebrain die in advanced Alzheimer's disease. It is possible that this is a secondary reaction to the formation of plaques in the cortex and hippocampus, pushing the acetyl choline containing nerve terminals away from their target cells.

What, then, does acetyl choline do in the cortex and hippocampus? Recent research in animals suggests that it switches neurons into a condition in which they are receptive to signals from other sources and can change their synapses, leading to the storage of memories.

There is now great excitement in the possibility of developing drugs (by analogy with L-DOPA for Parkinson's disease) that will help the remaining cells in the basal forebrain to make more acetyl choline. Barbara Sahakian at the Institute of Psychiatry in London is even finding that chewing gum laced with nicotine (which mimics acetyl choline in certain synapses in the brain) helps patients with Alzheimer's disease.

Again by analogy with the most recent, experimental attack on Parkinson's disease, a possible approach in the future may be the transplantation, into the brains of Alzheimer's patients, of groups of acetyl choline cells from the brains of aborted human fetuses. Though fraught with ethical as well as technical problems, this may one day be feasible. Anders Björklund at the University of Lund in Sweden has already laid the foundations of such an approach with experimental work in animals. Björklund has injected fragments of fetal brain, containing acetyl choline cells, directly into the region of the hippocampus of geriatric (21-23-month-old) rats. Three months later there was a clear improvement in the animals' ability to learn to swim to a platform hidden below the surface in a large tank of water. They also improved in their motor co-ordination and superficially appeared rejuvenated.

Fred Gage, formerly one of Anders Björklund's collaborators, now working at the University of California in San Diego, believes that it might even be possible to revitalise cells in the basal forebrain in the early stages of Alzheimer's disease before they actually die, by bathing them with a substance called nerve growth factor (NGF). This chemical occurs naturally in the brain and is thought (as its name implies) to stimulate the growth of nerve fibres, especially early in development. It turns out that NGF has a restorative effect specifically on acetyl choline cells. Gage cuts the fibres leaving the basal forebrain in normal rats, thus precipitating degenerative reactions in the cells, which would ultimately lead to their death. But when he injects NGF soon after inflicting the damage, the cells survive. 'One can think of a time when NGF could be introduced into early-diagnosed Alzheimer's patients to protect those cholinergic cells from death,' Gage suggests.

Exciting though this work is, Gage considers its future application to be limited. NGF itself cannot pass through the barrier that protects the brain from chemicals in the bloodstream, which means that it must be infused directly into brain tissue. And it is by no means certain that the cells which survive remain functionally intact and re-connect to their targets far away. 'The next step in demonstrating the potential clinical

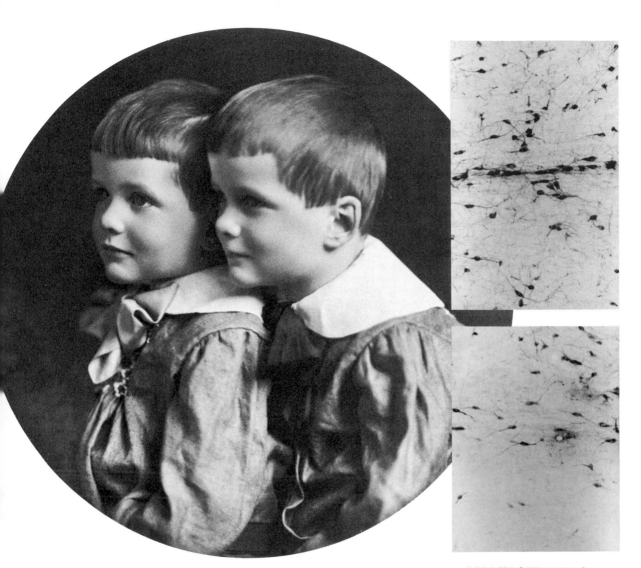

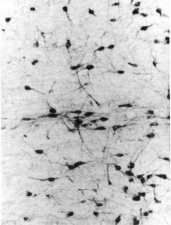

ABOVE *Bert and Hugh Bigelow as children.*

RIGHT *Microscopic sections through the basal forebrain of rats, prepared by Fred Gage, showing the neurons which use the transmitter acetyl choline. In humans this region degenerates in Alzheimer's disease. The nerve cells are normally quite densely packed (top) but they degenerate after the fibre bundles leaving this region have been cut (middle). However, if the animal is injected with nerve growth factor, degeneration is prevented (bottom).*

application of these approaches is crucial,' says Gage. 'We must show that, in fact, the surviving cells actually function in freely moving animals.'

• HOPE AND REALITY •

At no stage in life are the vicissitudes of fate so obvious as in old age. But there are many who believe that the 'seventh age' of life need not be the season of decay that Shakespeare portrays in *As You Like It*:

> *Last scene of all,*
> *That ends this strange eventful history,*
> *Is second childishness, and mere oblivion,*
> *Sans teeth, sans eyes, sans taste, sans everything.*

Many retirement communities and groups of elderly are investing their hope in an assumption that the ageing brain is like a muscle. 'Use it or lose it' is their guiding aphorism. They may not yet know of the work of William Greenough and Fred Gage but they have a simple trust in the notion that involvement, motivation, interest and activity might keep the brain 'young'.

One group, founded in Cambridge in 1982, has decided that old age is the third, not the seventh! They are the University of the Third Age, or U3A. U3A attempts to bring educational courses to the homebound. Its 800 volunteers travel throughout Britain, teaching subjects in which they have expertise. In addition, each member acts both as student and teacher, taking and giving classes. The educational opportunities offered are vast: they range from costumes of the nineteenth century to art, history, drama and mathematics, from discussions about the Bloomsbury Group to bridge, music, cooking and psychology. Speaking of her experience, one member of U3A said:

> It gives you an impulse to think each week. My brain is a tool, like my hands; and the same rules apply. The brain needs to be sharpened constantly. Since I joined the U3A, my brain seems to be working better now. My memory, especially, is nearly what it once was.

The promising results of U3A are far from scientific. It can be argued that the group which benefits most is self-selected – that those who profit from the experience might be just those who would have sought out stimulation on their own. But that perception seems, at best, a cynical one. Groups like U3A are giving the elderly access to experiences they might otherwise not have. For many who take part, the cognitive outlet provided has become a powerful tool in their efforts to remain healthy, constructive members of society.

We must accept that we shall not and cannot all be Charlie Chaplins or Herbert von Karajans; we cannot all expect to be both alive and alert into our eighties and beyond. But we can recognise the significance of such examples and take them as an encouragement to search for the kind of life that will give us the chance to make the best of our ageing brains.

The consequences of assuming that normal ageing inevitably means deterioration can be both sad and serious in a society that will soon be dominated by the predicament of the old. If a community perceives its elderly citizens as burdens, it fails to offer them constructive roles; they in turn experience declining prospects, a drabness of lifestyle, fewer comforts, less reason for living; they perceive themselves as second-class citizens and surely, as a result, become less active, less motivated, less involved. The vicious spiral continues to tighten. And society loses a precious, abundant resource.

If, on the other hand, there is a recognition of the special talents and interests of the elderly, of the contributions they can make, of the value they bring to so many strata of society, they will in turn strive to fulfil the expectations given to them. And society may continue to enjoy the fruits of their labours throughout their lives.

12

MODELS IN
THE MIND

Eight a.m. in the South Pacific. A dozen men, already sweating in the early morning heat, push a sleek, hand-built outrigger canoe down the sandy beach of their island. Six of them scramble aboard, check their provisions and bid farewell. The wind fills their sail; before them stretches a vast expanse of apparently featureless water. Hundreds of miles away lies their destination, a tiny island less than two miles wide. Without so much as a compass or a chart to guide them, these men must guide their vessel, barely 40 feet long, to its distant target.

Two p.m. in Norfolk, Virginia. The USS *Saipan*, a vast, glistening helicopter carrier, over 900 feet long, is casting off. Hundreds of minds focus on the problem of guiding the monstrous ship through the narrow, treacherous harbour and into the Atlantic ocean beyond. On land, the staff of the harbour master and of the US Coast Guard check their timetables, set their instruments and watch their radar screens. Out at sea, the other vessels of the US fleet, even hundreds of miles away, know of the imminent departure through operation plans and radio messages. On the *Saipan* itself, and in the pilot boat that guides it, the pitch of physical and mental activity slips into higher gear. Messages buzz from pilot to bridge, from bridge to engine room, from ships to shore. Commands are shouted, telephoned, radioed or sent wordlessly through the machinery of connections that steers the vessel.

The intrepid crew of the Micronesian craft are now alone, surrounded by the empty ocean with no radio, no radar, no Coast Guard or pilot. But their journey is by no means unplanned. The legendary skills of the Micronesian navigators have been acquired through thousands of years of practice and refined to perfection in the unforgiving academy of real life. The skill of navigation is passed from father to son; its only instrument is the mind of the navigator. He has no physical chart to guide him, but has, instead, the stored knowledge of the flight of birds, the positions of the sun and the stars, the form of the clouds and the direction and shape of the waves. In his imagined world, his canoe sits immobile – the centre of the universe – as the sea, the sun, the stars and the islands move around it.

The USS *Saipan* is emerging from the narrow channel of the naval base at Norfolk. On the wings of the ship, seamen take bearings on visible landmarks and telephone them to the bridge, where a committee of navigators receive the messages, read their radar screens, glance at the meteorological report and plot the progress of the ship on a huge chart – an abstract symbolic representation of the harbour, the vessel and the sea beyond. No single person is navigating. No single mind knows all the facts or makes all the decisions. The participants in this enormous task are atoms of mental responsibility bound together by technology into a vast social structure of thought.

The man at the helm of the Micronesian canoe, his eyes scanning the waves and the clouds, and the quartermaster on the bridge of the carrier, who looks not at the world but at his charts, seem to be doing utterly different things but they do have something in common – a system of thinking that we have inherited from our hominid ancestors. Those people may have travelled no more than a few miles each generation and may never have seen an ocean, but their brains contained the machinery of thought capable of sailing the seas and flying to the moon. Every decision that we take is built on a model of the problem in the mind. Like navigators, we must know where we have been; we must have ways of assessing our progress in the world and of perceiving where we currently stand; and we must conceive of our desired goal and have a plan to reach it.

• THOUGHT FOR FOOD •

In 1637, René Descartes, one of the most influential thinkers of the past millennium, published the *Discourse on Method*, a popular introduction to his philosophy. Ten years earlier, he had produced a book that gave an account of the state of man's scientific knowledge of the world, interpreted in mathematical terms. His *Geometry*, published in the same year as the *Discourse*, introduced the principles of Cartesian, analytical geometry. His knowledge of optics and his own observations on the structure of the eye enabled him to understand the way in which the eye focuses an image on the retina: indeed, he described these discoveries in *La Dioptrique*, which was published in the same volume as the *Discourse*.

René Descartes had an understanding of the nature of the world, of the mechanisms of the senses and of the power of science to explain, as full as that of any human being who had ever lived. Yet, in the *Discourse*, Descartes revealed a deep sense of unease that had permeated his philosophy. He knew that his senses could deceive him; he knew that his dreams were false images; in the face of such evident fraudulence in the mind, was there anything that he could truly believe? His solution was to adopt an attitude of extreme scepticism:

> I resolved to reject as false everything in which I could imagine the least doubt, in order to see if there remained afterwards anything that was entirely undubitable.

Descartes found that almost nothing in his experience survived this test of doubt. Indeed, all that remained after this censorship of scepticism was Descartes's certainty about his own existence as a thinking being, crystallised in his immortal phrase, *cogito ergo sum* – 'I think, therefore I am.'

For Descartes, thought is the product of a spiritual substance, the *res cogitans*, which, in its finest form, is uniquely human. Yet animals, which he believed were thoughtless machines, can perform such extraordinary feats of purposeful behaviour that it is hard to believe that human beings and animals operate in different universes of cogitation. However good the senses of an animal, they alone could guide no more than its immediate reactions to the world around it. To construct a piece of behaviour as rich, as prolonged and as purposeful as the homing of a pigeon, an animal must not only have knowledge of its immediate world but also have a view of its objectives and a plan to achieve them.

We shall never *know* for sure that animals think as we do, because thought (in the way that we normally use that word) lies in a domain of experience that can be communicated only through some direct linguistic statement about the nature of one's own conscious mind. But animals show us through their *actions* that, whether consciously thinking or not, they have the machinery in their brains to plan complex strategies that meet their needs. If thought is the weighing of evidence to arrive at conclusions, surely animals must have the rudiments of thinking, for their behaviour reveals the conclusions that they draw about the world around them.

The study of animals is now a major component of the science of psychology. But paradoxically the interest in animals grew out of the influence of a movement that denied any significance for consciousness in the production of the behaviour of any species, man or other animal. That movement was behaviourism, a school of thought that ruled psychology, at least in North America and Great Britain, from about 1920 until the mid-1950s. At the turn of the century, the young science of psychology, still widely known as experimental philosophy, was dominated by abstract speculation and by the introspective analysis of human thought. John B. Watson, whose mother was a fundamental Baptist and whose father ran away to live with two Indian women, was the founder of this new radical movement that joined animals and human beings in a union of mindless mechanism. Watson grew up to detest religion and learned, during his studies at the University of Chicago, to suspect philosophy too. His doctoral thesis *Animal Learning* was a remarkably original description of the tricks and tactics that animals use to solve problems. Watson rapidly acquired a reputation for his studies of animal learning, but his teachers and colleagues were alarmed at his suggestions that the powers of objective observation might be turned on the human species too. In 1912, Watson, then Professor of Psychology at Johns Hopkins University in Baltimore, gave a series of summer lectures at Columbia University which were to become the Sermon on the Mount of behaviourism.

The new school of behaviourism had a philosophical, even political zealotry right from the start. It is surely significant that Watson said in his famous lectures of 1912 that the theoretical goal of behaviourist psychology 'is the control and prediction of behaviour'. He imagined a pure science of psychology based on the neutral, objective analysis of cause and effect. This he hoped would give psychology as respectable a status within science as physics, whose aim is to invent laws that predict the behaviour of the inanimate world. If behaviour can be predicted, it can be controlled: and if behaviour can be controlled, life can be improved.

Watson and some of his behaviourist colleagues (most notably Burrhus F. Skinner) saw psychology as a true science of everyday life. But Watson himself was forced out of academic science at the age of only forty-two, after a divorce scandal, and was reduced to selling rubber boots; those who took up the behaviourist banner, most especially the American Clark Hull, sought academic respectability in the unnatural environment of the laboratory. The brain of the laboratory rat became the subject of a style of research as precise as the analysis of an unknown chemical compound or the description of a newly discovered galaxy. Hull's books were full of mathematical equations and precise, formal concepts that sought to explain behaviour in terms of the sensory information available to the animal and its own internal drives and habits. But in this battle between the brains of rats and men, the rats won! Clark Hull died in 1952 knowing that he had failed to construct a theory precise enough to predict in all circumstances the behaviour of even a laboratory rat.

Behaviourism (perhaps fortunately) has failed in its ambition of controlling human behaviour and it has left only a modest legacy of benefit in the therapeutic techniques of 'behaviour modification', which have had some impact in the treatment of neurosis, phobia and addiction. But behaviourism has carved a much deeper impression in the science of psychology. It has taught psychologists that there must be continuity of the principles of behaviour, no less than the principles of the structure of the body, from animals to the human species. Animals are our cousins; not because we all share the kind of clockwork machinery imagined in behaviourist theory, but because animals as well as humans use strategies of thinking that reveal their *understanding* of the world around them. As Herbert Terrace, Professor of Psychology at Columbia University, says: 'I think there is no longer a question: can an animal think? Now the question is: how does an animal think?'

A new movement has replaced behaviourism. This new school, cognitive psychology, attempts to account for behaviour in terms of the operations of a sophisticated, information-processing system of mind, whose actions reveal its *understanding* of problems in the world. Increasingly, cognitive psychologists are turning to animals to discover the seeds that have flowered into human consciousness and language.

The ability of an animal to discover inspired solutions to complex problems by thought alone surely implies that it has mechanisms for representing the problem it faces, for examining, without moving a muscle, the strategies that might be tried, and for coming up with a solution through imagination alone. These remarkable achievements imply that the animal has, within its head, a way of describing the arrangement of the world – a map of reality and of the problems to be solved. John O'Keefe of University College in London thinks that the hippocampus, the enigmatic structure tucked underneath the temporal lobe of the brain, is the site of this 'cognitive map'. Imagine the following situation. A hungry rat is placed in the middle of a large, open cage that consists of a central chamber with a number of alleyways that radiate out from it, like the legs of a spider. At the end of each alley is a single piece of food. The rat, familiar with this little puzzle, races from arm to arm collecting the food in random order, but almost never wasting its time by returning to an alley that it has already visited. If the hippocampus is damaged, the rat seems unable to remember where it has already been and it keeps returning again and again to arms of the maze that it has already cleared of food. It seems that the hippocampus contains some kind of record, in the activity of its cells, of where the animal is at any particular moment. This cognitive map may play a large part in the process by which the brain manipulates internal images of the world in its attempt to find solutions to problems.

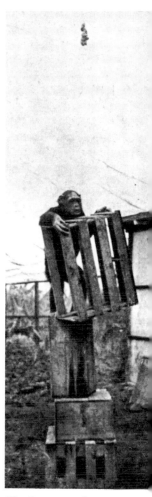

The German psychologist Wolfgang Köhler (1887–1967), studied the behaviour of apes on Tenerife during the First World War. He described the way in which they could solve problems, apparently through a flash of 'insight'. Here 'Grande' builds a four-storey structure to try to reach food hanging overhead.

The great achievements of science, technology and culture bear witness to the extraordinary power of human thought. Unless, like Descartes, we are reduced to a theory of frustration that ascribes thought to a spiritual 'thought substance' that lies outside the realm of conventional physical laws, we must have as our ultimate objective the explanation of thought in terms of the machinery of the brain. However, for the moment, the task of explaining thinking in terms of the myriad connections in the human brain is far beyond the scope of our knowledge of the nervous system. Instead, we search for metaphors; for systems that we *do* understand, which have some of the characteristics of human thinking. In the last century, the metaphors matched the technology of the time; the brain was a steam engine or a great system of magical clockwork. In this century the metaphors have shifted again and again, with each new leap of technology. The brain was 'an enchanted loom', a telephone exchange, a hologram or a chemical plant. But the most forceful and in some ways most frightening metaphor is that of the computer. The computer, in its broadest sense, is an engine of calculation, a device for processing information according to a program – a set of formal instructions. With such a compliant definition as this, the brain is not simply *like* a computer; it *is* a computer. In the immortal words of Marvin Minsky from the Massachusetts Institute of Technology, one of the founders of the new science of artificial intelligence, the brain is a 'meat machine'. John McCarthy, of Stanford University in California, who invented the term artificial intelligence, sees the equivalent of the highest aspects of the human mind – beliefs, thoughts and consciousness – in the operations of even the crudest kinds of machines: 'Machines as simple as thermostats can be said to have beliefs.... My thermostat has three beliefs – it's too hot in here, it's too cold in here, and it's just right in here!'

Surely John McCarthy was being deliberately provocative; but unless we propose that there is some indefinable magic in the brain, we must certainly conclude that the brain *is* a computing machine. In that case, can we find some clue to the mechanisms of human thought in the design of modern digital computers? People can solve logical problems, follow strategies in games such as chess, perform mathematical calculations. Computers can do all of these things, and, in many respects, they do them more efficiently. However, as in the fable of the hare and the tortoise, brains beat computers in so many ways because the cunning tricks they use outweigh the sheer speed and prodigious memories of man-made machines.

Despite the power of computers and the impact that they have had on our lives, their basic way of thinking is unbelievably naive. The archetypal universal computing machine, as envisaged by the remarkable

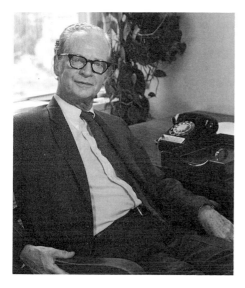

LEFT *Burrhus F. Skinner, the influential behaviourist who suggested that the richest aspects of mental life, including thought and language, might be explained by the formation of simple learned associations.*

BELOW RIGHT *Herbert Terrace, once a student of Skinner, now believes that chimpanzees and even much simpler animals are capable of forming internal representations of the world in their brains and using them as the basis of thought.*

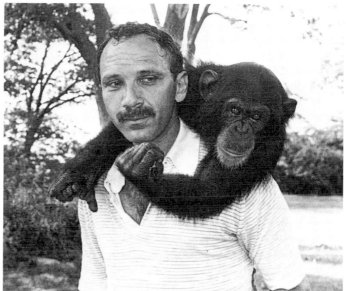

BELOW *Alan Turing (1912–1951) was a keen athlete and even trained for the Olympic marathon trials in 1947. He was persecuted because of his homosexuality but it is still not clear whether he took his own life or died as a result of a game that went wrong.*

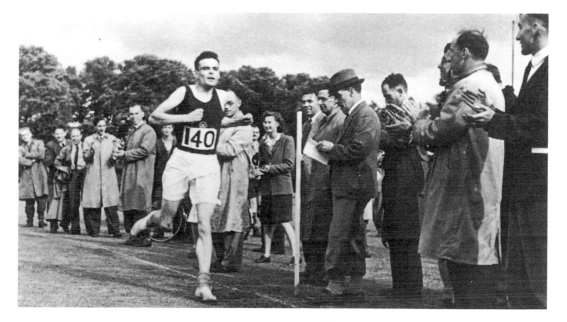

Cambridge mathematician Alan Turing, is nothing more than a system for reacting to a simple string of messages on a paper tape or some other form of serial presentation. Each step on the tape has on it a symbol or is blank. The computing machine is capable of moving the tape, one step at a time, backwards or forwards. It can erase a symbol or print a new one. That is all it can do. Yet by means of programs expressed in the simplest of instructions, consisting only of a string of zeros and ones, such a universal machine can, as Turing proved, tackle any problem that can be expressed in terms of a specific set of instructions or rules.

Alan Turing proposed this kind of architecture for a universal computer in a famous paper published in 1937, shortly after he graduated from Cambridge, almost ten years before a team led by the equally brilliant mathematician John Von Neumann in Philadelphia produced ENIAC, the world's first digital computer. Alan Turing was one of those eccentric but many-talented geniuses that science throws up from time to time. Some would say that Turing more than any other man was responsible for the defeat of Germany in the Second World War, for Turing designed 'Ultra', a kind of computer that cracked the code of a German cipher machine, called 'Enigma', which fell into the hands of British intelligence in 1939.

Turing died in 1954, at the age of only forty-one, after consuming cyanide that he had synthesised in his home laboratory. Four years before his death, he published what was perhaps his most provocative and controversial paper, entitled 'Computing machinery and intelligence'. In it he addressed a question that has become a central issue for cognitive psychology and philosophy, the question of whether machines might think. Remember that, at the time, the few digital computers that were in existence were monstrous, unreliable contraptions, with less memory than a good pocket calculator has today. Two years earlier, Turing resigned (or perhaps was dismissed) from the British project to build a computer at the National Physical Laboratory in Teddington, because of his impatience with the slow pace of progress. Nevertheless, in his seminal article, Turing had the prescience to ask questions about the relationship between computers and the human mind.

Turing realised that thought and consciousness are essentially private experiences. We can know about the thoughts of others only by the *actions* that reveal those thoughts (including the use of language to describe them). Although I assume that other human beings think in much the same way that I do, I have no direct evidence about their conscious minds. It is more difficult to accept that animals have thought processes like our own, unless they *look* or *behave* like people. Despite all the evidence that whales, for instance, are highly intelligent animals, with huge brains not very different in structure from our own, it is hard to imagine that whales think like us, yet very easy to believe that chimpanzees have something approaching human thought. The prejudice of appearance is even stronger when we consider the possibility that machines might think. No surprise that it is easier to empathise with the anthropomorphic. See Threepio robot from the movie *Star Wars* than with the infinitely more intelligent but immobile and bodiless *Hal* from *2001*.

Turing pointed out that it is no easier to 'get inside' other human beings to inspect the nature of their conscious cogitations than it is to penetrate the mental world of a computer. Instead of such mind-games, he proposed a practical test for recognising machine intelligence. In the imaginary Turing Test, an interrogator sits at a teletype, communicating with two other individuals, hidden from sight. The interrogator questions each of them about their mental experiences, and might try to guess which is a man, which a woman. The next step is to substitute a computer for one of the human beings. Can the interrogator now distinguish the machine from the remaining human being? If not, Turing concludes that the computer has passed the test of thinking like a person.

• INTELLIGENCE AND •
THOUGHT

The writings of Alan Turing have precipitated a debate about the nature of man no less heated than the public controversy that followed Darwin's *The Descent of Man*. Like Darwin, Turing was criticised as a heartless materialist with no sensitivity for the spiritual side of human beings. Nothing could be further from the truth. It is paradoxical that so exceptional a man, whose eccentricity no one would ever wish to mimic in a machine, could have been capable of such a detached and reasoned view of the nature of thought. In his amusing book on the early history of the computer, *Faster than Thought*, B. V. Bowden wrote: 'No machine is ever likely to undertake the work of those few extraordinary men whose dreams and whose efforts are responsible for the growth and the flowering of our civilisation.' Turing was surely such a man. Yet, to him, the computer was much more than a metaphor for mind; it was an instrument with the potential for true thought.

The death of Alan Turing was followed quickly by the birth of artificial intelligence, the new science created out of Turing's vision of machines with human-like thoughts. The march of technology was a million times faster than the slow progress of animal evolution. Over the course of just a few years, computers have changed out of all recognition, shrinking in size, while expanding in memory and speed, like some silicon version of *Alice in Wonderland*. The memory capacity of John Von Neumann's first computer, in 1946, was only twenty 'words'; but memory soon leapt to thousands, then millions, and now billions of 'words' of information.

As the machines themselves became ever more powerful, the languages and techniques for programming them increased in sophistication. For the first few years of the artificial intelligence revolution, from about 1957 to the mid-1960s, the prophets of this new semiconductor religion were wildly optimistic. They set themselves to teach machines to do the things that we admire most as the pinnacles of intelligence in human beings – doing mathematics, solving logical problems, playing chess. The sheer speed, the prodigious memory and the uncanny accuracy (on a good day) of the modern digital computer gives it the sheer brute force to tackle problems like these with considerable success. Within two or three years of the start of the artificial intelligence project at the Massachusetts Institute of Technology, there was a computer program that could do calculus as well as most graduates in mathematics. In a few more years, the world backgammon championship was won by a computer program written by Hans Berliner. It looked as if computers were winning hands down over the human mind. But in the following twenty years, the optimism has lost its shine, and even the most enthusiastic of the artificial intelligentsia realise that computers are still a long way from imitating all the achievements of human thought. It is clear that computers have done so well in certain tasks only by virtue of their spectacular speed and their immense memories. They are far from mastering the more cunning tricks of human thought. And it turns out that the goals set in the early days of artificial intelligence – the mathematics, the logic and the chess – were *not* the most impressive things that we do with our brains.

The most profound computations in the brains are the ones that everyone does effortlessly and unconsciously. Recognising individual objects from the unbelievable jumble of shapes in the retinal image; deciphering the torrent of sounds that makes up human speech; standing up on two legs, walking to a door and opening it. These are the real miracles of human thought that make the achievements of even the grandest computers look like the intellectual efforts of a worm.

There are people who can, in a sense, make their brains work with the sheer number-crunching precision of a computer. The distinguished mathematician from Edinburgh University, Professor A. C. Aitken, used to give a good imitation of a pocket calculator as a party trick. The psychologist I. M. L. Hunter described Aitken's reaction to being asked to express the fraction 4/47 as a decimal:

> He is silent for 4 seconds, then begins to speak the answer at a nearly uniform rate of 1 digit every three-quarters of a second. '0-8-5-1-0-6-3-8-2-9-7-8-7-2-3-4-0-4-2-5-5-3-1-9-1-4, that's about as far as I can carry

it.' The total time between the presentation of the problem and this moment is 24 seconds. He discusses the problem for 1 minute and then continues the answer at the same rate as before. 'Yes, 1-9-1-4-8-9, I can get that.' He pauses for 5 seconds. '3-6-1-7-0-2-1-2-7-6-5-9-5-7-4-4-5-8, now that is the repeating point. It starts again at 085. So if that is 46 places, I am right.'

Professor Aitken's extraordinary skill derived partly from great natural capacity for mental arithmetic but more from his expert knowledge of the nature of numbers. More remarkable are those rare individuals whose minds seem to work with the precision of a computer but who cannot explain or articulate their skills and whose intelligence in every conventional sense is very low. A classic case was an eleven-year-old boy, described in 1945, whose intelligence quotient or IQ (that much-maligned measure of intelligence) fell in the range of the mentally retarded. However, he could, at a moment's notice, name the day of the week for any date from the year 1880 onwards. His recall of the dates of birth of hundreds of people was equally remarkable. People of this sort are often called 'idiots savants' or calculating geniuses. They are living proof that the skill of truly intelligent thought is quite different from a simple feat of memory or calculation. But intelligence does have *something* to do with the power of memory and the speed of mental processes. Indeed, the simple reaction time of a person – the time that it takes to press a button when a light flashes on, for instance – is a remarkably good predictor of the same person's IQ. It may be that one factor that limits the capacity for the kind of thought measured by intelligence tests is merely the speed with which nerve impulses can buzz around the brain. But real intelligence is so much more than the simple storage of information and the frenzied clicking of nerves.

The characteristics of genius and the achievements of human creativity cannot be captured in a single number. How could we design an IQ test that would discover with equal facility the genius of Shakespeare, of Newton or of Beethoven? Different minds flourish in different ways. Human life is a panoply of skills; a giant in one may be a simpleton in another. Sir Arthur Conan Doyle, Henry James and Schubert were practically innumerate; Charles Darwin and William Wordsworth were considered so idle and so stupid that they were virtually disowned by their families; Sir William Osler, the Oxford physician who was the father of modern medicine, was expelled from school; Albert Einstein hardly spoke a word until he was nearly four.

• LESSONS FROM •
A GAME OF CHESS

It is no wonder that chess has become a favourite subject for the artificial intelligentsia; a game of logic and strategy, with a strict but rich set of rules and no space for luck. The quality of chess-playing programs has steadily increased in the past thirty years. You can now buy off the shelf in a toy shop tiny, battery-driven boxes that play chess at the level of a reasonable club player. The biggest and most successful of the chess-playing programs are creeping up on the world's grand masters; their success is a direct product of the increasing speed and memory of modern computers. But do these programs actually simulate the mind of a master?

The number of possible configurations that might occur in a chess match has been estimated at more than 10 000 million million million million million million million! In 1985, the North American Computer Chess Championship was won by Hans Berliner's program *Hitech*, which is able to look at 20 to 30 million positions for each move. But according to those who have analysed the play of human chess masters, they remember between 30 000 and 50 000 basic patterns of play – a huge number, but trivial compared with the capacity of *Hitech*. Moreover, the human grand master rarely considers more than twenty or thirty positions for each move. When the great grand master Richard Reti was asked how many moves ahead he considered, he replied, 'One; the right one!'

Even the most massive of present-day computers is not sufficiently large or fast to allow a complete and exhaustive survey of every possible move before it makes a decision. The best chess programs use a variety of tricks for searching through a classified network of hundreds of thousands of possible moves each second and using a scoring system to determine which strategy is best. But however clever the chess programs are at finding short cuts through the forest of possibilities, they shrink into insignificance compared with the capacity of the human brain to squeeze the blood of genius from the stone of its mere neurons. People think so very differently from computers – and much more efficiently too.

In the Roberto Clemente Middle School in the South Bronx, chess master Bruce Pandolfini sits with his back to the chess board, playing, without looking, against an entire class of excited schoolchildren, who pit their collective minds against that of the master. They lose; but they admire Pandolfini – not for his physical force but for the strength of his mind. Pandolfini describes the skills that children learn from the challenge of chess:

> In a superficial sense, chess gives children many attributes. It improves their memory, their concentration skills; it gives them discipline, makes them more logical, having to arrange their ideas in logical sequence.

They learn to look for analogies and to spot patterns. Perhaps more importantly than anything, though, it enables them to determine what's truly relevant about a situation, and to devote all their energies to solving a problem.

But what is this factor of 'relevance' which children can learn from a game of chess? Can this be the clue to the distinctive difference between human and computer thought?

• THROUGH THE EYES OF UNDERSTANDING •

Daniel Kahneman, from the University of California in Berkeley, sees a lesson about the everyday business of thinking in the abstract world of chess:

> The chess master is in some ways an example of the way we think in general. And what's come to light in the studies of chess playing is the very close link between cognition and perception. That is, when the chess master looks at a complicated position he sees the potentialities in it; he recognises patterns, and he assembles those patterns into a meaningful whole.

Through the eyes of a good chess player, the simple chequered board and the pieces on it actually take on *meaning*. When the pieces are placed in sensible positions, corresponding to a snapshot of a real game, the whole board assumes a life of its own; the little scene of plastic shapes has sense and significance, immediately stimulating thoughts of possible moves. If the same pieces are arranged in a nonsensical pattern, one that could not represent a true position in a real game, the *lack* of meaning is immediately obvious to a skilled player. When we look at any scene, we do not just see the present; we infer a past and we anticipate a future. We search in our interpretation of the situation for its origins and its potentialities.

The Swiss developmental psychologist, Jean Piaget, suggested that children go through a crucial stage in their cognitive development between the ages of about six and eleven. The world is transformed from a place of simple certainties, of yes or no, to a universe of *probability*, in which the concept of chance is discovered. As Daniel Kahneman put it, 'Uncertainty is a fact with which all forms of life must be prepared to contend.... At all levels, action must be taken before the uncertainty is resolved.' The classical rules of logic, relatively easily incorporated into the program of a computer, deal with the world of absolute truth or falsehood. A conclusion either follows or does not follow from the premises stated. However, the clues to the future that the world around us provides are usually full of uncertainty. If an animal on one occasion discovers food in a particular place, what conclusion can it draw? A *single* experience can tell it nothing. If the food lies in one of the arms of a radial maze, of the type used by John O'Keefe in his experiments, the rat will soon learn that the *other* arms of the maze contain the rest of the food. On the other hand, if the rat is in a simple maze, in which food is always put in the same place, it will realize that it must return again and again to the arm in which the food lies.

Animals learn, then, on the basis of the statistical nature of their experiences. However, the hope that the strict rules of statistical theory might be used to account for the everyday judgements of animals and human beings proved unfounded. Daniel Kahneman and Amos Tversky studied the 'natural statistics' of human thought and discovered that people were influenced in their judgement of likelihood, by their prejudices, by their expectations and by their prior *knowledge* of the real world. In the experiments, volunteers were given a little character sketch and then asked questions about the person involved:

Linda is 31 years old, single, outspoken, and very bright. She majored in philosophy. As a student, she was deeply concerned with issues of discrimination and social justice, and also participated in anti-nuclear demonstrations.

After reading such a statement, the subject of the experiment was asked whether it was more probable that Linda is a bank clerk, or that she is a bank clerk who is an active feminist. Over 80 per cent of college students chose the *second* statement, even though it is obvious that the chance of one thing being true cannot possibly be greater than the chance of that thing *and* something else simultaneously being correct. Evidently, the factor that contaminates the natural sense of statistics is the *expectation* that people have of the world around them. Daniel Kahneman argues that people judge likelihood in terms of representative idealised models of the way that they think the world should be.

We have all grown accustomed to the evidence of statistics. We read with interest about the likelihood that cigarette smokers will die of lung cancer, that commercial aircraft will crash, that the weather will be fine and sunny. Yet we are much more influenced in our judgements of such things by our own very limited (and therefore unreliable) experience of them, or by the vividness of our recollection of *single* instances. Every confirmed cigarette smoker clings to the fact that *he* knows of a 50-a-day man who lived to be more than ninety years old. No amount of publicity about the safety of air travel can erase from the mind the horror of a news story about the crash of a jumbo jet. And one freak storm does more to influence our confidence in the weather forecasters than a decade of 70 per cent correct prediction! What seems to intervene between evidence and interpretation is the power of *personal* experience.

The same is certainly true in the mental machinery that controls the behaviour of animals, especially their reactions to *unpleasant* situations. The vast majority of animal species show a remarkably rapid and permanent form of learning, aptly called one-trial learning, in which they will avoid, sometimes for the rest of their lives, a situation in which they have been frightened or hurt just once. Such a strategy makes no sense at all from a statistical point of view. But why take the risk of thinking in terms of *probabilities* when the alternative is the *certainty* of never being hurt in the same way again? People and animals are built to pay particular attention to single, vivid experiences. The endorsement of a product in an advertisement by a popular movie star or athlete can obliterate the solid good sense of a thousand reports in consumer magazines. Joseph Stalin once pointed out that a single Russian death was a tragedy; a million deaths just a statistic.

Daniel Kahneman believes that the *mistakes* that people make (which a computer would be unlikely to make) reveal the special nature of human thought. The currency of behaviour is certainty; no animal (human or otherwise) can plan its actions with the half-hearted indecision of statistical theory. Yet we base our firm convictions on fragmentary evidence; and we play the gambler's strategy of sticking with the winning line until a conflicting experience makes us change our minds.

• THE FRAGILE NATURE OF TRUTH •

The influence of expectation and experience reaches down to the roots of thought – to our very perception of the world, and to the things that we remember. We are able to capture as long-term remembrances only a minute fraction of the experiences that wash through our short-term memory. Every second of our waking lives is a frantic decision about what to remember and what to forget. No wonder, then, that especially vivid and emotional events are trapped for ever in the net of long-term memory, while the humdrum sprats of everyday experience slip through and are lost. Just as important as the selection of memories on the basis of their vividness is the process of organisation, based on expectation and prejudice, to which those memories are then subjected.

The Cambridge psychologist, Sir Frederic Bartlett, working in the 1930s, made a study of the way in which people forget and the manner in which they organise and distort the memories that they retain. In Bartlett's experiments, one person read a story to another, who in turn tried to repeat it, from memory, to a third, and so on. No surprise that the stories became more cryptic than the original. However, they also became distorted to fit the conventions and cultural expectations of the successive listeners and story tellers. The same kind of thing happened when a single person tried time after time to reproduce the original story (in some cases years after hearing it). Bartlett suggested, with extraordinary prescience, that people do not simply remember scattered but accurate fragments of their original experiences. Rather, they actively construct an abstract representation or mental schema, which distorts the original information according to the person's existing beliefs, knowledge and emotions. Ominously, the errors that are injected into our memories through the prejudice of expectation take on the same cloak of certainty as the accurate features of the memory.

Needless to say, the discovery that memory is not only fallible but is a creation of our mental prejudices is of great concern to the world of the courtroom, in which witnesses swear to tell the whole truth using brains that are designed to manufacture their own version of the truth. Elizabeth Loftus of the University of Washington studies the reliability of eye-witness testimony. She finds that both *previous* experiences and snippets of information learned *after* an event has occurred can colour the recollection of that event. Her experimental subjects look at a series of photographs, representing glimpses that someone might have seen during the course of an accident or a crime. Loftus showed that subsequent suggestive questioning can slip into the memory of a witness an object as big as a barn! 'How fast was the car going past the barn when it hit the other car?' she asks (even though there was no barn in the original photographs). Immediately the subject conjures up an imaginary barn, and answers the question confidently!

• MODELS IN THE MIND •

Ever since Plato, philosophers and mathematicians have searched for rules of logic that allow unequivocal conclusions to be drawn from the premises available. The beauty and precision of pure logic spilled over from philosophy into mathematics and the physical sciences and even into psychology. Indeed, Jean Piaget went so far as to propose that there is a strict *mental* logic, which children construct for themselves during their development by taking their own actions and the consequences into their minds, and reflecting on them. The mental machinery created by this reflective process was thought to lead to logical thinking.

But anyone who has lived with children knows that they *change* and expand their ways of thinking as they grow up. Thinking is surely just as much a learned skill as is riding a bicycle. And, in any case, the strategies of thought that we learn are far from the rarefied dogma of classical logic. The inferences that we draw about the world are not abstract exercises in

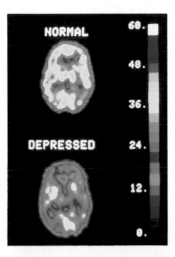

LEFT PET *scans* (*forehead at the top*), *showing activity in the normal brain* (*above*) *and the brain of a depressed person* (*below*). *The most active regions appear red, the least active blue. The entire cerebral cortex appears relatively inactive in the depressed patient.*

RIGHT *A patient is prepared for* ECT, *which seems particularly effective for the rapid treatment of potentially suicidal patients, though the deleterious effect on memory and the possibility of long-term complications still cause many worries.*

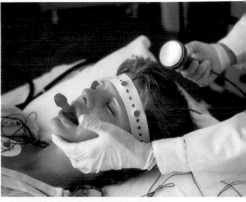

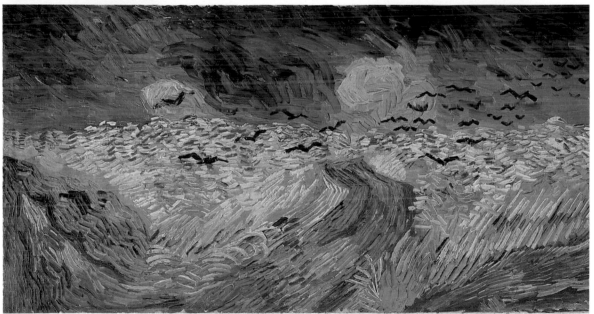

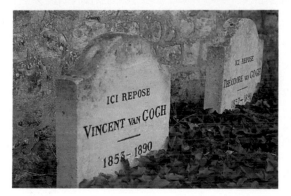

Van Gogh painted Crows over the Wheatfield (*above*) *in Auvers just two weeks or so before his death. He wrote to his brother Theo about it:* '*I did not need to go out of my way to express sadness and extreme loneliness.*' *Theo died only five months after Vincent and their graves lie side by side in the cemetery at Auvers* (*left*), *covered with ivy transplanted from Dr Gachet's garden.*

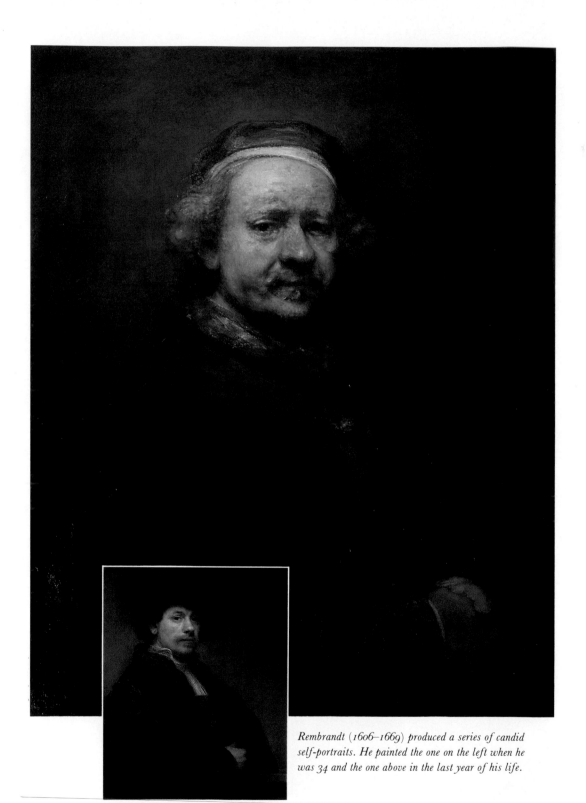

Rembrandt (1606–1669) produced a series of candid self-portraits. He painted the one on the left when he was 34 and the one above in the last year of his life.

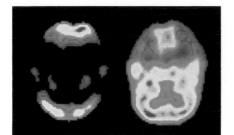

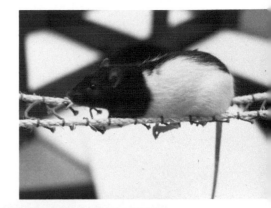

LEFT *PET scans, showing horizontal slices (forehead at the top) through the brain of a normal person (right scan) and an elderly person suffering from advanced senile dementia (Alzheimer's Disease). Regions of highest activity appear red, those that are least active appear blue and black. Activity is very low throughout the brain in Alzheimer's Disease.*

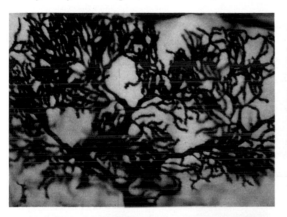

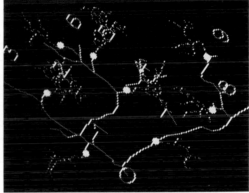

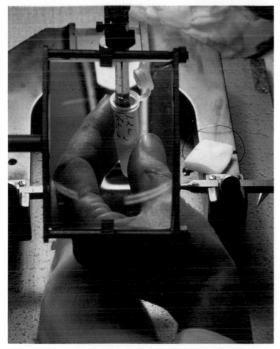

Active stimulation can cause anatomical changes in the brains of elderly rats. William Greenough at the University of Illinois studied the dendrites of large nerve cells in the cerebellum (above left), producing computer reconstructions (above right) to show all the fine 'spines' on which nerve fibres terminate. When old rats that had previously been housed in small cages were transferred to large open cages with much opportunity for social contact and exploratory activity, there was a large increase in the number of spines and therefore, probably, of the number of synaptic contacts on these nerve cells.

LEFT *Brain tissue transplantation might one day offer hope for the treatment of Alzheimer's Disease. Anders Björklund and his colleagues in Sweden take immature nervous tissue from the region of the embryo rat brain that is known to degenerate in Alzheimer's Disease and then inject it into the brains of aged rats. When such grafts are made close to the hippocampus, the animals improve their performance in tests of memory and cognitive ability.*

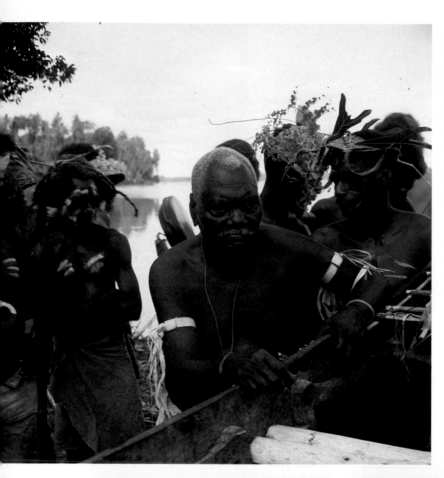

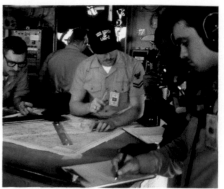

Navigation involves the construction of 'mental models' including the knowledge of space and time. In the Solomon Islands (left) navigators use their understanding of the movements of sun, clouds, waves and birds to guide them. On the USS Saipan (above), they have a host of modern instruments to help them.

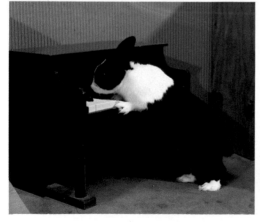

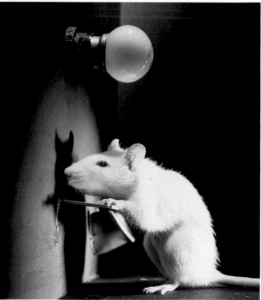

A simple learned sequence can make a rabbit look intelligent (above)! In the 'Skinner box' (right), animals learn to press a lever in response to signals, such as a light flashing.

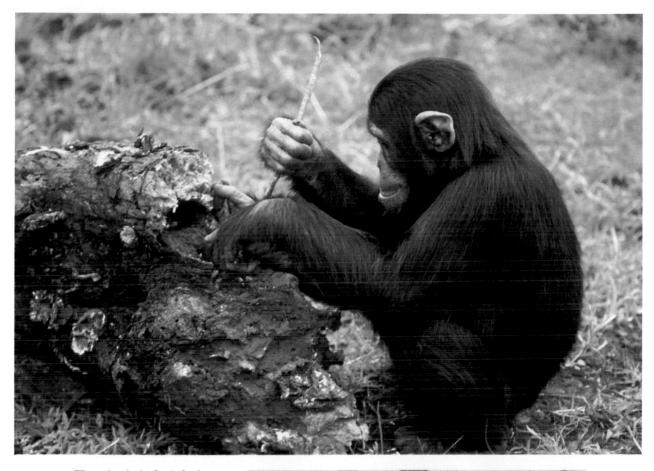

The archaeologist Louis Leakey once defined human beings as 'tool makers', believing that the capacity to conceive and construct tools was uniquely human. But in 1960 Jane Goodall saw chimpanzees cleaning grass stems and twigs, and poking them into termite nests to collect the juicy insects (above). Chimpanzees apparently have the ability to form 'models' of problems and solve them by mental manipulation.

RIGHT The phrenologists thought that the human brain was fundamentally different from those of animals because of the development of 'organs' of intellectual and moral sense distributed over its surface.

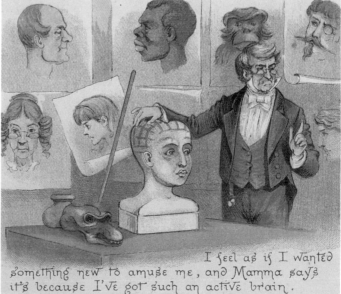

I feel as if I wanted something new to amuse me, and Mamma says it's because I've got such an active brain.

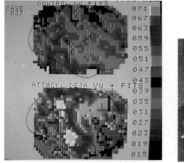

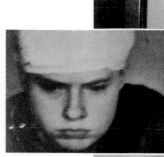

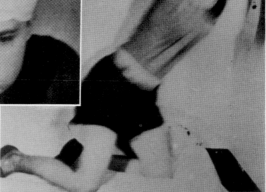

'Julie' photographed just after remote-control stimulation through an electrode implanted in her amygdala. She suddenly attacked the wall (far right).

The computer-generated diagrams (above left) show measurements of blood flow (reflecting the level of activity of nerve cells) in the right cerebral hemisphere of an epileptic patient, viewed from the side. Colour, from blue and green to red and white, indicates increasing levels of blood flow. The upper diagram shows the brain in its normal state, the lower one the massive activity just after an epileptic seizure. The patient was experiencing 'déjà vu' – a feeling that the past is being re-lived – which is commonly a symptom of temporal lobe epilepsy.

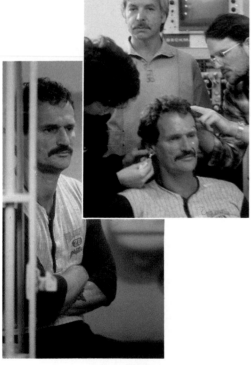

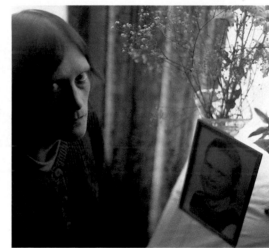

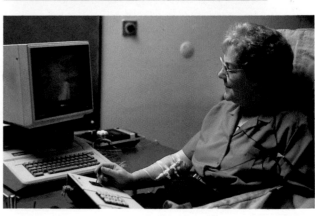

ABOVE *Al Ross, being tested in the laboratory of Bob Hare, and in gaol.* ABOVE RIGHT *Sandie Craddock.* RIGHT *Dawn Stanton.*

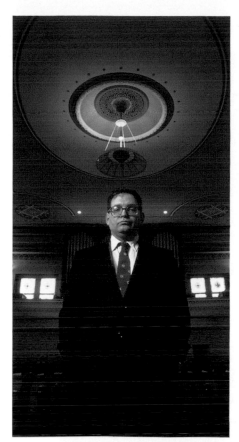

LEFT *Jay Centifanti, in the Old Pine Presbyterian Church, where he hid after the attack on his wife.*

RIGHT *An angry wife beats her husband with a distaff in this illustration from the Luttrell Psalter, written in East Anglia about 1340. Even today most violence probably takes place in the home.*

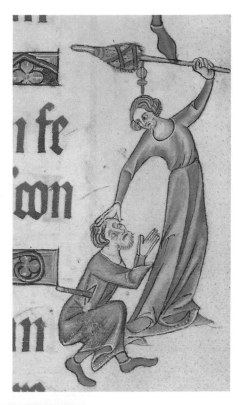

BELOW *Throughout history, much that has passed for sport and entertainment has been little more than ritualised violence.* The Divided Arena *by Francisco de Goya (1746–1828).*

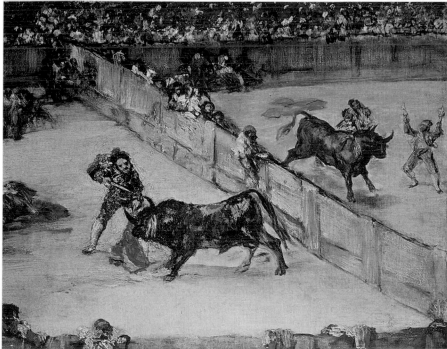

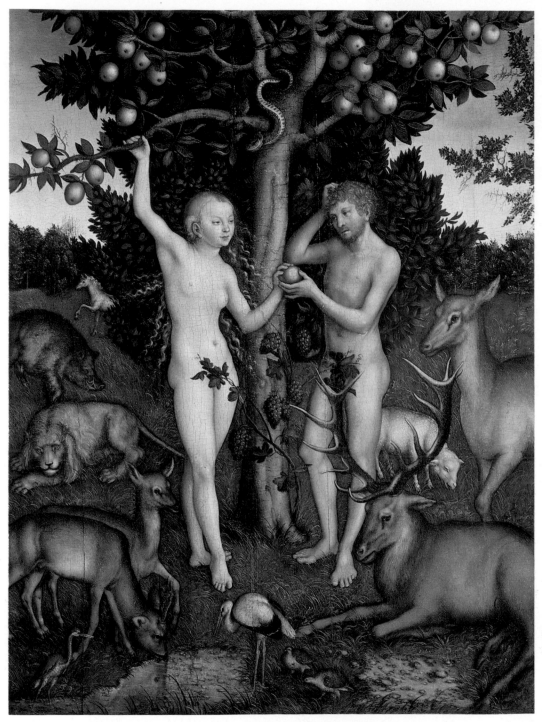

Adam and Eve in the Garden of Eden *by Lucas Cranach the Elder (1472–1553).*
Some see Adam's temptation as the loss of a perfect state; others might view it as the triumph
of free will. But what do we really mean by the concept of choice?

deduction, like a logician's equations of symbols. They depend on *general knowledge* about the nature of the problem in mind. And the more that children learn about the real world, the more knowledge they are able to bring to bear on any problem of thought.

The Cambridge psychologist Phil Johnson-Laird and his students have studied the thought processes of children. Faced with the following sentence, 'The Smiths saw the Rocky Mountains flying to California', young children have great difficulty in drawing the obvious conclusions about its meaning. Equally, when confronted with the sentence, 'The man stirred his cup of tea', a young child will not immediately see that a spoon must have been involved! The reading skills of children seem to depend on their ability to fill in the missing gaps in a story. The best readers are those who, without knowing it, are using their general knowledge to pad out the story and hence make it easier to understand as a whole.

Another Cambridge scientist, Kenneth Craik, who was killed in a road accident at only thirty-one, gave an important clue to the process that might underlie human thinking. Craik had studied psychology under Frederic Bartlett and, in his pitifully short career, he established himself as one of the most original of thinkers about thought. Although he had started by studying philosophy, he was also a practical man – a talented designer and model-maker, even from an early age. A set of miniature steam engines, each one smaller than the last, which he made when he was still a schoolboy, is on display in the Royal Scottish Museum in Edinburgh. This interest in technology blossomed when he did applied research during the war. In his most important piece of writing, the book *The Nature of Explanation*, Craik argued that the brain is a *predictive* device that has to capture the rules of the world in the same way that a predictive anti-aircraft gun-sight must do. He saw that the brain could achieve its predictive skill through incorporating a *model* of the external world, just as a structural engineer models the forces that will act on a building as he or she tests whether an architect's design will stand the test of the real world. Craik was the first to propose clearly that thinking is a manipulation of internalised models of situations or problems in the world. As Johnson-Laird puts it:

> The notion of a *model* here is very akin in function to an architect's model; that is to say it allows you to anticipate how something will occur. But, of course, the architect's model is a physical thing out there in the real world, whereas a mental model is something that is constructed computationally by the brain.

Perhaps this theory – the idea that thinking is the manipulation of a model in the mind – explains why the abstract intellectual skills of mathematics and reasoning, which we feel to be the most difficult forms of thinking, are so easy to do better with a computer. For most of us, it is impossible to relate the recondite problems of mathematics or quantum mechanics to any kind of everyday experience. If the first requirement for explaining something is that you should *understand* it, no wonder that most of us have difficulty in thinking of things that we cannot imagine. Perhaps the skill that distinguishes an Einstein or a Newton from the rest of us is a very rare ability to translate the most abstract of concepts – gravity, time, infinity – into models that can be manipulated in the mind. An important point here is that the models that we make are enriched by our general knowledge of the world around us: the more that we already know, the more that we are able to know how to know. And the operations that we perform on the models that we make in our mind can be far from the cold rules of logic and statistics. Tolstoy once wrote that if human beings controlled their lives on the basis of pure reason, all chance of spontaneity would be lost.

• A PYRAMID OF THOUGHTS •

In computational terms, the brain constructs models of the problems it solves. Not a *single* model of the whole of existence, but a playroom full of models, all clustered together and interconnected like the houses and farmyards of a giant mental Lego Land. And most of these models of reality lie below the surface of consciousness. Every step that you take depends on a model of the ground in front of your feet (and of the force of gravity; and of the kind of shoes that you are wearing; and of the time of the appointment that you are hurrying to keep). The models are built, in part, on the evidence of the senses; but also, to a large extent, on understanding and expectation about such things as rubber soles and rain-soaked cobblestones. The model must, in the jargon of computers, run in real time, and it must be *predictive*. It would be no use understanding everything about the step that you made two minutes ago; what matters is where you are about to put your foot.

Not only must the models in the brain make up for the delay in sensory signalling: they must also keep up with the inexorable, irreversible march of time in the real world. What use would vision be if it took half an hour to analyse the meaning of every glance? And how could an animal move freely in the world if its brain could compute only one step every hour? We know from the attempts of the artificial intelligentsia to program huge computers to interpret images or to control the movements of robots that these things are unbelievably complicated, in computational terms. Yet our brains achieve them effortlessly, continuously, in perfect step with the world that rushes on around us.

Most of the model-building in the brain goes on in subconscious mental workshops, far below the uncluttered world of conscious experience. We, the conscious architects of our lives, know little of the labours of the model-building draughtsmen. Their creations come to us in the form of the glittering jewels of perception, the flashes of insight into problems, as the recognition of a melody or the conscious desire for food or sex. The laborious computations in our brains that underlie these simple, conscious sketches of reality are all but hidden from view. In the terminology of the computer world, the high-level operating system that is the conscious mind cannot reach down and inspect the internal operations of the huge, hierarchical array of parallel processors that make up the rest of the computational machinery of the brain. Phil Johnson-Laird wrote:

> Even in the most deliberate of tasks, such as the deduction of a conclusion, you are not aware of how you carried out each step in the process. Similarly, you are not aware of the underlying nature and mechanism of mental representations: you are conscious of what is represented and of whether it is perceived or imagined, not of the inherent nature of the representation itself.

One model, however, often comes into the view of the conscious mind. That is the model of the mind itself. The very act of being conscious, particularly self-conscious, implies that the brain has the capacity to construct a model of the person to whom that brain belongs, and to fit this mental puppet into a theatre of the mind – a world of other people, sharing the same kinds of minds and intentions. And it is here, in the domain of self-awareness and the modelling of social existence that the capacity of the brain to *anticipate* reaches its peak. Taking a step or hitting a cricket ball requires a tiny peep into the future; but choosing a subject to study, a job, a mate, a religious philosophy – these involve models that look forward through the whole of life, and even, sometimes, to an imagined world beyond. The more that the model in the mind races ahead from the prison of the moment, the more that it depends on the power of invention and speculation. As Johnson-Laird puts it: 'The essence of human thinking that distinguishes it from other sorts of thinking is that we can think about things that are not real. Hence, we love to tell each other stories.'

• THE TEMPLE OF THOUGHT •

Even the lowliest corners of the nervous system have the capacity to form models of their own little worlds of action. But where in the brain might the grandest model makers live? Where is the machinery that can build the models that allow us to see *ourselves* as part of a complex social world, that enable us to form purposeful plans, to anticipate the future, to make critical judgements?

Bill Muzzall from Oregon graduated in 1983 in the top 10 per cent of his class at law school and passed the bar examination at the first attempt. Six months later, at the age of twenty-six, as he sat watching television, a blinding pain flashed through his head. An aneurism – a fragile, ballooning blood vessel – had burst, bleeding into Bill's frontal lobes. A scan of his brain now shows the havoc caused by that stroke. Yet, to the untutored eye, Bill does not seem handicapped by the death of a huge portion of his cerebral hemispheres. His perception and memory are virtually unaffected. His understanding and use of language seem quite normal. Even his intelligence is little changed. Bill himself, remarkably perceptive and articulate, describes the problem:

> My wife would always say 'I'm not going to be happy until I have the old Bill back. The same old Bill.' She's never going to have the old Bill back; I think we've both grown to know that, because something has changed me. It's not just a little problem with my memory or problem of motivation or whatever. The stroke caused a fundamental change in *me*.

Bill reported back for work with his law firm after the stroke, but within a day it became clear that he was a different man. He remembers being told to do some research on a client's file that first day – a job that should have taken him half an hour:

> I went to the law school and I spent about four and a half hours there. I forgot what I was supposed to do. I looked at my notes; they didn't make any sense. I read three or four cases and completely forgot them as I read, so at the end of the day at about 4 o'clock I got back over to the firm and I said 'Well, I sort of forgot what I was supposed to do.'

Bill's promising career died with the death of the neurons of his frontal lobe. Yet, 20 000 people around the world had their frontal lobes deliberately damaged by well-meaning surgeons in the 1940s. The Nobel Prize for Medicine in 1949 was awarded to a Portuguese neuropsychiatrist, Egas Moniz, for devising the surgical technique of pre-frontal lobotomy – the deliberate destruction of the major part of the frontal lobes, connected with the emotional centres of the limbic system below. How could it be that an injury that is considered a tragedy when it is accidental could have been performed deliberately and with the best of intentions on so many thousands of people?

The extraordinary story of lobotomy, and indeed of the field of 'psychosurgery' that has followed it, stems from a research conference held in London in 1935. John Fulton, the eminent American neurologist, who had studied with Sir Charles Sherrington at Oxford, reported the results of his latest experiments in which he investigated the possible involvement of the frontal lobes (previously an enigmatic area of the brain) in learning and memory. He had trained two chimpanzees to remember where a piece of food was hidden and then surgically removed parts of the frontal lobes to see whether they had difficulty remembering this simple task. Egas Moniz listened with growing excitement as Fulton described the unexpected effects on the emotional behaviour of one of the chimpanzees, called Becky. Before the surgery, Becky was temperamental and became angry and disturbed whenever she failed the experimental test. But after her frontal lobes were damaged she was much more placid and less concerned.

Moniz sprang to his feet and asked, 'If frontal lobe removal prevents the development of experimental neuroses in animals and eliminates frustration behaviour, why should it not be feasible to relieve anxiety states in man by surgical means?' The following year Moniz and the surgeon Almeida Lima started to operate on aggressive and neurotic human patients. Their enthusiastic reports of the success of this technique led others to take it up and simplify it.

Although psychosurgery, in a more cautious form, still plays some part in the treatment of the most severely ill, the heyday of lobotomy is remembered with embarrassment by most psychiatrists and neurologists of today. It gradually became clear that, rather than curing the illness, damage to the frontal lobes merely changed the patient into a different person. Far from being the appendix of the brain – a useless vestige left by the progress of evolution – the frontal lobes are the part of our brain that, more than any other, makes us human.

Although the frontal lobes are vastly enlarged in human beings, comprising fully one-third of the entire cerebral cortex, they are impressive structures in the brain of a monkey too. The study of the structure, connections and activity of nerve cells in the frontal lobes of monkeys is helping to unravel the complexity of this mysterious part of the brain.

A rhesus monkey sits, looking at three small wells set in the table in front of it. A peanut is dropped into one of the wells, to the evident interest of the monkey, and all three are covered up. A screen drops in front of the monkey; when it is raised again about twenty seconds later the monkey has the chance to reach out, uncover the well and to take the peanut. A trivially easy task; on a good day, he gets it right every time. What is happening in the monkey's brain during that twenty-second period of remembering, planning and anticipating?

Pat Goldman-Rakic of Yale University has been testing monkeys in this way while a tiny microelectrode, implanted painlessly into the anim-

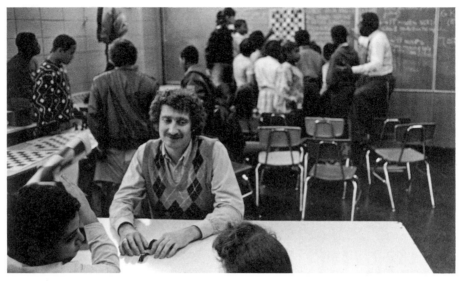

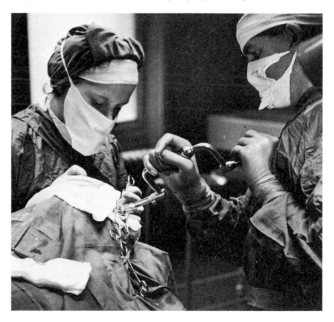

ABOVE *Bruce Pandolfini plays chess against a class in the Roberto Clemente Middle School in the South Bronx, with his back to the chess board.*

BELOW *A neurosurgical operation in 1946, of the type used to gain access to the brain in the early days of lobotomy.*

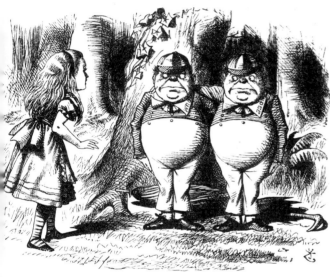

ABOVE *Behind the Looking Glass, Alice encountered Tweedle Dum and Tweedle Dee ...*

'*I know what you're thinking about,*' *said Tweedle Dum;* '*but it isn't so, nohow.*'
'*Contrariwise,*' *continued Tweedle Dee,* '*if it was so, it might be; and if it were so, it would be; but as it isn't, it ain't. That's logic.*'

al's brain, listens in on the impulses of nerve cells in the frontal cortex. Cells in the foremost part of the frontal lobe – the pre-frontal cortex – suddenly become active, pouring out torrents of impulses, whenever the monkey tries to keep some hidden scene in mind. When the screen comes down, and the monkey can no longer see the food-wells, nerve cells in its pre-frontal cortex start to fire, as if those cells were storing vital information about the position of the hidden peanut until the screen is lifted and the monkey has the chance to act. Sure enough; if the frontal lobes of a rhesus monkey are damaged, it has the greatest difficulty in this kind of delayed response task, as if it can no longer keep its mind on things, can no longer build and manipulate a mental representation of the problem and of what it wants to achieve.

This simple test soon sorts out the mental sheep and goats. A primitive prosimian monkey, the Galago, lower down the evolutionary scale than the rhesus and with much smaller frontal lobes, often fails to remember where the food is hidden, even with a delay of just a few seconds. Out of sight, out of mind.

It seems that the frontal lobes, the most highly evolved regions of the cerebral hemispheres, are the last part of the cortex to mature in the growing child. Parents are, for much of the childhood of their infants, surrogate frontal lobes, warning their offspring what will happen if they do this or that, helping them learn from their own experiences, substituting for their inability to piece together the meaning of the things that they see and assemble from them a plan of their lives.

The pre-frontal cortex is strategically placed in the complex network between the sense organs and the nerves that control the muscles. Pat Goldman-Rakic has recently found that this apparently anatomically bland, homogeneous area of the brain is, in reality, a fine mosaic of little regions, each one receiving fibres from one or more of the specialised sensory regions that lie scattered in the rear two thirds of the cerebral hemispheres. It may be, then, that the nerve cells in each of these frontal islands are concerned with the task of clinging to the memory of a particular aspect of the sensory scene that the monkey (or man) has just had in view. Many of the fibres that leave from the cells of the frontal cortex pass down to the basal ganglia, massive structures that are known to be an important part of the complex pathways for the control of movement.

Thinking, pure thinking, is the most private thing we do. Time and again, in the course of history, oppressive dictators and regimes have suppressed the explicit machinery of expression of dissent – broadcasting, the press, trade unions, opposition parties. But time and again, those despotic governments have been overwhelmed by an irrepressible medium of debate and defiance – the medium of human thought. What happens in our brains as we indulge in the purest ritual of consciousness – an isolated thought detached from the reality of the world or the need for action? How can we explain this mental equivalent of wallowing in a bath merely for the sake of the pleasure it gives?

To René Descartes, pure reflection, detached from the stimulation of the environment or the need of the individual, would presumably have been interpreted as the flexing of spiritual muscles by the soul within the body, perhaps through gyrations of the pineal body, which Descartes thought of as the seat of the soul. But to a materialist (who eschews such a dualist interpretation as capitulation to the forces of obfuscation) thought must have its origin in the causal connectivity of nerve cells in the brain. The dualist rejoices in the evident ability of the human mind to range spontaneously through the whole universe of thought without a single stimulus from the outside world to set it off. Just close your eyes and sit perfectly still in a quiet room; despite the lack of sensory stimulation, your thoughts can race wherever you send them, back through your life to your birth, or forward, in anticipation, even to your death; from a mental exploration of your own home, out to the boundaries of your town or even, in imagination, to the edges of the universe. But is it right to think of these mental gymnastics as a product of a purely spiritual mind?

It is surely naive to think of the brain as merely a giant set of reflex connections between sense organs and muscles, or to see behaviour as if it were as simple as the mindless scurrying of one of those clockwork toys that turns itself and moves in the opposite direction whenever it hits an obstacle. The brain is full of its own mechanisms for generating activity. First, it has the ceaseless, irreducible stream of information from sensory systems within the body that constantly taste and monitor the contents and pressure of the blood, that sense the length of all the muscles, that detect the posture of the joints and the direction of gravity. But also, there are the internally stored memories of the past, trapped as circuits of constantly firing neurons and as molecular changes in the synapses between them. The brain is always active, never at rest, even in the depths of sleep.

Some years ago, Per Roland, now working in Stockholm, set out with his colleagues to try to detect the work done by the brain during the purest of thoughts. They used one of the many methods now available for detecting the metabolic activity of nerve cells in the brain, the measurement of local cerebral blood flow. A human volunteer lies, motionless, in a warm room, with his eyes covered and his ears plugged. His head rests against a pillow of technology – an array of 254 detectors that can pick up minute levels of radioactivity. The signals from these detectors are passed to a computer and are converted to an image of the distribution of radioactivity across the surface of the volunteer's brain. A tiny injection of a solution of the radioactive inert gas xenon 133 is made, without disturbing the person in any way, into the blood in his internal carotid artery, which passes directly to the brain. For forty-five seconds after this injection, the radioactive blood permeates through the vessels of the cerebral cortex. In each part of the cortex, the *volume* of blood flow (and therefore the local level of radiation) is influenced by the *activity* of the nerve cells in that region. The more highly active is any part of the cerebral cortex, the more blood will flow through it, and therefore the more radiation will be given off. The computer image, then, produces a picture of the distribution of activity amongst the billions of nerve cells of the cerebral hemispheres.

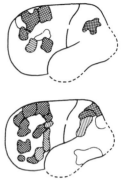

Illustrations of the side of the left hemisphere of the human brain, showing (top) small islands of increased activity during the 'minus 3' thinking task and the 'route-finding' problem (bottom). Many of the islands lie in the frontal lobe, on the left.

Imagine that the volunteer is asked to try to think of nothing, to clear his mind completely and to lie perfectly still during the forty-five seconds of analysis. Not surprisingly, blood flow is relatively low through the whole of the sensory areas that cover the back of the brain and through the areas that directly control movement, at the very back of the frontal lobe. But, even in the deepest state of mental relaxation, the whole of the pre-frontal cortex is more active than the rest of the brain, presumably keeping up a constant dialogue with the systems of memory, need and emotion in the limbic system, to which the frontal lobe is so strongly connected.

Now, the volunteer is deliberately asked to think during the forty-five seconds of analysis. In fact, he is given one of three different kinds of thought work to do. In the 'minus 3' thinking task, he is asked to do mental arithmetic, silently subtracting 3 from 50, then 3 from the result and so on. In the 'jingle' task, he has to imagine in his mind a familiar Danish jingle – a string of nonsense words – and to jump mentally to every second word in the jingle. The final task, the 'route-finding' problem, requires the subject to imagine that he steps out from the front door of his house and turns left, then walks to the first junction and turns right, then to the next junction and turns left, and so on.

The patterns of activity set up in the brain by these three mental tasks, detected by the local blood flow, were remarkably specific and quite different from each other. Each kind of thought was revealed as a characteristic patchwork of highly active regions, each between 2 and 9 square centimetres in area. Typically, the 'minus 3' task caused activity in sixteen of these small fields (though one or two of the volunteers had a couple of extra fields of their own). The 'jingle' and 'route-finding' tasks activated more fields, up to about thirty of them. Most significantly, the majority of these little thinking areas were in the pre-frontal cortex. Although a few of the areas seemed to be participating in all three thinking tasks, some of them appeared to be used for only one of the types of thinking. These remarkable experiments have allowed us to glimpse the world of introspection with the technology of modern science. But still the view is a hazy one, crude in localisation and very slow compared with the speed of a thought.

To move a finger; to conjure up nonsense in one's mind; these are merely the tiniest threads compared with the magnificent tapestry of human thought. But these experiments are at least the first step in building a neurology of thought. Perhaps we shall never really know what goes on in the mind of a chess master, a great mathematician, or a violinist converting dots of ink on a page into music which is a pure compound of inspiration and ecstasy. But without such simple beginnings, there is certainly no chance that we shall discover the origins in our brains of our rich capacity for thought. As Joseph Kovach, survivor of the Russian Gulag puts it, 'We have a way of creating worlds from ourselves, in our heads, and sharing that world'.

It is the task of the scientists who study thought to explain how the jelly of cells that is the human brain can create its own world and can imagine the future. To René Descartes, to think was to exist; *cogito ergo sum*. But human thought gives us so much more than existence alone; it provides us with hope for the future.

Cogito ergo ero; I think therefore I will be!

THE VIOLENT MIND

T HE HUMAN BRAIN is a machine, which alone accounts for all our actions, our most private thoughts, our beliefs. It creates the state of consciousness and the sense of self. It makes the mind.

That, in three sentences, is the central thesis of this book. To my mind, there is no other rational foundation on which to base the study of the brain. But what makes sense in the rarefied world of science can contradict the most fundamental beliefs of everyday life. To accept that the earth moves around the sun, that life cannot be generated spontaneously, that we are descended from ape-like creatures – those changes in conception, each born out of a scientific revolution, took decades, even centuries to settle within the popular understanding of the world. The view that our very mind – the inventor of the world as we know it without the help of science – is not what we feel it to be is the ultimate challenge to our system of belief. And it raises a monstrous paradox; it requires us to use our minds to accept that our minds are not what our minds tell us they are!

Woven inextricably into the fabric of our invented world is the belief that each of us contains an agent – an actor who speaks our lines and plays our part in life. The actor is the self in the mind-made model of the world. This self is the focus of an egocentric universe, the spectator of perception, the thinker of thoughts, the target of emotions. Above all it is the guardian of *will*, that most-cherished of all our mental possessions. To accept that our brains are machines, do we have to abandon the most fundamental beliefs that we have – that we are free to *choose* and are responsible for our choices? The answer is yes, but no.

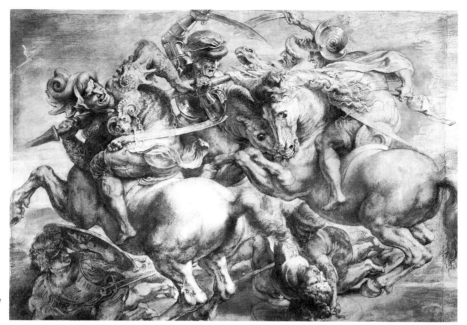

RIGHT Aggression, distilled in a design by Rubens (1577–1640)

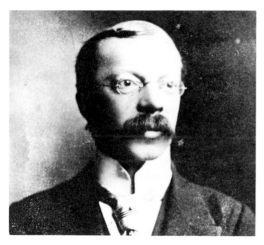

ABOVE For some people the deep streak of aggression in human nature becomes the focus of their lives. Dr Hawley Harvey Crippen poisoned his wife in London, was arrested on board ship to the United States, and hanged in England in 1910.

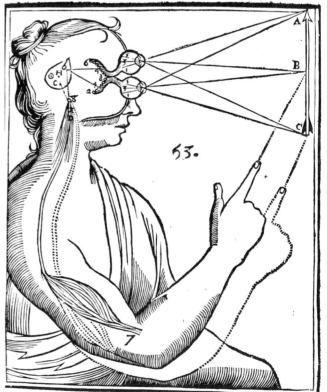

ABOVE RIGHT In the Traité de l'Homme *of 1664, René Descartes imagined that free will was due to the influence of the soul on the machinery of the brain through the tiny pineal gland (the pear-shaped organ). Here it directs the finger to point at different parts of the arrow seen by the eyes.*

To help me explain what I mean, I want you to imagine that you are an utterly impartial member of a jury. You are to judge the actions and feelings of other people; but also on trial are both the concept of free will and the rational science of mind. The cases are real; real people and real events, all involving violence or aggressive intentions. To commit violent acts against others (outside the sanctioned arenas of aggressive sport, war or self-defence) is the deepest offence against the order of society.

To put someone on trial for kicking out with their leg when the tendon of the knee is tapped, or for constricting the pupil of the eye when a bright light is shone into it would make no sense; not just because those actions break no legal code, but because they are quite obviously merely reflex products of the machinery of the nervous system. But where, along the spectrum of action, does choice intervene? Under what circumstances can people be said *not* to be responsible for their actions?

Those are questions that are of great concern to the courts because the judicial system must decide not only whether individuals have committed acts but also whether they were responsible for their actions. In 1723 the 'Wild Beast Test' was established in English law to decide what kind of person should not be punished for an offence:

> It must be a man that is totally deprived of his understanding and memory and doth not know what he is doing, no more than an infant, than a brute or wild beast; such a one is never the object of punishment.

The outcome for those who were so insane that they passed this harsh test was complete freedom. But in 1800 an attempt on the life of George III by James Hadfield, a soldier who had received a head wound in the war against the French, led to a change in the law. Hadfield was clearly deranged, but he was considered so dangerous that he could not be released. An Act of Parliament was passed allowing 'the safe custody of insane persons charged with offences'. When a madman, Daniel McNaghten, killed Robert Peel's secretary while attempting to shoot the prime minister in 1843, the House of Lords again revised legal procedure, allowing judges to find someone 'not guilty by reason of insanity' only if it can be proved that the person at the time of the act was 'labouring under such defective reason from disease of the mind as not to know the nature and quality of the act' and did not know that it was wrong. McNaghten was acquitted (and detained in a mental institution) and, ever since, a 'McNaghten defence' has become a regular feature of trials for violent crime. The courts have come to rely on 'expert witnesses' to provide evidence of 'defective reason' and ignorance of right and wrong.

But after the public outrage when John Hinkley was found 'not guilty by reason of insanity' after attempting to kill Ronald Reagan in 1981, legislators in half the states of America removed this defence from the statute books, or severely limited its application. In Britain, four psychiatrists pronounced the Yorkshire Ripper, Peter Sutcliffe, schizophrenic at his trial in 1981 – but intense pressure from press and public ensured a guilty verdict.

With this in mind, and with evidence and experts to help you, consider the following cases.

• DAWN STANTON •

The knife became a rather powerful symbol to me, a symbol of destruction. And I was afraid, I really was afraid that I might start reacting in a kind of insane way.

Mrs Stanton is a British school teacher who has never committed a crime. What you must consider are not her actions but her inclinations. A few years ago she began to have strange thoughts.

On one occasion, Dawn experienced 'an amazing sense of power ... I was totally convinced I was in charge of everything and that all I had to do was think and the thing would happen.' On another, she became certain that a bluebottle was a terrorist and she threw a radio at it in self-defence. On a third she went into the garden and took all her clothes off. 'At the time I was totally without inhibition and I didn't care that I was sitting there naked.'

Once when she was preparing a meal in the kitchen she suddenly felt strangely drawn to a set of knives. 'I was being extremely tempted by the knives I had about me ... and especially the thin knife which it seemed would be very easy to stick into somebody ... I was introduced to an idea I'd never had before and it all became a powerful symbol, a symbol of destruction.' Her husband arrived, and fortunately he realised what was going on and took the knives away.

What was going on was that Dawn was hypoglycaemic – the level of glucose in her blood was abnormally low. Dawn discovered ten years ago that she has diabetes; her pancreas does not secrete enough insulin (a hormone that is needed to assist the entry of glucose into most of the cells of the body). The treatment is, in principle, straightforward; simply inject insulin to replace the missing hormone. But in practice it is more complicated. Inject too much insulin and the body takes up so much glucose that the level in the blood falls and the brain is starved of fuel. The quantity of insulin needed to produce such hypoglycaemia depends on the amount of glucose in your bloodstream, which in turn depends on what you had for your last meal, when you had it and how much exercise you have taken.

Hypoglycaemia usually leads quickly to unconsciousness, but, as blood glucose falls, there is a window of experience between sanity and coma in which self-control is lost and that precious feeling of conscious choice disappears. 'When you're in that state, there's absolutely no ability to reason with yourself or tell yourself that such and such an act would be pointless,' says Dawn. 'You have no possibility of controlling your own actions; your body behaves on its own.' A small number of diabetics experience feelings of aggression during the state of hypoglycaemia.

The brain is an extraordinarily active organ and since it cannot break down fat and protein, it uses almost 75 per cent of the glucose in the blood. A fall in glucose rapidly causes a failure of the function of the most active nerve cells. One of the first areas of a rat's brain to be affected by hypoglycaemia is the hippocampus, which is thought to play a role in allocating significance to incoming sensory information and making associations with previously stored memories. When it runs out of energy, it may begin to trigger inappropriate associations. The extraordinary behaviour and loss of will that hypoglycaemia precipitates may become understandable in such physical terms.

Dawn's experiences were similar to those described by people suffering from schizophrenia, many of whom have obvious damage in and around the hippocampus. In hypoglycaemia, as in schizophrenia, raw emotions can be released from normal control. 'I've actually felt what it must feel like to be in a state of total aggression, total animal aggression,' says Dawn. Luckily, nowadays she can easily avoid hypoglycaemia. All it takes is a pin-prick of blood and a small portable meter to give an accurate measure of blood sugar. And once the level is within normal limits again, a feeling of normality returns – and with it that familiar illusion of free will.

Hypoglycaemia is well known, and its implications are recognised by the law in the form of the special defence of 'sane automatism'; the body is said to have done the deed without the mind's consent.

• DAVID GARABEDIAN •

It just happened so fast. I didn't know who was doing this. I didn't feel in charge.

Brought up in a respectable and leafy suburban town near Boston, Massachusetts, David never raised his voice in anger or got involved in fights; and he was well liked by his sisters and by his friends, who described him as a 'peacemaker'. He sometimes had problems concentrating, but had no significant medical conditions. Then, in March 1983, he got a job with Old Fox Lawn Care company, mixing concentrated pesticides and spraying them on clients' lawns. He had not been well trained in the safe handling of these chemicals and as he mixed them, he certainly inhaled the fumes and splashed the liquid on his skin.

Within days David started to feel unusually thirsty; he needed to urinate a lot and had diarrhoea. He suffered from chest pain, headaches and bad nightmares. He coughed a lot and was nervous and tense. He had difficulty focusing his eyes. A finger twitched uncontrollably. He giggled inappropriately, had quick mood changes and some paranoid ideas, and his memory became poor.

On 29 March 1983, David was surveying a lawn not far from his own home. He felt the need to urinate and was discovered doing so by the owner of the house, Eileen Muldoon. She threatened to report his behaviour to his employers and during the argument that ensued he took a piece of string from his pocket and strangled her. He then threw several large rocks at her face, mutilating it severely. Covered in blood, he drove home, went to bed and slept. At 2.00 a.m. police came to arrest him, guns drawn. He went with them without protest.

At the trial, psychiatrist David Bear, then of Boston University, gave evidence in his defence. He told the court that the principal ingredient in the insecticide that David mixed was chlorpyrifos, a substance that acts as a nerve gas and, in high doses, can kill. It is a so-called anticholinesterase drug: it inhibits an enzyme, the function of which is to destroy the transmitter substance acetyl choline, preventing it building up in the synapses between certain nerve cells.

In sub-lethal doses chlorpyrifos disturbs transmission in many parts of the brain, including the hypothalamus, which is known from much research to be involved in regulating aggressive behaviour in animals. Many of David's odd symptoms – his desire to urinate and his difficulty in focusing, for instance – were almost certainly due to the build-up of excess acetyl choline. And in animals, drugs that affect synapses that use acetyl choline can turn placid animals into vicious killers.

Peter Spencer, a toxicologist also called in by the defence, concluded that 'the behavioural changes caused by involuntary intoxication with chlorpyrifos played a role of indeterminable magnitude in the action that resulted in the death of Mrs Muldoon.' But, by the time it was checked, the acetyl choline level in David Garabedian's blood was within normal limits and the jury was not persuaded that the chemical had abolished David's control over his own actions. He is now serving a life sentence. David Bear gave his view of the verdict:

I think it is a tragedy. But there's another side to this. What happened to Mrs Muldoon is awful and I think we need to understand it, just as we want to understand the crash of an airplane. If we get angry at the pilot and shake our fists, while the real problem was a cracked wing, we've made an awful mistake; another plane is going to crash.

On the night of 31 August 1983, Korean Airlines Flight 007 strayed over Soviet territory and was shot down with the loss of 269 lives. A small autopilot mode selection switch was set on the wrong notch. Like that aircraft, David Garabedian may have been set for an almost inevitable rendezvous with disaster.

• SANDIE CRADDOCK •

When I look back, I have nightmares – and I think to myself, a person in their right mind, male or female, wouldn't do the things that I've done in the past.

Sandie Craddock's parents gave her a good home, love and affection, but she became a problem child at about the age of fifteen. From then on she suffered from black moods in which she was violent and aggressive. Often she just walked out of the house and disappeared for several days, ending up in the local magistrates' court. By the time she was twenty-eight, Sandie had received twenty-six convictions for offences ranging from criminal damage, theft and trespass, to the possession of dangerous weapons.

But Sandie was no ordinary criminal. Even hardened lawyers regarded her behaviour as bizarre. She often waited at the scene of the crime until the police arrived. On several occasions she actually telephoned the police to give herself up, although she was rarely taken into custody without a struggle. Once, it took six policemen to hold her down. Sandie's own recollections of these episodes are rather hazy, as though she had periods of transient amnesia. She would simply wake up, wandering around the streets of London, or in a police station or hospital ward, with very little idea of how she had got there.

Like many violent offenders she also turned her aggression on herself; her scarred arms testify to more than twenty attempts to take her own life. Over the years, Sandie developed paranoid fears that fed on the reactions of an increasingly hostile world. Then an event took place that changed the whole picture – Sandie found herself on a murder charge. She was accused of stabbing Karen Hillier, a nineteen-year-old barmaid, six times with a kitchen knife after an argument. Sandie was convicted of manslaughter.

During the trial her father read a newspaper article about a Harley Street doctor who ran a clinic for people who suffered from premenstrual tension. The story described Sandie's strange moods with an uncanny clarity. Could hormone changes associated with the menstrual cycle have been the cause of Sandie's problems? Sandie had kept a diary, which confirmed her father's hunch; Sandie's behaviour had a pattern.

Katharina Dalton, an expert in hormonal disturbances at University College, London, agreed to testify on Sandie's behalf and began to make enquiries about her conduct while in detention. The prison records documented regular monthly episodes of disturbed behaviour; arson, smashing windows, attempted hanging and wrist-slashing, assaults on other inmates and staff. A statistician analysed the data – it fitted a twenty-nine day cycle.

The evidence was so compelling that the judge agreed to postpone sentencing for several months while Katharina Dalton treated Sandie with injections of progesterone, a hormone involved in the regulation of the menstrual cycle. Sandie became a different person. The testimony of prison staff convinced the judge that the diagnosis was correct and the treatment effective. Sandie was released on probation, with the stipulation that she receive regular progesterone injections indefinitely. Since then there have been only two minor incidents and both occurred after nurses failed to give Sandie the prescribed dose of hormone.

The link between the so-called premenstrual syndrome and irresponsible violent behaviour is well established. A survey conducted by Katharina Dalton showed that almost half of all women entering psychiatric hospital are admitted just before menstruation, that half of all crimes leading to imprisonment of women are committed during that stage in the menstrual cycle, and that more than half of all suicide attempts among women occur around the time of a period.

Just prior to menstruation or after giving birth, progesterone levels fall precipitously. This sudden fall seems to trigger dramatic mood swings in some people. Studies of rats and mice show that females become markedly more aggressive soon after giving birth, which not only helps the mother to protect the young, it also influences the male's behaviour and his hormone system. For a period the female becomes more dominant than the male and thus has increased access to food.

Was such a mechanism once important to humans? We don't know, but progesterone does have a definite calming effect on the brain, and it has been used as an anaesthetic. Its mechanism of action is not fully understood but some recent evidence suggests that progesterone may be broken down to produce chemicals that work like the tranquillisers, Valium and Librium, which act selectively on benzodiazepine receptors and cause the damping down of activity in various parts of the brain.

Sandie and others like her may be predisposed to their particular problems by their genetic make-up. Very recently another important receptor system in the brain has been shown to be influenced by progesterone. The hallucinogenic drug PCP ('angel dust') stimulates these particular receptors and produces strange, aggressive and paranoid behaviour. Progesterone has the opposite effect; it reduces the activity of the receptors. If an error in Sandie's genes has caused her brain to produce excessive numbers of these receptors, she might need to produce larger than normal amounts of progesterone to keep them under control.

In Sandie's case, the judge decided that hormones were responsible for her actions, not Sandie's *self* – the kind of self that we all presume is resident within our bodies.

• 'JULIE' •

This strange feeling would come over me, stranger and stronger than hell.
A frightening feeling. . . . You had no control over how your body reacted.

Julie's birth was difficult, but she grew up in New England as a normal, creative and musically gifted child. She developed an allergy to chocolate, which made her suddenly aggressive and disobedient, but otherwise she was consistently good-natured. Then, in her teens, she began to suffer minor lapses of consciousness, and later she had convulsions accompanied by panic and aggression. She was diagnosed by psychiatrists as psychotic, and endured some sad visits to the back wards of mental hospitals.

In those days, Julie carried a small knife for protection, in case she found herself in a dangerous part of the city during one of her panic attacks. One day, while at the cinema with her father, she began to feel an attack coming on. She had the familiar sense of fear in the pit of her stomach, and she walked into the ladies' toilet, taking out the knife as she went. This time, unusually, she did not run away but stood transfixed in front of the mirror, believing she saw a disfigurement on one side of her body. To her horror, part of her face and hand seemed to be changing in shape and size.

At that moment another young girl entered the room, came towards the washbasin, and brushed up against Julie, on the side she thought was disfigured. Julie struck out at the girl's chest and drove the knife into her heart. There was a scream and Julie's father rushed into the women's lavatory; he administered first aid to the victim, saving her life. The police held Julie in custody for three days, before releasing her to the care of psychiatrists. It was later that Vernon Mark, a well-known but controversial Boston neurosurgeon, became involved in the case.

Mark recognised that Julie had a rare form of epilepsy with symptoms similar to those of patients described over a hundred years ago by Henry Maudsley in London. He suspected, because of the extreme aggression that accompanied her attacks, that the epileptic focus was in the amygdala (a region of the emotion-controlling limbic system, which is involved in regulating aggression in animals). He decided to use an experimental

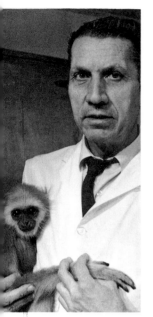
José Delgado.

procedure, previously developed in animals, to locate and destroy the guilty piece of brain. Walter Hess, working in Switzerland in the late 1950s, had introduced techniques for painless stimulation of the brain through implanted electrodes in freely moving animals. He had shown that stimulation of parts of the hypothalamus (to which the amygdala is connected) would make a placid, purring cat extend its claws, lash its tail, spit and growl as if faced with an attack from a dog. The moment the stimulation stopped the cat would resume its reverie as if nothing had happened. José Delgado in Spain had even turned brain stimulation into a spectator sport by showing that an aggressive bull charging him in a bull ring could be stopped in its tracks by stimulation through a radio-controlled electrode implanted in a different part of its hypothalamus.

Vernon Mark and his team inserted electrodes in and around Julie's amygdala and found that one group of electrodes picked up strong, rhythmic 'epileptiform' discharges. Then, he fixed on Julie's head a radio receiver connected to the electrodes and watched her while she moved around freely. He sent a signal at random intervals to stimulate different sites in her brain. At one spot only, the stimulation caused her to strike out with her fists and her guitar against the wall.

Mark was certain that he had located the home of Julie's evil self and he destroyed it by passing radio-frequency currents to boil the tiny piece of brain. Afterwards her appetite increased, she had difficulty playing music and there were a few temper tantrums. But within six months her weight was normal, her musical ability returned and the aggressive episodes ceased. That was nineteen years ago, and now Julie is in her forties, living independently and happily. She has been able to take university courses and record songs, and she is a volunteer worker for the local epilepsy society. Vernon Mark says:

> When we look at violent behaviour, we have to look at two factors: the environment and the brain, and we have to evaluate which is playing a part in generating abnormal behaviour. In some cases, the environment is almost completely responsible, in other cases, such as Julie's, it is the brain.

• JOSEPH B. CENTIFANTI •

I could not have stopped what began that evening and continued through that whole period of my being a fugitive, no matter what I did, until it was over, until the process burnt itself out.

On 15 August 1975, 'Jay' Centifanti, a lawyer in Pennsylvania, took a thirty-eight calibre revolver and went in search of his estranged wife and her boyfriend. He had drunk a good deal, and smoked some marijuana too. He lay in wait for the couple at Philadelphia's 30th Street station and when he saw them on a train, he boarded it. He says now that he just intended to frighten them, but a 'higher power' took over. He claims that he received messages spelt out in lights. 'Shoot her now!', the first message said. He fired at her head. 'You don't want to kill her!' said the second, causing him to aim the next three shots at her back rather than her head. He charged through the carriages, terrifying the other passengers, and forced the driver to stop the train. He received another message. 'Run.' He ran to the Old Pine Presbyterian church and hid there undetected in the dark attic for six weeks, stealing food from the church refrigerator. He could look down through a grille and see his wife (who had survived the shooting) sitting in the pews on Sundays, protected by policemen because Jay was still a fugitive, and nobody knew where he was. When his pastor, Bill Pindar, thought Jay must have killed himself, he delivered a eulogy about him which Jay could hear from the attic. Then, one day Jay accidentally left a copy of a book Bill had loaned him in the aisle of the church. The police were called; Jay was found and taken to the Norristown State Hospital.

Jay Centifanti had known since he was a teenager that his unpredictable swings of mood came from inside him. He was manic-depressive and he claims that his mania drove him to commit that act. He described what a manic episode is like:

> You have an engine in your chest and you can't stop it, and it goes on and on. I can easily believe Handel wrote the Messiah in eighteen days without stopping, first draft! That's what I felt like most of the time.

All those who had to deal with Centifanti – a judge, the police, the psychiatrists – were convinced that he was psychotic and could not be held responsible for his acts. On 22 July 1976 Jay was given a two-and-a-half year sentence, but he was held in a secure mental institution rather than a prison. On the order of the court he was treated with lithium and psychotherapeutic counselling. Since his release he has lived a normal life without any further episodes of aggression, but he is not permitted to resume his practice as a lawyer, even though he never went to jail. Now he serves as a volunteer adviser to Project Share (a support group for the mentally ill), and he is a bright and intense person. As a hobby, he conducts a traditional jazz band. He still has to take lithium to control the peaks and troughs of his manic depression.

Bob Sadoff, the psychiatrist who first saw Jay after he was captured, is certain about the validity of psychiatric evidence in court:

Legally a crime is composed of two parts: *actus reus*, the act itself, and the *mens rea*, the mental state. What we come into court for is to help the court decide about what guilty intent there may or may not have been connected with the act. Otherwise, you'll just find people guilty of acts, and not crimes.

But if Jay's wife had died it is by no means certain that he would have been found not guilty by reason of insanity. After all, he put the gun in his pocket, got drunk, smoked a couple of joints, and waited at the station for his wife in a state of extreme jealousy. His action appeared to be fully premeditated. But what does 'meditation' mean when you have the chemical engine of mania in your brain?

• AL ROSS •

I did a number of violent acts in my youth, and I don't think at any time I felt any remorse or concern about the individuals I'd beaten.

Al Ross, a child of the rough Lower East Side of Vancouver, has had forty-six convictions – for drug offences, thefts, assaults and bank robbery. Inside and outside jail, he deliberately cultivated his image as a hard man. He still seems to take some pride in his skill at lying. At times, his violence was extraordinarily indiscriminate. In prison once he stabbed a fellow inmate simply because the man refused to change a radio station.

Al himself says, 'I'm accountable for all the things I have done in my life.' He blames his early environment for twisting his life: 'I believe, when we place people, especially youngsters, in de-humanising institutions and facilities, we foster and we nurture anti-social and violent behaviour.' He was placed in his first tough adult jail at the age of fifteen.

Others believe that Al Ross is a 'psychopath' and that this ugly word has meaning in terms of the organisation of the brain. Bob Hare, a psychologist at the University of British Columbia has studied extremely anti-social criminals for twenty years and realised at the start of his work that a diagnostic system was desperately needed. He devised a seventeen-point scale to help define who is a psychopath. He believes that the following characteristics are definitive: a persistent pattern of anti-social behaviour, a disregard for social mores and conventions, impulsive behaviour, egocentricity, irritability, hostility, an ability to manipulate and control others, superficial charm, a lack of empathy and conscience. Some individuals with Bob Hare's list of characteristics deal well with perfectly legal jobs, including high finance. Many turn to violent crime.

Recently Bob Hare's team has come up with intriguing findings about the way psychopaths use and process language. First, unlike most normal right-handed people (whose language functions are concentrated in the left hemisphere), most psychopaths seem to process language evenly on both sides of the brain. In the latest experiment, real words and non-words are flashed up on a screen and the subject has to press a button to say which is which. Most people give a quicker response to emotional words ('love', 'kill', 'baby') than to neutral words ('train', 'handle', 'green'). But psychopaths respond, robot-like, at exactly the same rate to all kinds of words. Again, if shown three words, such as 'warm', 'loving' and 'cold', and asked to choose the pair that belong together, most people will look at the words in terms of emotion and metaphor, and group 'warm' with 'loving'. But psychopaths usually take the dictionary meanings as important, and group 'warm' with 'cold'.

'Conscience is partly internalised language, and if I say that I shouldn't do something, I actually *feel* that I shouldn't do it,' says Bob Hare. 'The psychopath can say the same thing but he doesn't *feel* that he shouldn't. The emotional components of conscience seem to be absent.'

But is the absence of an active conscience in simple laboratory tests a product of some genetic or developmental 'fault' in the brain; or is it just because the psychopath has *decided* not to be concerned about issues of conscience? Hare is unsure of the scientific, let alone the philosophical and legal implications of his findings and he will not appear as an 'expert witness' in court, for either the defence or the prosecution.

Al Ross came out as 'psychopathic' in the seventeen point rating scale and in most of the laboratory tests, but he rejects the label and believes that his actions are determined by free will. Indeed he says that he has *chosen* to leave his criminal career behind. Today, he is a volunteer social worker, trying to stop teenagers from taking to the life of crime he once knew.

• WHAT IS WILL? •

These examples are hardly representative of the run-of-the-mill aggressive personality or the average violent crime. The British courts are clogged with football hooligans, small-time muggers and the young thugs for whom gratuitous violence in town centres seems to have become a way of life. It would be foolish to pretend that the science of the brain can explain such anti-social behaviour, let alone excuse it. But the vivid, even bizarre cases that you have considered here were chosen because they bring into sharp focus the issue of responsibility and the nature of free will.

Surely no one could believe that violent thoughts or actions committed by otherwise model citizens while their blood glucose is very low or their amygdala is exploding with epileptic discharges were *intended* by the person involved. There would clearly be more debate about a killing or near-killing committed after handling insecticide, or just before a menstrual period, or during a manic, drunken high. And I suspect that there will have to be much clearer scientific evidence before the public or the courts will accept that a violent psychopath who has no overt brain injury and whose behaviour has been unremittingly criminal is merely the victim of genetic predisposition and a difficult childhood.

The problem comes when we try to mix the judicial system with medical science and expect them to use the same language. The courts are concerned with questions of both action and guilt. But science has no simple place for right and wrong; it seeks causal explanations for events. No one would try to assign *responsibility* for the fact that the earth orbits the sun. Nor is it the job of science to decide whether people are responsible for actions that society judges to be wrong.

Morality is not absolute; details of moral and legal codes vary from culture to culture. To the extent that systems of ethics are a phenomenon in the world, science is entitled to try to analyse them and give a functional interpretation of them. Indeed the field of 'sociobiology' (to the annoyance of many sociologists and political theorists), led by its champion Edward Wilson of Harvard University, has tried to account for such apparently biologically disadvantageous behaviours as homosexuality, voluntary celibacy and altruism in terms of the benefits that they might bring to whole families or related groups. But however powerful its theories of behaviour, science is surely not entitled to dictate the *contents* of a moral code, any more than it should force on society a perfect language or an ideal religion.

The judicial system has two tasks (crystallised in the distinction between *actus reus* and *mens rea*); it must enforce a generally agreed moral code by deciding whether individuals have committed acts that are judged to be wrong; and it must then decide on an appropriate sentence. If violence or extreme anti-social behaviour are involved, the question of the future protection of society is an important factor. But there is little evidence that life in prison is less pleasant than in a mental institution or that it has any particular strong deterrent effect on those who are judged to be responsible for their acts. Surely what matters is not so much where those whom society decides to lock away should be housed, but whether there are explanations for their behaviour that can be tackled in more fundamental ways.

All our actions are products of the activity of our brains. It seems to me to make no sense (in scientific terms) to try to distinguish sharply between acts that result from conscious intention and those that are pure reflexes or that are caused by disease or damage to the brain. We *feel* ourselves, usually, to be in control of our actions, but that feeling is itself a product of the brain, whose machinery has been designed, on the basis of its functional utility, by means of natural selection.

We are machines, but machines so wonderfully sophisticated that no

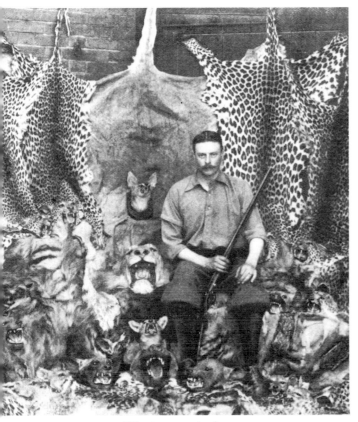

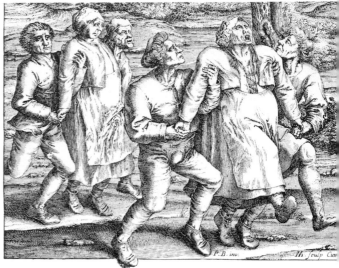

ABOVE *Epileptics being carried during their fits; line engraving (1642) by Hendric Hondius, after Pieter Brueghel the Elder. Some people with epilepsy are violent during their fits but this is so clearly a product of their disease rather than their will.*

ABOVE *Why do some gain pleasure from the ritual slaughter of animals?*

BELOW *The tragedy of football hooliganism at the Heysel Stadium in Brussels in 1985. Is gratuitous violence a statement of independent will or the complex product of inheritance, upbringing, education and social structure?*

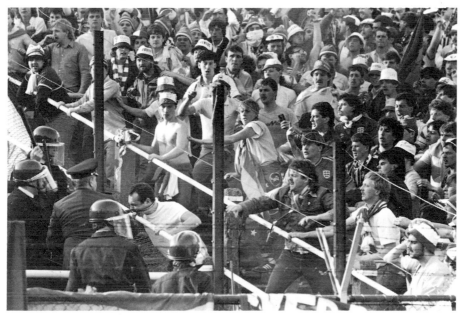

one should count it an insult to be called such a machine. Our actions are not the intentions of a spiritual self that lurks among the synapses of the brain, but nor are they the outcome of machinery as simple as clockwork.

The brain is built by instructions in the genes, but modified by events throughout life, from the uterus to the death-bed. In those terms our actions are the combined results of the information that constantly bombards the senses, of the stored memories of past events, of desires and ambitions (partly inherent, partly learned), of childhood experiences captured in their effect on the structure of the brain, of the education that we have received, of our knowledge of conventions of right and wrong and, indeed, of our understanding of the existence of courts and methods of punishment. In such a rich universe of cause and effect, what need is there for pure will?

The *sense* of will is an invention of the brain. Like so much of what the brain does, the feeling of choice is a mental model – a plausible account of how we act, which tells us no more about how decisions are really taken in the brain than our perception of the world tells us about the computations involved in deriving it. To choose a spouse, a job, a religious creed – or even to choose to rob a bank – is the peak of a causal chain that runs back to the origin of life and down to the nature of atoms and molecules. It is a chain with a million influences and a little statistical variability thrown in. But we should not search in textbooks of quantum mechanics for the nature of intention. Why look to *indeterminacy* in search of self-determination?

People often reject deterministic accounts of behaviour because of the fear that they reduce human beings to mere predictable puppets. But there is so much complexity in the history of any individual that it would surely be a daunting, not to say unrewarding task to try to predict their every action. I should be uncomfortable to feel that I was not in control of my life or to feel that I was not responsible for my actions. But I believe that the 'I' in me is the operation of a mind, which is itself the operation of a brain, constructed solely by genes and environment. I find that notion just as wonderful as, and in many ways more satisfying than, the empty illusion of a spiritual self.

INDEX

Italic page references refer to illustrations

PICTURE CREDITS